Cryosurgery

Paola Pasquali
Editor

Cryosurgery

A Practical Manual

Springer

Editor
Paola Pasquali
Department of Dermatology
Pius Hospital de Valls
Tarragona
Spain

ISBN 978-3-662-43938-8 ISBN 978-3-662-43939-5 (eBook)
DOI 10.1007/978-3-662-43939-5
Springer Heidelberg New York Dordrecht London

Library of Congress Control Number: 2014950821

Printed on acid-free paper

Springer is part of Springer Science+Business Media (www.springer.com)

There are beings whose very existence made this project possible. This book is dedicated to them:

My mother, for whom nothing is impossible

My father, for whom even the impossible must be written down and communicated

My husband, whose love and companionship make possible the impossible

My brother Arnaldo, long gone but always present, from whom I learn to infuse all actions with some good

My daughter, whose very existence justifies any such actions

Foreword

The aging of populations in first-world countries and the expansion of medical care in third-world countries have increased the worldwide burden of dermatologic diseases. While an array of treatment options for many of these diseases exists, the one most commonly employed may be cryosurgery. The aged and infirm can be treated with cryosurgery in nursing homes and other extended care facilities without the need to transport the patient to the medical center. The portability of cryosurgery in comparison with other forms of treatment means that cryosurgery will be performed in areas with limited health-care delivery systems. Thus, there is a need for a manual for practitioners to be able to deliver care more efficiently and effectively.

Dr. Paola Pasquali gathered 28 of the foremost cryosurgeons to render a truly readable and practical manual for practitioners. The content of the manual ranges from basic concepts, e.g., cryoanesthesia prior to performing a skin biopsy, to advanced concepts, e.g., using high-frequency ultrasound (22 MHz) to determine the shape and volume of the area to be treated. Cryoanesthesia, which can obviate the discomfort of the injection of local anesthesia with the stinging sensation caused by the acidic pH of the anesthesia, could be beneficial for millions of patients having diagnostic skin biopsies. High-frequency ultrasound can determine if the basal cell carcinoma is superficial or if it has a deep component within the tumor. Trans-cryosurgical high-frequency ultrasound enables the depth obtained by the freezing front to be visualized. By assuring that the temperature at the periphery of the tumor is sufficient to kill the tumor cells, the cure rate for thousands of patients with skin cancers will be improved. The potential reach of this manual, which depends upon readers implementing the concepts, could be from several thousands to millions of patients.

Chapters are devoted to each of the following conditions commonly treated by dermatologists with cryosurgery: warts, skin cancers, and eyelid lesions. Additional contributions about vascular lesions and oral lesions provide the information to be able to expand cryosurgical treatment to these areas. An excellent chapter focuses on the use of cryosurgery to provide palliative care. Commentary about other imaging techniques that are not yet in widespread clinical use, e.g., reflectance confocal microscopy, is provided to give a perspective about future improvements in cryosurgical treatment. And two atlases nicely complete this work.

The reader will be well served with the concise descriptions and illustrative figures of this manual.

June K. Robinson, MD
Research Professor of Dermatology
Northwestern Feinberg School of Medicine
Chicago, IL, USA

Preface

I sit down to write about why and how this book came to be. I have spent countless evenings going over images, papers, and surgical experiences (those of others and personal ones). I am trying to keep a cool head as I try to find one concept to wrap it all up.

Finally, I find one sentence that, taken out of context, might sound like a weather forecast or a global warning from a panicky futurologist: Cold is here to stay.

No other conclusion is possible when one sees the broad spectrum of conditions for which cryosurgery has been, is, and will be used. Cryosurgery is probably the most common procedure used by dermatologists, nurses, family physicians, gynecologists, and veterinarians, among others. It was started formally some 120 years ago, and it still stands as one of the safest, most versatile, least expensive, and most time-efficient surgical methods.

And still, not many manuals on this subject are available. In proportion to the immense number of procedures done with this method, very little has been written. Wondering why this is so, one finds that part of cryosurgery's popularity is its simplicity. It is so simple to perform that it may seem unnecessary to have formal training. It is so simple that most dermatology programs do not teach it. But it is just in such routine work, in the seemingly simple, that we should not let our guard down.

A manual of procedures becomes mandatory. There is a definite need for a body of knowledge on this subject written in a concise manner. And thus this book.

This is not the first book on the subject, and I hope it is not the last. But it is the book that has reunited those of us who have made cryosurgery part of our lives. We have all worked with and for cryosurgery. We have applied it for conventional sites and in conventional manners. We have applied it in original ways on nonconventional sites. As a whole, we have wanted to transmit the evidence-based knowledge together with our own know-how, with the help of many images and two atlases, to those of you who are now opening these pages for the first time.

I welcome you to this amazing journey into the realm of the cold. I hope that you will come out of it transformed, loving cryosurgery as much as we do or more, and with the desire to blaze a new path for this amazing specialty.

Tarragona, Spain　　　　Paola Pasquali

Acknowledgments

There is an old tradition in Catalonia of building towers several levels high, consisting entirely of people. They are called *castell* (castle). These human monuments are the most compelling visual representation of teamwork.

Similarly, this book has been built through the efforts of many visible and not-too-visible people. All of them have worked hard, dedicated much of their time, and, most of all, done it with passion.

A special acknowledgment goes to the contributors, the most visible part of this team effort, who have generously contributed from their lifetime of expertise. All of them share with me a lifelong love for cryosurgery. Their contributions have been wonderful and their friendship and solidarity priceless.

To all the patients who have participated through the presence of their images in this book: They have been our best teachers.

To my committed Senior Editor, Sverre Klemp, the man behind the project, who made it possible for this book to come to fruition.

To Liz Corra, my patient development editor, who did bear with me and my endless list of questions for many months.

To the librarians of the Biblioteca Hospital Universitari Joan XXIII of Tarragona, always available to provide to me all the information I requested, in the fastest way possible.

To Jennifer McGillan, archivist from the Archives and Special Collections, Augustus C. Long Health Sciences Library, Columbia University Medical Center, for her thorough historical research.

To all of them, my sincere and deepest gratitude. Together, we built our own *castell*.

Contents

Contributors

Christina A. Banzhaf, MD Department of Dermatology, Roskilde Hospital, Roskilde, Denmark

Health Sciences Faculty, University of Copenhagen, Roskilde, Denmark

Ioannis D. Bassukas, MD, PhD Department of Skin and Venereal Diseases, Faculty of Medicine School of Health Sciences, University of Ioannina, Ioannina, Greece

David Buckley, MB, BCh, NUI, MRCGP Solas Dermatology and Laser Clinic, The Ashe Street Clinic, Tralee, County Kerry, Ireland

Joseph Chao Department of Dermatology, University of Arizona Medical Center, Tucson, AZ, USA

Melissa Chu Three Bridges, NJ, USA

Clara Curiel-Lewandrowski, MD Section of Dermatology, Department of Medicine, University of Arizona Cancer Center, Tucson, AZ, USA

Angeles Fortuño-Mar, MD, PhD, MBA Eldine Patologia Laboratory, Tarragona, Spain

Georgios Gaitanis, MD, PhD Department of Skin and Venereal Diseases, Faculty of Medicine, School of Health Sciences, University of Ioannina, Ioannina, Greece

Consuelo Garcia Silva, MD Department of Cryosurgery, Dr. José Barba Rubio Dermatological Institute of Jalisco, Zapopan, Mexico

Eleni A. Georgakopoulou, MD, DDS, MSc Department of Histology and Embryology, Medical School of Athens, Athens, Greece

Mildred J. Gutiérrez, MD Department of Dermatology, Hospital Central Universitario Dr. Antonio María Pineda, Barquisimeto, Venezuela

Mercedes Hernández-Torres, MD Department of Dermatopathology, Dr. José Barba Rubio Dermatological Institute of Jalisco, Zapopan, Mexico

Rainer Hofmann-Wellenhof, MD Department of Dermatology, Medical University Graz, Graz, Austria

Gregor Jemec, MD, DMSc Department of Dermatology, Roskilde Hospital, Roskilde, Denmark

Health Sciences Faculty, University of Copenhagen, Roskilde, Denmark

Jānis Ķīsis, MD, PhD Department of Infectology and Dermatology, Riga Stradins University, Riga, Latvia

Aleksandar L. Krunic, MD, PhD Department of Dermatology, University of Illinois College of Medicine, River Forest, IL, USA

Nikoforos Kollias, PhD Department of Dermatology, University of British Columbia, Vancouver, BC, Canada

Olle Larkö, MD Department of Dermatology, The Sahlgrenska Academy, Sahlgrenska University Hospital, University of Gothenburg, Gothenburg, Sweden

Gun Lindgren, MD, PhD Department of Ophthalmology, Sahlgrenska University Hospital, Mölndal, Sweden

Miguel Alejandro Lopez Blanco, MD Department of Dermatology, Hospital Militar Carlos Arvelo, Caracas, Venezuela

Panagiota Loumou, MD, DDS, PhD Second Department of Dermatology, University Hospital Attikon, Athens, Greece

Mette Mogensen, MD, PhD Department of Dermatology, Bispebjerg Hospital, Copenhagen, Denmark

Health Sciences Faculty, University of Copenhagen, Copenhagen, Denmark

Peter Nordin, MD Läkarhuset Hospital, Dermatology Clinic, Gothenburg, Sweden

Anthony Panagiotopoulos, MD Department of Cryosurgery, Hospital Andreas Syggros, Athens, Greece

Paola Pasquali, MD Department of Dermatology, Pius Hospital de Valls, Tarragona, Spain

Raimo Suhonen, MD, PhD Department of Dermatology, Ikioma Medical Center, Mikkeli, Finland

Lotte Themstrup, MD Department of Dermatology, Roskilde Hospital, Roskilde, Denmark

Health Sciences Faculty, University of Copenhagen, Roskilde, Denmark

Aleksejs Zavorins, MD Department of Dermatology, Private Practice of Prof J. Kisis, Riga, Latvia

Miroslava Zolano Orozco, MD Department of Dermatology, Civil Hospital of Guadalajara Fray Antonio Alcalde, Guadalajara, Mexico

Part I

The Basics

A Short History of Cryosurgery

1

Paola Pasquali

Contents

P. Pasquali, MD
Department of Dermatology, Pius Hospital de Valls, 43800 Tarragona, Spain
e-mail: pasqualipaola@gmail.com

Key Points

- The discovery of and handling of cryogens with sufficient low temperatures made possible the destruction of tumors.
- The modern history of cryosurgery started in the physical chemistry laboratories and later developed with the expert contribution of engineers and physicists engineers, physicists and physicians.

1.1 Introduction

Human beings have always been obsessed with controlling extreme temperatures and apparently all for one purpose: eating. At one end of this thermic spectrum, man's discovery of fire marked a crucial turning point in human evolution. For some authors, cooking made man [1]. Control of fire allowed man to cook and feed himself with new products to nourish his body and mind. Control of cold helped humans with food preservation: there is evidence in ancient China and India that man knew how to preserve ice. But then ice got into the medical cabinet. It has been the oldest analgesic and anti-inflammatory treatment, back even to the times of the Pharaohs and the ancient Greeks. An Egyptian papyrus document describes the use of cold as an anti-inflammatory, and Hippocrates, back in fifth century BC, recommended cold for reducing bleeding, bruising, and swelling [2]. Ice was known as a cooling agent for many centuries,

P. Pasquali (ed.), *Cryosurgery: A Practical Manual*,
DOI 10.1007/978-3-662-43939-5_1, © Springer-Verlag Berlin Heidelberg 2015

but low temperatures had to be controlled. In the ninth century, the Tang dynasty used potassium nitrate (saltpeter) mixed with sulfur and coal to make gunpowder, while saltpeter and water were combined to created a cooling agent. The Spanish physician Blasius Villafranca in his "Methodus refrigerandi ex vocato sale nitro vinum aquamque" [3], published in 1550, uses the word "refrigerant" for the first time, mentioning some of its uses.

However, if cold was to be used to cure diseases, lower temperatures were needed. This marked the beginning of the cold race: the quest for the perfect refrigerant had begun.

1.2 When Ice Met Salt (−20 °C): Arnott, the First Crusader of Cryosurgery

The first record of a formal medical application of controlled freezing to destroy tissues is found by James M. Arnott (Scotland, 1797–1883), an English physician who used a technique that allowed him to reduce tissue temperature to the proximity of −20 °C. Between 1819 and 1879, he published on the use of cold as a medical treatment [4, 5]. Arnott designed his own cold equipment that used a mixture of crushed ice, water, and salts as refrigerant. He placed a waterproof bladder in contact with the lesion, while two hoses circulated the freezing fluid in and out of the bladder with the help of a pump. Incredible as it might sound, this medical invention was exhibited by Arnott at the 1851 Great Exhibition of London [6] where he won a prize medal (Fig. 1.1). He wrote that very low temperatures would stop any inflammation process as long as it was kept in close contact with the cold source for a long enough period of time. Although he started using cold for palliation of tumors, he ended up using it for many skin, breast, and uterine cancers; he was afraid of the pernicious side effects of chemicals used as early anesthetics and preferred the anesthetic power of cold for reducing pain.

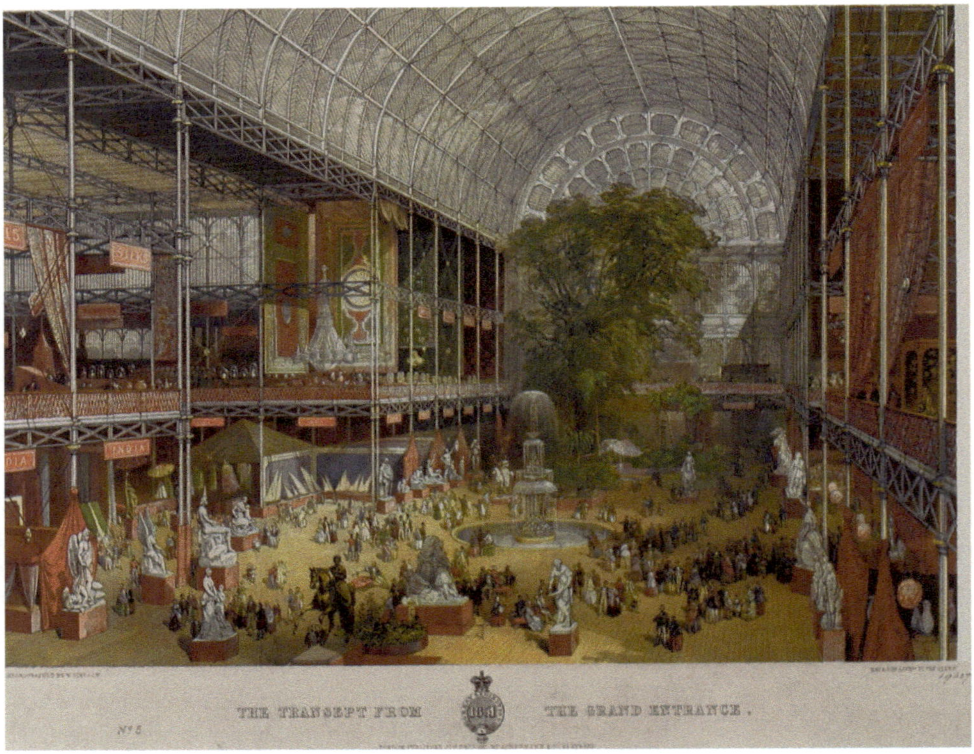

Fig. 1.1 General view of the Great Exhibition of London of 1851, where Arnott received the prize medal for original equipment that allowed reducing tissue temperature to −20 °C (*Source*: http://upload.wikimedia.org/wikipedia/commons/e/eb/Crystal_Palace_interior.jpg. With permission of collections.vam.ac.uk. Artist: McNeven J. Lithographer: William Simpson. The transept from the Grand Entrance, Souvenir of the Great Exhibition. Publisher: Ackermann & Co: 1851)

1.3 End of the Nineteenth Century: The Race for Liquefied Gases Begins

Mixtures of crushed ice with salts were, however, not capable of reducing tissue temperature enough to destroy tumor cells. Lower temperatures were needed, and they were finally attained in the last part of the nineteenth century thanks to the discovery of the necessary technology to liquefy gases. First it was oxygen and then nitrogen. Raoul-Pierre Pictet (Switzerland, 1846–1929) (Fig. 1.2) [7] was the first person to liquefy oxygen. On December 22, 1877, the Academy of Sciences in Paris received a telegram from Pictet in Geneva reading as follows: “Oxygen liquefied today under 320 atmospheres and 140 degrees of cold by combined use of sulfurous and carbonic acid.” Two days later – and following the paradigm of multiple independent discoveries – the French scientist Cailletet announced having liquefied oxygen by a completely different process [8]. Louis-Paul Cailletet Laperouse (1832–1913) (Fig. 1.3) [9] demonstrated at the French Academy of Science that oxygen and carbon monoxide could be liquefied [10]; he built an apparatus that allowed him to produce droplets of liquid oxygen (Fig. 1.4) [11]; he was also the first to liquefy carbon monoxide [12]. Pictet and Cailletet share credit of being the first men to liquefy an atmospheric gas.

Carl von Linde (Germany, 1842–1934) (Fig. 1.5) [13] had achieved the first liquefaction of gases at the end of the nineteenth century [5]. By 1871, he built his first ammonia compression machine, and by 1905 he obtained pure oxygen and nitrogen. He was the first to create a continuous process for liquid gas production. Linde became an expert in refrigeration and gas separation technologies and was the founder (1879) of what is today a leading multinational gases corporation.

In 1891 the physical chemist James Dewar (Scotland, 1842–1923) (Fig. 1.6) [14] built a

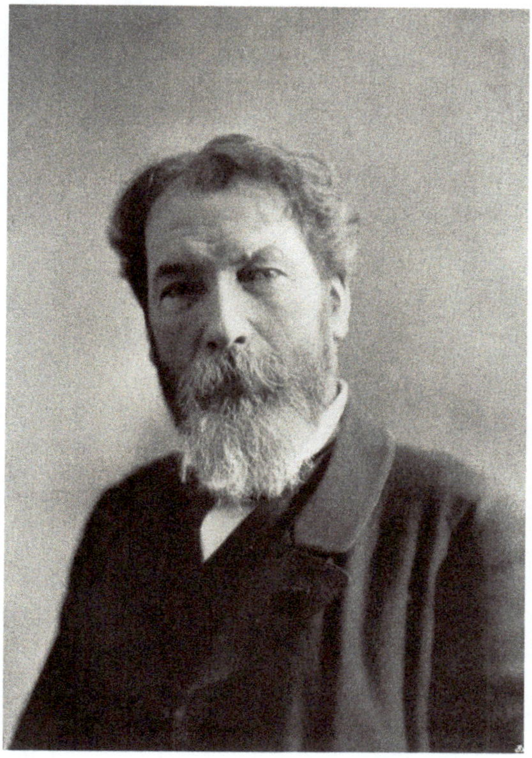

Fig. 1.2 Raoul-Pierre Pictet (Geneva, Switzerland, 1846–1929) (*Source*: Edgar Fahs Smith Collection, University of Pennsylvania Libraries. http://sceti.library.upenn.edu/sceti/smith/imagedetail.cfm?PictureID=1303&position=1&keywords=pictet&subcoll=scientist. In Public Domain)

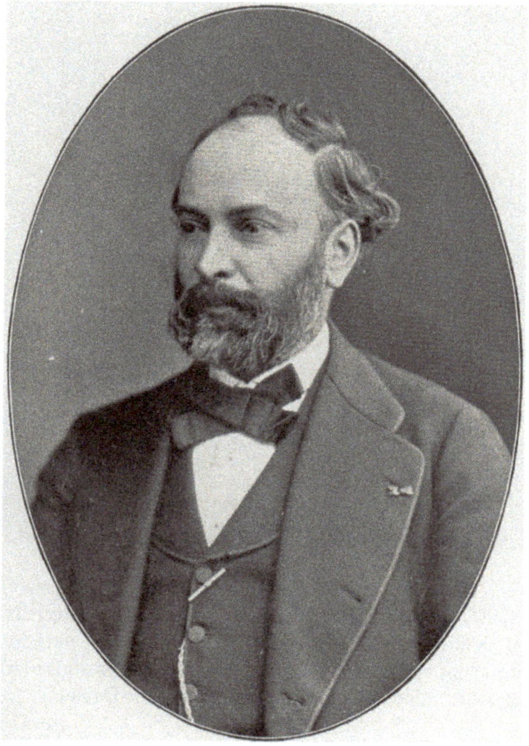

Fig. 1.3 Louis-Paul Cailletet Laperouse (Châtillon-sur-Seine, Côte-d’Or, France, 1832–1913) (*Source*: Edgar Fahs Smith Collection, University of Pennsylvania Libraries. http://sceti.library.upenn.edu/sceti/smith/imagedetail.cfm?PictureID=1390&Position=2&keywords=cailletet&subcoll=scientist. In Public Domain)

Fig. 1.4 Image of Cailletet's gas liquefaction apparatus (*Source*: http://upload.wikimedia.org/wikipedia/commons/1/1e/PSM_V12_D635_Cailletet_gas_liquefaction_apparatus.jpg. *The Popular Science Monthly*, No 12, Nov 1877 to April 1878. New York: D. Appleton and Company, 1879. https://archive.org/details/popularsciencemo12newy; In Public Domain)

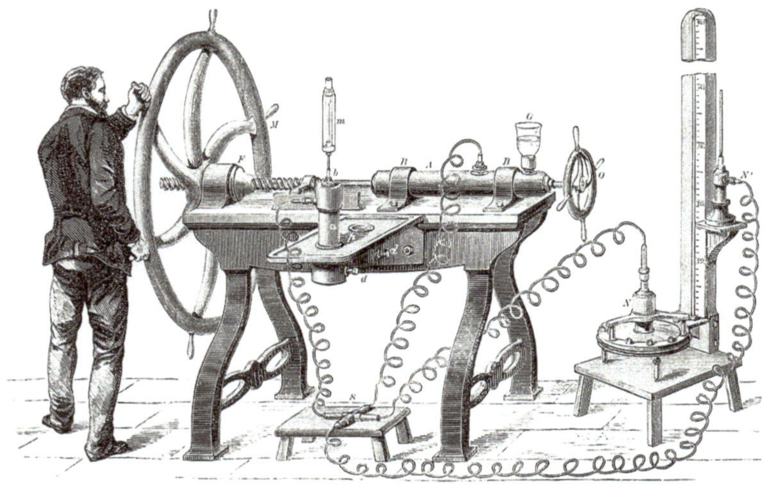

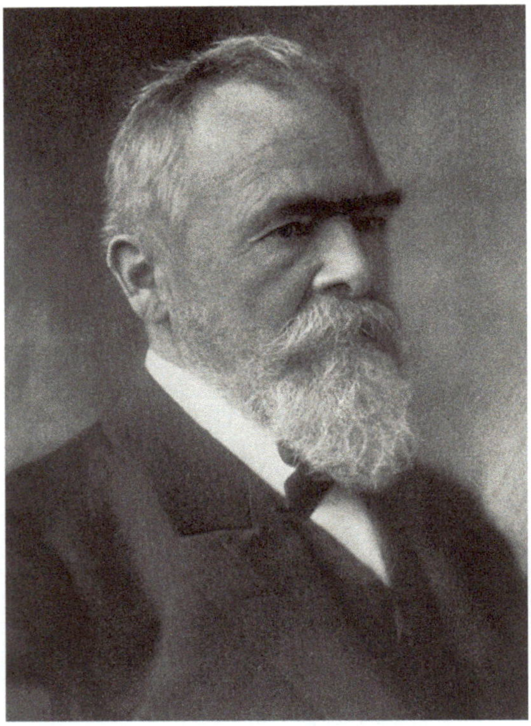

Fig. 1.5 Carl von Linde (Upper Franconia, Germany, 1842–1934) (From Edgar Fahs Smith Collection, University of Pennsylvania Libraries. http://sceti.library.upenn.edu/sceti/smith/imagedetail.cfm?PictureID=271&position=1&keywords=linde&subcoll=scientist. In Public Domain)

machine capable of making liquid oxygen in large quantities. Dewar worked throughout his life on the behavior of gases at very low temperatures.

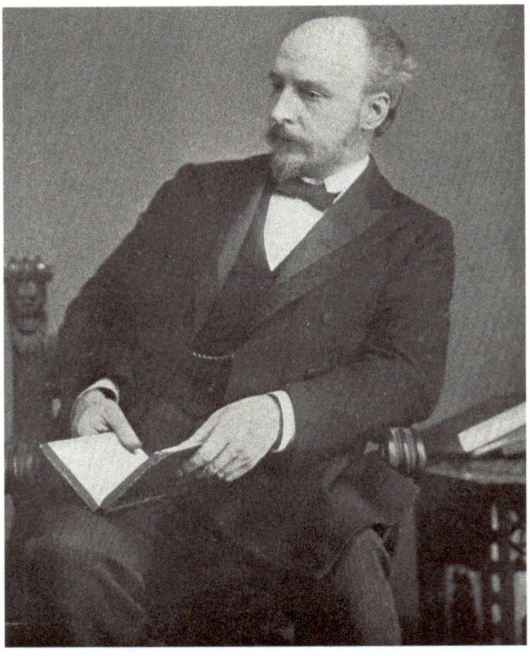

Fig. 1.6 James Dewar (Kincardine-on-Forth, Scotland, 1842–1923) (From Edgar Fahs Smith Collection, University of Pennsylvania Libraries. http://sceti.library.upenn.edu/sceti/smith/scientist.cfm?PictureID=611&ScientistID=477. In Public Domain)

He made liquid forms of many gases and designed many devices to produce them or to store them. In 1898, Dewar condensed liquid hydrogen with the help of one of the devices he had invented, the Dewar flask. He needed a place to store the

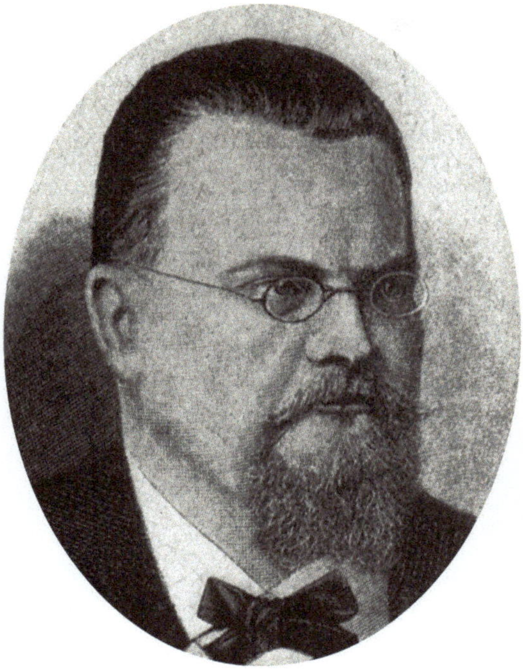

Fig. 1.7 Zygmunt Florenty Wróblewski (Russian Empire, presently Belarus, 1845–1888) (*Source*: http://commons.wikimedia.org/wiki/File:Zygmunt_Florenty_Wroblewski_Polish_physicist.jpg. Polish "Problemy" monthly, May 1964. In Public Domain)

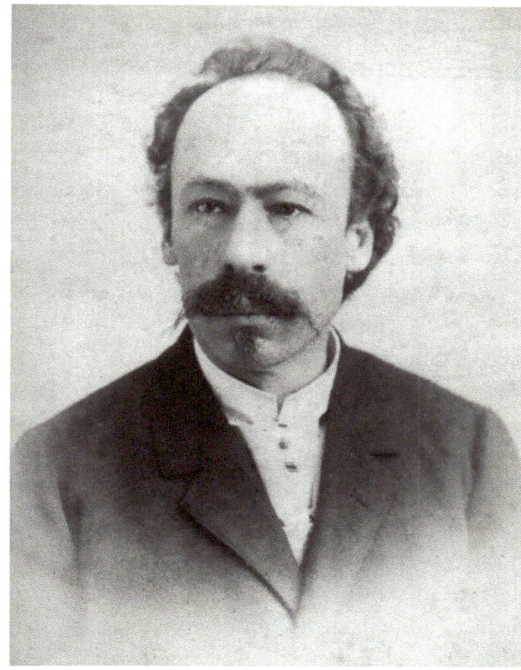

Fig. 1.8 Karol Stanisław Olszewski (Broniszów, Poland, 1846–1915) (*Source*: http://en.wikipedia.org/wiki/File:Karol_Olszewski.jpg. In Public Domain)

liquefied gases he produced. In 1892, he developed the idea of a flask with two silvered walls separated by an evacuated air chamber, thus insulating the inside from the outside of the flask. He knew heat transfer occurred by three physical phenomena: convection, conduction, and radiation. Vacuum eliminated convection, since there are no moving molecules in the gas to transfer heat, and also greatly reduced conduction, as there would be far fewer adjacent gas molecules. Dewar's invention allowed for the first time the use of liquid gases outside the laboratory, thus making liquefied gases accessible to physicians. In his honor or perhaps unknowingly, the insulating storage vessel commonly used to keep liquid nitrogen is still called Dewar flask.

Zygmunt Florenty Wróblewski (Russian Empire, today Belarus, 1845–1888) (Fig. 1.7) [15] and Karol Stanisław Olszewski (Poland, 1846–1915) (Fig. 1.8) [16] were the first scientists reporting liquefaction of oxygen, nitrogen, and carbon dioxide in a stable condition (1883). At the Jagiellonian University in Krakow, where the two scientists met as professors, Olszewski had started his experiments compressing and condensing carbon dioxide. In 1884, Olszewski was the first to liquefy hydrogen in a dynamic state at −225 °C. Wróblewski died of severe burns (1888) during an experiment to study the properties of hydrogen. Olszewski liquefied argon in 1895, but he failed at liquefying helium. In 1886, just a few days after learning about Wilhelm Röntgen's work on X-rays, Olszewski replicated the experiment.

1.4 The Day Air Became Liquid and Available to Physicians (−195 °C)

Although part of the physical chemical laboratories, liquefied gases were not yet available for medical use. Archibald Campbell White

(New York, USA) at Vanderbilt clinic, Columbia University, was the first one to use liquefied gas in medicine. Although he died at the age of 39 [17], he left a significant legacy in the form of the medical use of liquefied gases. White had worked together with Thurston G. Lusk and his associates at Roosevelt Hospital at Columbia University and with George M. Fox, a renowned dermatologist.

In 1899, he reported successful use of liquid air for the treatment of dermatologic pathologies such as lupus erythematosus, herpes zoster, chancroid, nevi, warts, varicose leg ulcers, carbuncles, and epitheliomas [18–20]. He reported positive results by using liquid air for the treatment of skin cancer [21, 22]. To get the liquid air sprayed, he used a glass flask with two glass tubes going through a double pierced cork. One tube went down to the bottom of the flask, finishing on the outside end on a spout with a small hole the size of a pencil point; the other tube was shorter, being used with a thumb to control the entrance of free air from the outside. The flask acted as a liquid air sprayer, becoming the first handheld cryosurgery device (Fig. 1.9) [23]. Sometimes he rolled a glass flask partially filled with the refrigerant over the lesion (Fig. 1.10) [24, 25] as in the doorknob probe used today for vascular hypertrophic lesions. At other times, he used a cotton swab dipped in the liquid air.

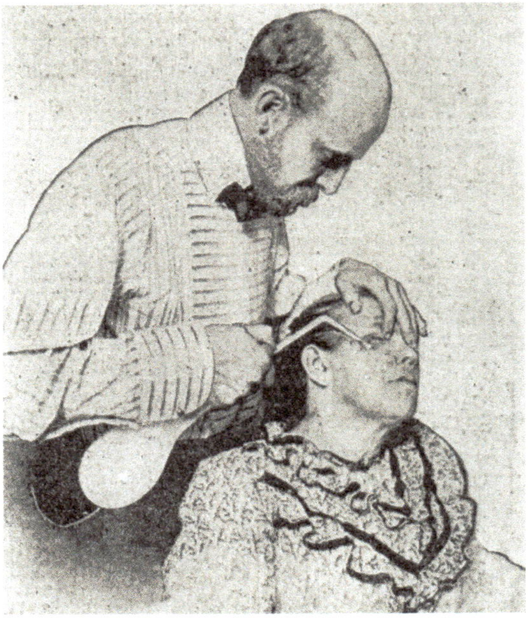

Fig. 1.9 White treating a skin lesion with sprayed liquid air as it appeared in the New York Tribune (October 25, 1900). The title reads: "Uses of Liquid Air: The vast possibilities of the new force" (*Source*: http://chroniclingamerica.loc.gov/lccn/sn83030214/1900-10-25/ed-1/seq-22/. *Chronicling America: Historic American Newspapers*. Library of Congress, Washington, DC. New-York Daily Tribune, October 25, 1900, Page 8, Image 22. In Public Domain)

White used cold application to "allay or abort an acute inflammation" while "not neglecting to treat the cause." He sprayed liquid air with the same technique used today in acne: "I would completely freeze it, possibly pricking it while frozen here and there with a needle, in order to relieve any subsequent congestion.... only one application is necessary." His description of the postoperative effects of cryosurgery is identical to that of liquid nitrogen treatment, in a manner that is impressively similar to the postoperative events with today's liquid nitrogen cryosurgery: "after freezing, the carbuncle should be dressed with a dry absorbent dressing, so that discharge, which will be abundant and accompanied with considerable bleeding, can be readily absorbed." White treated inflammatory conditions such as lupus or chronic ulcers with superficial spraying technique, as well as "nevi and other hypertrophies." In cancer, as a curative treatment he mentions "the great good liquid air has done in these cases." "I believe that epithelioma, treated early in its existence by liquid air, will always be cured by its application." White also praised the palliative effect "even in cases in which the treatment has failed to cure." "The great good done in the relief of pain and the destruction of bad odor, both so characteristic of this disease, places liquid air in efficiency far above any other treatment we have today" [26, 27]. White was the first one to use liquefied gas and deep freeze (−195 °C) as a medical treatment, thus giving birth to deep-freeze cryosurgery.

Liquid air used by White was supplied by Charles E. Triplet, the inventor of the process to produce low-cost liquid air. Triplet was a New York entrepreneur who helped White to promote the medical use of liquid air. Before the White and Triplet collaboration, liquid air and

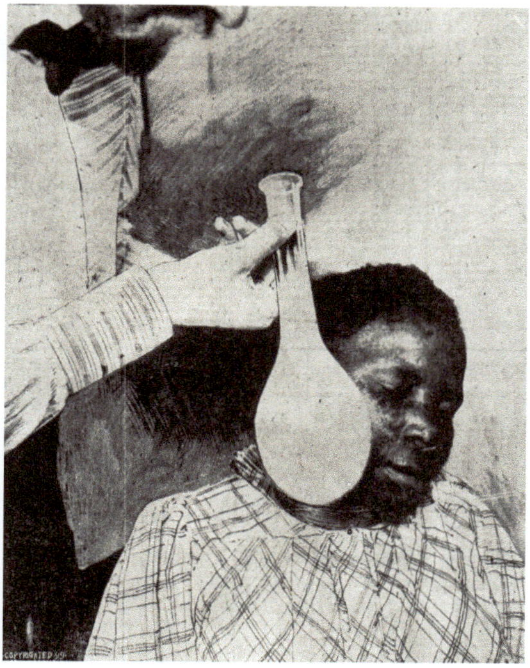

Fig. 1.10 White treating a skin lesion with liquid air as it appeared on the San Francisco Call (August 6, 1899). The title reads: "Curing cancer by freezing with liquid air. Remarkable surgical experiments by Dr. A. Campbell White of Vanderbilt Clinic, Columbia University, in which liquid air has superseded x-rays as the newest marvel how it is applied and reasons why it effects such wonderful cures" (*Source*: http://cdnc.ucr.edu/cgi-bin/cdnc?a=d&d=SFC18990806.2.205.19. California Digital Newspaper Collection, Center for Bibliographic Studies and Research, University of California, Riverside, http://cdnc.ucr.edu. San Francisco Call, Volume 86, Number 67, August 6, 1899. In Public Domain)

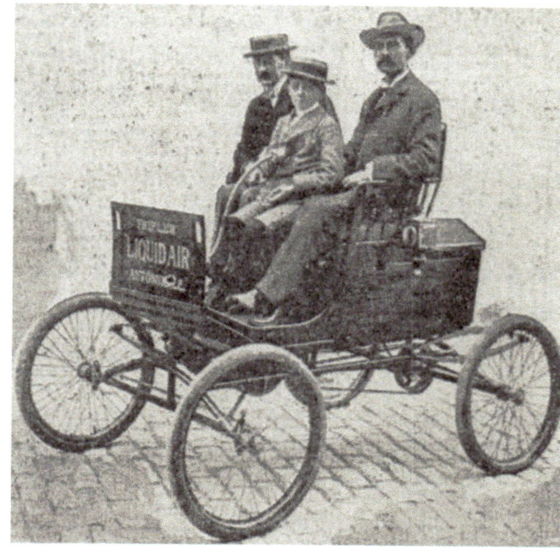

Fig. 1.11 Triplet automobile on the streets of New York (1900), the first car that moved by means of a liquid air engine (*Source*: http://chroniclingamerica.loc.gov/lccn/sn83030214/1900-10-25/ed-1/seq-22/. *Chronicling America: Historic American Newspapers*. Library of Congress, Washington, DC. New-York Daily Tribune, October 25, 1900, Page 8, Image 22. In Public Domain)

other liquid gases were not available for medical use; Triplet also promoted liquid air as an energy source for transportation, building the first automobile powered by liquid air (Fig. 1.11) [23]. Thanks to the commercial interest of Triplet to promote different uses for liquid air, White could have enough liquid air for experimenting and treating patients. Although liquid air was announced by Triplet as a cheap product – "the cost being hardly more than that of mineral water" [28] that could be delivered to the clinic in an insulated one-gallon tank – it was never widely used due to its poor availability.

The first known combination treatment in cryosurgery was performed in 1907. H. Whitehouse (New York, USA) used sprayed liquid air combined with radiotherapy to treat a wide variety of skin conditions that ranged from epitheliomas to lupus erythematosus to vascular nevi. He froze recurrent tumors previously treated with radiotherapy. He found that this combination gave better results than repeating radiotherapy [29]. He later stopped using the spray technique in favor of a cotton swab.

In 1907, Bowen and Towle reported the successful use of liquid air for vascular tumors [30]. They also used liquid air for the treatment of pigmented hairy nevi and lymphangiomas.

1.5 Liquid Oxygen (−183 °C)

Because of a similar boiling temperature (−182.9 °C), liquid oxygen was used as a cryogenic agent in a similar way to liquid air, particularly during the 1920s and 1930s. It was mainly used to treat acne. In 1929, Irvine and Turnacliff reported good results with some skin conditions such as warts and lichen planus. Liquid oxygen soon became obsolete as a cryogenic agent because of its high combustibility [31]. One of the last reports on liquid oxygen as cryogenic agent is the one by Kile and Welsh (1948); they published the results of a study on approximately 1,000 patients of a diversity of nonmalignant tumors that included warts, hemangiomas, mucosal diseases, and leukoplakia [32].

1.6 Solid Carbon Dioxide (−79 °C)

Arnott was the first to suggest that solid carbon dioxide might be used to achieve a more effective cold treatment in patients [5], but there is no evidence that he might have tried it. Solid carbon dioxide did not become commercially available until the end of the nineteenth century, thanks to the then new advances in gas physical chemistry.

Solid carbon dioxide was first described in 1830 by French inventor Adrien-Jean-Pierre Thilorier (1790–1844) (Fig. 1.12) [33], who published the first account of the substance [34]. According to the official Bulletin of the Laws of the Kingdom of France, Thilorier, still an employee of the postal office of Paris, obtained in 1832 legal protection for his invention of a gas compression machine [35]. He had filed for a patent back in May 1831, but not until 5 years later was he identified as the inventor of a gas compression machine (Fig. 1.13) [36]. He was the winner of the French Academy of Sciences' Montyon Prize for Mechanics (1829) [37].

Major John Hall-Edwards (Birmingham, England, 1858–1926) described in 1911 his carbon oxide (CO_2) collector and compressor. He later detailed the methods of collection and uses for CO_2 (1913). He was a renowned radiotherapist in the Midlands who understood well the advantages and disadvantages of carbon dioxide in contrast to radiotherapy [38], a victim himself of the effects of chronic exposure to X-rays that eventually led to the amputation of his left arm [39].

R. Cranston-Low, a physician at the skin department of Edinburgh and contemporary of Hall-Edwards, also promoted the use of carbon dioxide [40]. Solid CO_2 sublimates at −78.5 °C at Earth's atmospheric pressures. By 1924, Thomas B. Slate applied for a US patent to sell solid carbon dioxide commercially.

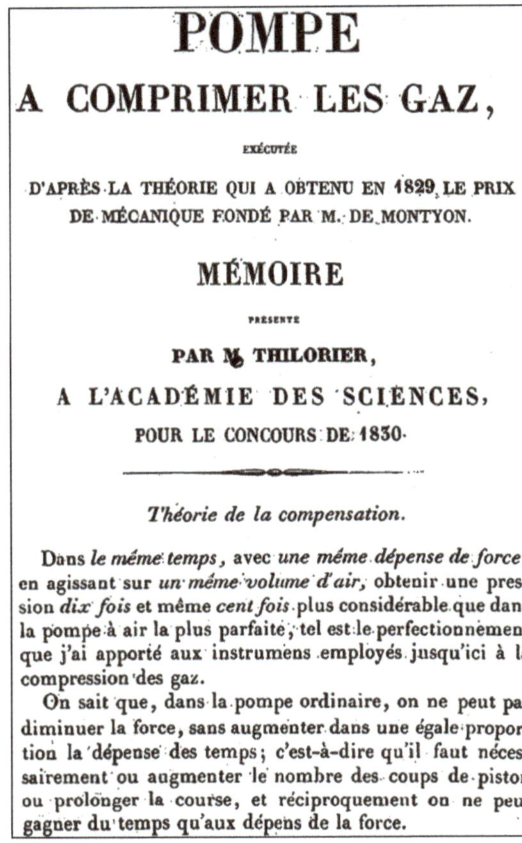

POMPE

A COMPRIMER LES GAZ,

EXÉCUTÉE

D'APRÈS LA THÉORIE QUI A OBTENU EN 1829 LE PRIX DE MÉCANIQUE FONDÉ PAR M. DE MONTYON.

MÉMOIRE

PRÉSENTÉ

PAR M. THILORIER,

A L'ACADÉMIE DES SCIENCES,

POUR LE CONCOURS DE 1830.

Théorie de la compensation.

Dans *le même temps*, avec *une même dépense de force*, en agissant sur *un même volume d'air*, obtenir une pression *dix fois* et même *cent fois* plus considérable que dans la pompe à air la plus parfaite, tel est le perfectionnement que j'ai apporté aux instrumens employés jusqu'ici à la compression des gaz.

On sait que, dans la pompe ordinaire, on ne peut pas diminuer la force, sans augmenter dans une égale proportion la dépense des temps; c'est-à-dire qu'il faut nécessairement ou augmenter le nombre des coups de piston ou prolonger la course, et réciproquement on ne peut gagner du temps qu'aux dépens de la force.

Fig. 1.12 The description of solid carbon dioxide by Adrien-Jean-Pierre Thilorier presented at the academy of science in 1830 (*Source*: http://gallica.bnf.fr/ark:/12148/bpt6k33093/f576.image. Biblioteque National de France. In Public Domain)

Subsequently, he became the first successful CO_2 industrial manufacturer [41]. By 1925, this solid form of was trademarked by DryIce Corporation of America and sold commercially for refrigerating purposes [41] for the first time as "dry ice," a metonymy still in use [42].

In parallel to the investigation on the medical use of liquid air, William Allen Pusey (USA, 1865–1940) (Fig. 1.14) [43] made popular the use of solid carbon dioxide in the form of carbon dioxide snow (or carbonic acid snow) in preference to the mixture of ice and salts [8]. After 1910, liquid air was seldom used, and solid CO_2 became the most popular cryogenic agent because it was cheaper and more readily available than liquid air. Pusey liberated carbon dioxide gas from a pressured cylinder, creating a drop in temperature (the Joule-Thomson effect; 1852), thus producing carbon dioxide flakes.

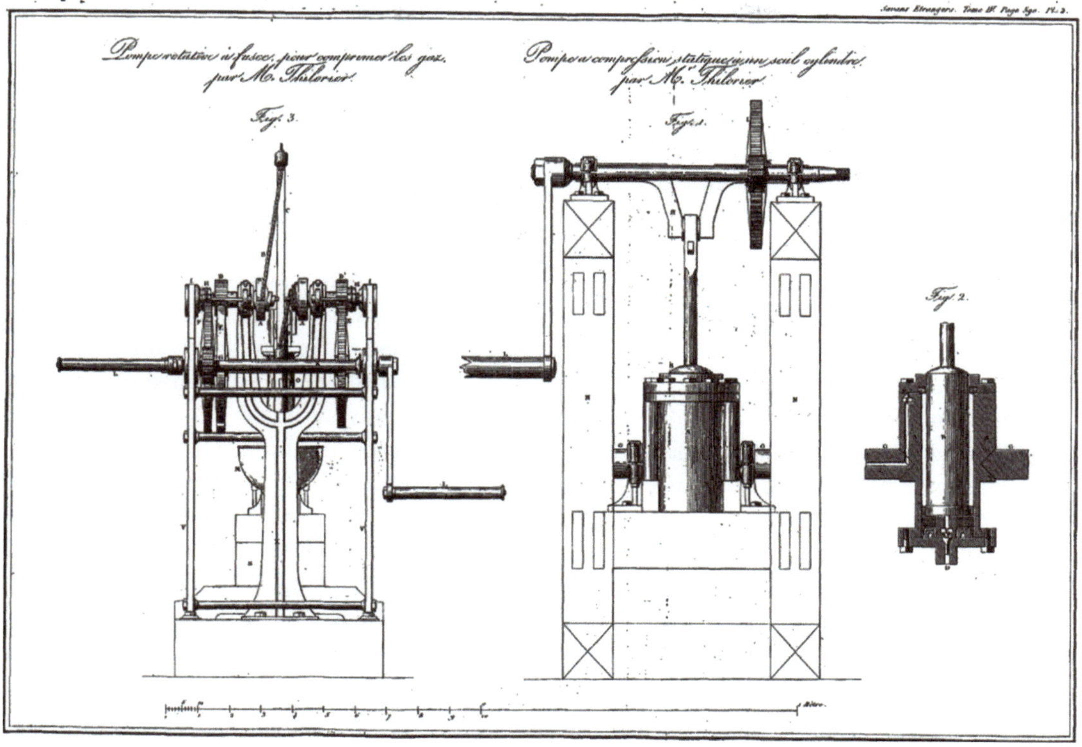

Fig. 1.13 The gas compression machine invented by Thilorier (*Source*: http://gallica.bnf.fr/ark:/12148/bpt6k33093/f603. Bibliotheque National de France. In Public Domain)

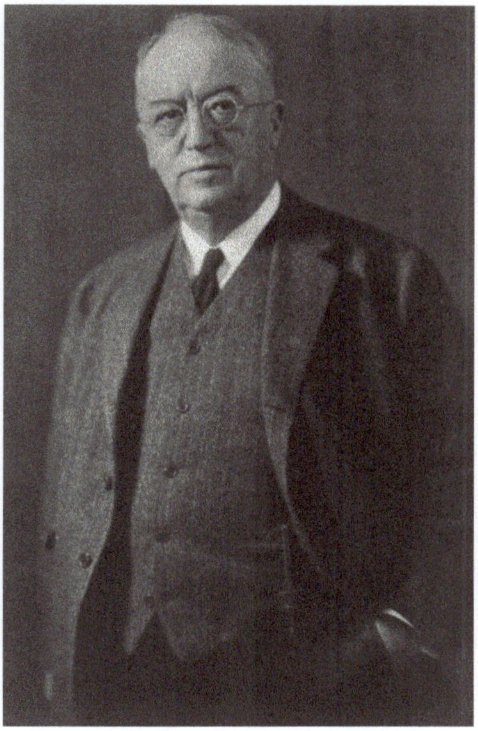

Fig. 1.14 William Allen Pusey (Hardin County Kentucky, USA, 1865–1940) (Used with permission of University of Illinois College of Medicine)

This CO_2 snow (or carbonic acid snow) was then shaped into forms (mostly pencils) suitable for treating tumors. Pusey's first reported case was the treatment of a black hairy nevus on a young girl's face; this was probably the first demonstration of the extraordinary sensitivity of melanocytes to cold. Pusey treated warts, vascular nevi, lupus erythematosus, lupus vulgaris, and epitheliomas [44].

1.7 Liquid Nitrogen (−196 °C)

After the end of the Second World War, liquid nitrogen (LN) became a commercial product. Acknowledging that the cryogenic characteristics of liquid nitrogen were similar to those of either liquid air or liquid oxygen, Herman V. (Ray) Allington started using it in the USA in 1950, by application on a saturated cotton swab. Until 1962, LN was used by the saturated cotton swab technique on benign and premalignant lesions. It was Allington who introduced its highly effective use for the treatment of selected skin lesions, and it was he who – having worked with Frederick Mohs at the University of Wisconsin in Madison – brought an improved modification to the micrographic surgical technique [45].

A main step forward in the development of modern cryosurgery occurred with the work of physician Irving S. Cooper (1922–1985) (Fig. 1.15) [46] and engineer Arnold Lee. They developed a cryosurgical probe (1961) that has inspired other probes that were developed afterward. Cooper and Lee's probe was made of three concentric tubes: the inner tube allowed the flow of liquid nitrogen out toward the tip of the probe; the space between the inner tube and the middle tube made possible the return of nitrogen in gas state from the tip of the probe; the space between the middle tube and the outer tube was air-evacuated, thus allowing thermal insulation of the two inner tubes [47]. Cooper developed chemopallidectomy and cryothalamectomy as surgical techniques for primary control of tremor in patients with Parkinson's disease [48].

1.8 Handheld Spray Apparatus

A more widespread use of liquid nitrogen in medical practice came with the design of devices suitable for use in the physician's office. Back in 1900, White had developed the first rudimentary device for spraying liquid gas on a small area, but its use ended with the end of liquid air for medical treatment. The first modern patented handheld device was by engineer Michael Bryne (Fig. 1.16) [49] (US Pat. 3,534,739A and 3,651,813) (1969) (Fig. 1.17a, b) [50, 51], later founder of the Brymill Corp. Other handheld units by Setrag Zacarian (US Pat 3,702,114A,

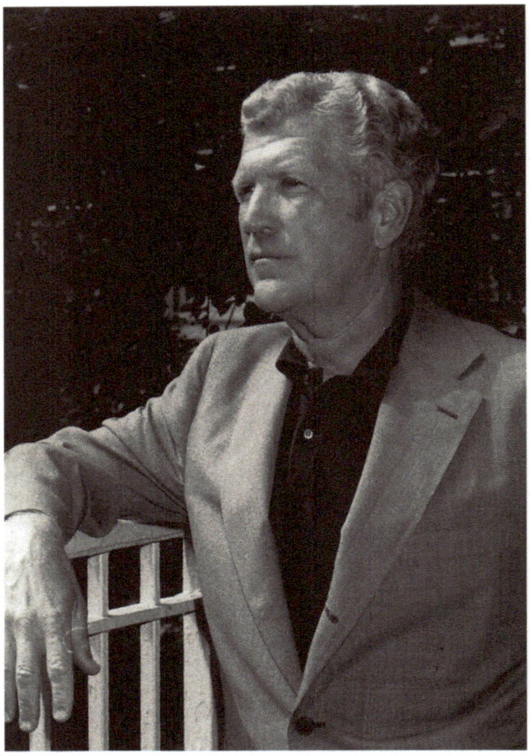

Fig. 1.15 Irving S. Cooper (New York, NY, USA, 1922–1985) (Reproduced with permission of the family of Irving Cooper)

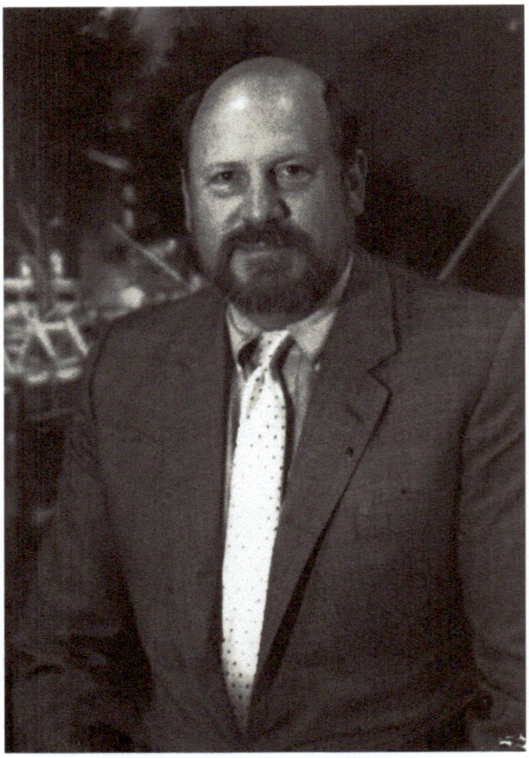

Fig. 1.16 Michael Bryne (Harford, CT, USA, 1938–1992) (Reproduced with permission of the family of Michael Bryne)

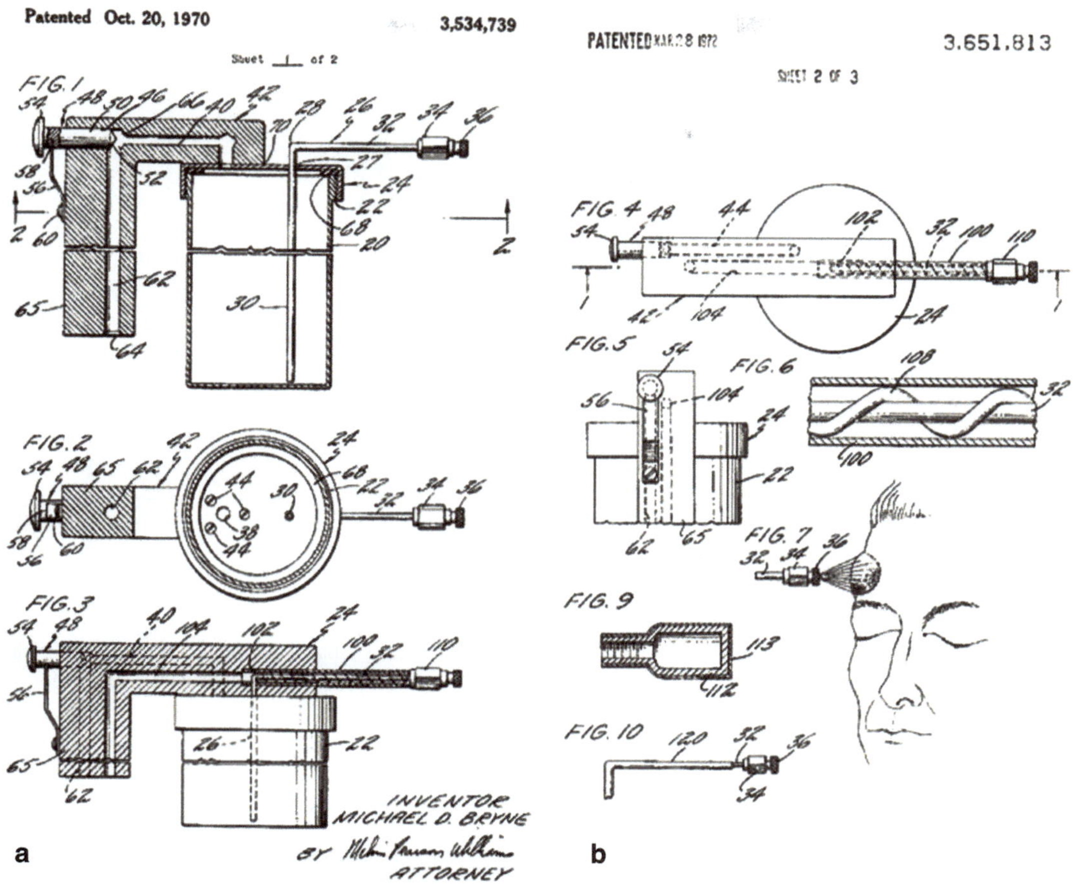

Fig. 1.17 (**a, b**) First patented handheld unit by Michael Bryne (US Pat. 3,534,739, US Pat. 3,651,813) (*Source*: http://www.google.es/patents/US3534739A and http://www.google.com/patents/US3651813. In Public Domain)

Fig. 1.18) [52], Theodore Tromovitch (US Pat. 3,823,718, Fig. 1.19) [53], and Douglas Torre (US Pat. 4,313,306, Fig. 1.20) [54] followed.

Setrag Aram Zacarian started working and reporting his research and clinical data in 1969 [55], becoming a leading reference in the field [56, 57]. The term "cryosurgery" is used by him for the first time.

In the USA, educational programs for cryosurgery were conducted by Zacarian, Torre, Gage, Kuflik, Graham, Lubritz, Elton, and Spiler. In 1988, Torre, Lublitz and Kuflik coauthored a book on the practical aspects of cryosurgery in dermatology [58]. In the UK, during the late 1970s and following years, cryosurgery training was popularized by Dawber et al. who published a successful textbook that already has three editions. In the meantime, a Venezuelan dermatologist, Gilberto Castro-Ron (Fig. 1.21) [59], who had trained in Philadelphia, learned about this specialty, brought it back home, and set up a dermatologic unit at the Hospital Oncologico Luis Razetti (Caracas, Venezuela), which became a significant reference for most Spanish-speaking countries. He was the first one to treat large vascular tumors. His numerous Latin American students themselves started new centers of teachings in their own countries or origin, such as in Mexico, Colombia, and Peru, among others.

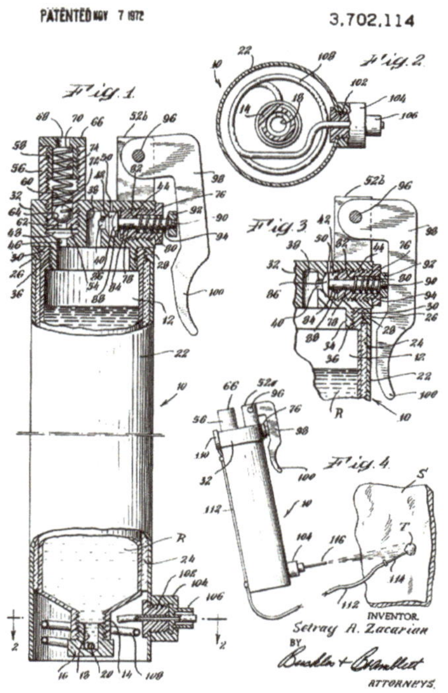

Fig. 1.18 Zacarian's handheld unit (US Pat. 3,702,114) (*Source*: http://www.google.com/patents/US3702114. In Public Domain)

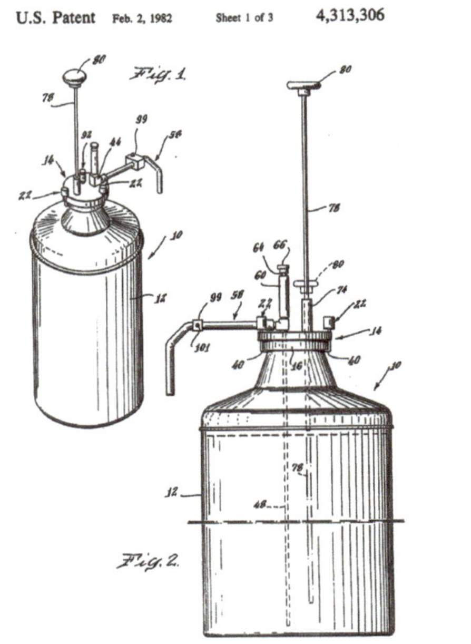

Fig. 1.20 Torre's handheld unit (US Pat. 4,313,306) (*Source*: http://www.google.com/patents/US4313306. In Public Domain)

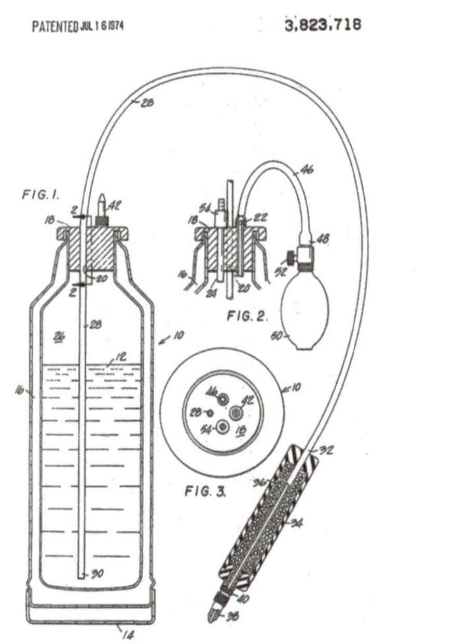

Fig. 1.19 Tromovitch's handheld unit (US Pat. 3,823,718) (*Source*: https://www.google.com/patents/US3823718. In Public Domain)

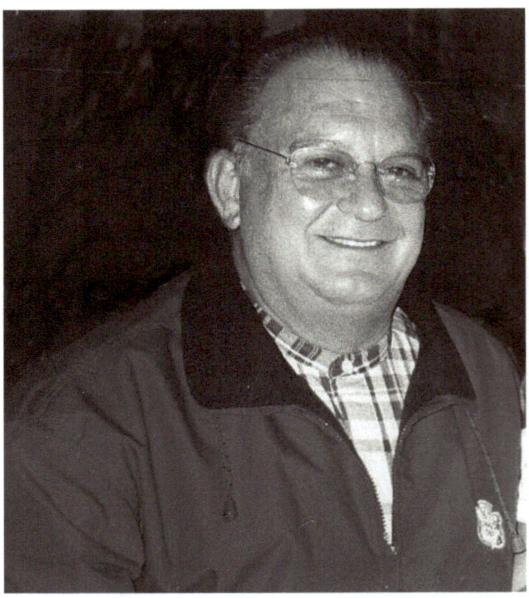

Fig. 1.21 Gilberto Castro-Ron (Zaraza, Venezuela, 1937–2004) (Reproduced with permission of the family of Gilberto Castro-Ron)

1.9 Other Specialties

Cryosurgery is very popular for the treatment of skin conditions among dermatologists, family physicians, and specialized nurses. It is by no means an exclusive domain for skin surgeons; other specialties that use it extensively are gynecology, urology, cardiology, thoracic surgery, orthopedics, and ophthalmology. Among the most commonly used cryogens are liquid nitrogen, argon, and argon-helium.

In the subsequent chapters of this book, we will review and discuss current practice of cryosurgery, showing its multiple and versatile uses. A timeline is shown in Table 1.1.

Table 1.1 Timeline for cryosurgery

Ancient world. Ice is used as an anti-inflammatory and to reduce bleeding, bruising, and swelling
1835 – Thilorier observes solid carbon dioxide
1851 – Arnott uses a mixture of crushed ice and salt to reduce tissue temperature to −20 °C
1851 – Arnott suggests that solid carbon dioxide might be better than ice
1877 – Pictet and Cailletet independently obtain liquid oxygen by different methods
1882 – Dewar invents what today is the Dewar flask for storing liquid gas
1883 – Wróblewski and Olszewski liquefy oxygen, nitrogen, and carbon dioxide in stable condition
1884 – Olszewski liquefies hydrogen in a dynamic state
1891 – Dewar creates a machine to produce liquid oxygen in large quantities
1892 – Dewar designs the first vacuum-insulated flask to store liquid gases
1895 – Linde produces oxygen and nitrogen in a continuous process
1899 – Triplet commercially produces liquid air as a source of energy as well as for medical treatments. He collaborated with Archibald Campbell White and other New York physicians
1899 – White is the first to use liquid gas (liquid air) for medical practice. He developed the first handheld device to spray liquid air for cryosurgery. He was followed by Lusk and Fox
1907 – Whitehouse uses sprayed liquid air for treating dermatologic pathologies. In the case of cancer, he combined cold with radiotherapy
1907 – Bowen and Towle use liquid air for vascular tumors
1907 – Pusey makes solid carbon dioxide popular in the form of snow (carbonic acid snow)
1910 – From this date on, liquid air is seldom used
1911 – Hall-Edwards in England designs a carbon dioxide collector and compressor
1911 – Cranston-Low promotes the use of carbon dioxide in Scotland
1913 – Hall-Edwards detailed the method of collection and use for carbon dioxide
1924 – Slate applies for a US patent on carbon dioxide
1925 – Solid carbon dioxide is trademarked in the USA as dry ice
1929 – Irwin and Turnacliff use liquid oxygen for warts and lichen planus
1945 – With the end of the Second World War, liquid nitrogen becomes a commercial product
1948 – Kile and Welsh report the use of liquid oxygen in more than 1,000 patients with different tumors
1950 – Allington uses liquid nitrogen with the saturated cotton swab technique
1962 – Liquid nitrogen is still used with the saturated cotton swab technique on benign and premalignant lesions
1961 – Cooper and Lee develop the cryosurgical probe
Mid-1960s – First use of thermocouple to measure temperature at the depth of the tumor
1965 – Torres develops liquid nitrogen spray equipment with interchangeable tips
1966 – Bryne (Brymill) develops and patents the first handheld cryosurgical device
1967 – Zacarian presents results of the handheld cryo-spray
1970 – Dawber in the UK starts popularizing cryosurgery
1969 – Book. Zacarian S. *Cryosurgery of Skin Cancer, and Cryogenic Techniques in Dermatology.* Springfield, IL: Charles C Thomas (Publisher)
1970 – During the following years, educational programs on cryosurgery were conducted in the USA by Zacarian, Torre, Gage, Kuflik, Graham, Lubritz, Elton, and Spiler
1973 – Book. Zacarian S. *Cryosurgery of Tumors of the Skin and Oral Cavity.* C. C. Thomas (Publisher)
1974 – Foundation of International Society of Cryosurgery
1977 – Foundation of American Academy of Cryosurgery
1985 – Book. Zacarian S. *Cryosurgery Skin Cancer.* Mosby (Publisher)
1988 – Book. Torre D, Lubritz R, Kuflik E. *Practical Cutaneous Cryosurgery.* Appleton & Lange (Publisher)
1990 – Book. Breitbart EW, Dachow-Siwiec E (Editors). *Advances in Cryosurgery (Clinics in Dermatology).* Elsevier Science (Publisher)

(continued)

Table 1.1 (continued)

1990 –	Book. Kuflik E, Gage A. *Cryosurgical Treatment for Skin Cancer*. Igaku-Shoin Medical (Publisher)
1992 –	Foundation of Colegio Iberoamericano de Criocirugía
1992 –	Book. Rodney P. R. Dawber, Graham Colver and Arthur Jackson. *Cutaneous Cryosurgery: Principles and Clinical Practice*. First Edition. Taylor & Francis Ltd. (Publisher)
1997 –	Book. Pringle F, Colver G, Jackson A, Dawber R. *Cutaneous Cryosurgery: Principles and Clinical Practice*. 2nd edition. CRC Press (Publisher)
1998 –	Criocirugía y Radiofrecuencia en Piel y Mucosas (CD-ROM). Stolar E, Turjansky E (Authors). McGraw Hill Interamericana (Publisher)
2004 –	Book. Mintzias P. *Cryosurgery in Dermatology*. Dimopoylos Panagos (Publisher)
2005 –	Book. Colver G, Jackson A, Dawber R. *Cutaneous Cryosurgery: Principles and Clinical Practice*. Third Edition. Taylor & Francis (Publisher)
2007 –	Marketing of the first equipment capable of measuring and recording temperature (Cry-Ac® TrackerCam™ by Brymill) during the freezing procedure

Essential Tidbits

- Liquefying gases and developing machines to produce them in large quantities, to store them, and to transport them safely were all essential steps in bringing cryosurgery into physicians' offices.
- In the timeline of events that brought us to what we know as modern cryosurgery, Archibald Campbell White stands as the first modern cryosurgeon.
- Handheld units simplified and standardized liquid nitrogen delivery. A series of different designs have brought us to what we use nowadays: small, handy, light, and versatile equipment.

References

1. Cordón F. Cocinar hizo al hombre. 1st ed. Colección Los 5 Sentidos. Spain: Tusquet Ed.; 1980.
2. Hippocrates. Aphorisms. Section V. Available from: http://classics.mit.edu//Hippocrates/aphorisms.html [Accessed: 14th Jan 2014].
3. Wexcombe A. Reviving the use of saltpetre for refrigeration. A period technique. Available from: https://www.academia.edu/1136936/Reviving_the_Use_of_Saltpetre_for_Refrigeration_a_Period_Technique.
4. Arnott J. On the treatment of cancer by the regulated application of an anaesthetic temperature. London: Churchill; 1851.
5. Bird H. James Arnott, MD (Aberdeen), 1797–1883, a pioneer in refrigeration. Anaesthesia. 1949;4:10–7.
6. McNeven, J. (draughtsman (artist)), William Simpson (lithographer). The transept from the grand entrance, Souvenir of the Great Exhibition (Print). 1851. Printed and published: Great Britain, United Kingdom: Ackermann & Co. Available from: http://upload.wikimedia.org/wikipedia/commons/thumb/e/eb/Crystal_Palace_interior.jpg/640px-Crystal_Palace_interior.jpg.
7. Raoul-Pierre Pictet. 1914. http://sceti.library.upenn.edu/sceti/smith/imagedetail.cfm?PictureID=1303&position=1&keywords=pictet&subcoll=scientist.
8. Cooper SM, Dawber RPR. The history of cryosurgery. J R Soc Med. 2001;94(4):196–201.
9. Cailletet LP. 1910. http://sceti.library.upenn.edu/sceti/smith/imagedetail.cfm?PictureID=1390&Position=2&keywords=cailletet&subcoll=scientist.
10. Cailletet L. Recherches sur la liquéfaction des gaz. Ann Chemis Physique. 1878;15:132–44.
11. Cailletet gas_liquefaction_apparatus. http://upload.wikimedia.org/wikipedia/commons/1/1e/PSM_V12_D635_Cailletet_gas_liquefaction_apparatus.jpg.
12. McKetta Jr JJ. Encyclopedia of chemical processing and design, vol. 6, Calcination equipment to catalysis. CRC Press; 1978.
13. Carl Linde (1842 – 1934). http://sceti.library.upenn.edu/sceti/smith/imagedetail.cfm?PictureID=271&position=1&keywords=linde&subcoll=scientist.
14. Sir James Dewar (1842 – 1923). http://sceti.library.upenn.edu/sceti/smith/scientist.cfm?PictureID=611&ScientistID=477.
15. Zygmunt Florenty Wroblewski. http://commons.wikimedia.org/wiki/File:Zygmunt_Florenty_Wroblewski_Polish_physicist.jpg.
16. Karol Olszewski. http://en.wikipedia.org/wiki/File:Karol_Olszewski.jpg.
17. Archie Campbell White. Deaths. JAMA. 1908;L(12):984. doi:10.1001/jama.1908.02530380055028.
18. White AC. Liquid air: its applications in medicine and surgery. Med Rec. 1899;56:109–12.
19. White AC. Possibilities of liquid air to the physician. JAMA. 1901;36:426–9.
20. ProQuest Historical Newspapers: Chicago Tribune (1872–1922); 26 Jul 1899. p. 6 – Liquid air in surgery.
21. CDNC.ucr.edu. Weblog. [Online]. San Francisco Call, vol 86(67), 6 Aug 1899 – Curing cancer by freezing with liquid air. [Article] Available from: California Digital Newspaper Collection, Center for Bibliographic Studies and Research, University of California, Riverside. http://cdnc.ucr.edu/cgi-bin/cdnc?a=d&d=SFC18990806.2.205.19.

22. Sacramento Daily Union, vol 98(10), 31 Aug 1899 – Liquid air.
23. Chronicling America: Historic American Newspapers. Library of Congress, Washington, DC. New-York Daily Tribune, 25 Oct 1900, p. 8, Image 22. http://chroniclingamerica.loc.gov/lccn/sn83030214/1900-10-25/ed-1/seq-22/.
24. Hannah Strom LL, Madison D, Madison J. Am J Nurs [Letters to the editor]. 1904;4(8):657–9. Published by Lippincott Williams & Wilkins. http://www.jstor.org/stable/3401762.
25. http://cdnc.ucr.edu/cgi-bin/cdnc?a=d&d=SFC18990806.2.205.19. California Digital Newspaper Collection, Center for Bibliographic Studies and Research, University of California, Riverside, http://cdnc.ucr.edu. San Francisco Call, vol 86(67), 6 Aug 1899.
26. White AC. Possibilities of liquid air to the physician. JAMA. 1901;426–9. Originally presented to the section on Diseases of Children at the 55th annual meeting of AMA, Atlantic City; 5–8 June 1900.
27. Dr. Campbell A. Curing cancer by freezing: remarkable surgical experiments with liquid air. ProQuest Historical Newspapers: The Atlanta Constitution (1868–1945); 30 Jul 1899. p. A6.
28. Freezing out cancer: wonderful results of the use of liquid air in surgery. ProQuest Historical Newspapers: Los Angeles Times (1886–1922); 30 Jul 1899; p. 4.
29. Whitehouse H. Liquid air in dermatology: its indications and limitations. JAMA. 1907;49:371–7.
30. Bowen JT, Towle HP. Liquid air in dermatology. Med Surg J. 1907;157:561.
31. Irvine HG, Turnacliff DD. Liquid oxygen in dermatology. Arch Derm Syphilol. 1929;19(2):270–80.
32. Kile RL, Welsh AL. Liquid oxygen in dermatologic practice. Arch Derm Syphilol. 1948;57:57–60.
33. Pompe a comprimer les gaz . http://gallica.bnf.fr/ark:/12148/bpt6k33093/f576.image.
34. Thilorier. "Solidification de l'Acide carbonique". Comptes Rendus (in French) 1835;1:194–6. See also: "Solidification of carbonic acid," The London and Edinburgh Philosophical Magazine. 1836;8:446–7.
35. The Bulletin des Lois du Royaume de France (Bulletin of the laws of the kingdom of France), 9th series, part II, no. 92, p. 74 (Feb 1832).
36. Thilorier´s gas compression machine. http://gallica.bnf.fr/ark:/12148/bpt6k33093/f603.image.
37. French Ministry of Commerce. Pour le perfectionnement d'une machine à comprimer le gaz, description des machines et procédés consignés dans les brevets d'invention. 1836;30:251–67.
38. Edwards JH. The therapeutic effects of carbon dioxide snow: methods of collecting and application. Lancet. 1911;II:87–90.
39. Major John Hall-Edwards. http://www.birmingham.gov.uk/xray.
40. Cranston-Low R. Carbonic acid snow as a therapeutic agent in the treatment of disease of the skin. Edinburgh/London: William Green; 1911.
41. Killeffer DH. The growing industry-dry-ice. Ind Eng Chem. 1930;22(10):1087.
42. The Trade-mark Reporter (v. 20). United States Trademark Association. 1930. ISBN 1-59888-091-8.
43. William A. Pusey. http://chicago.medicine.uic.edu/departments___programs/departments/dermatology/history/.
44. Pusey WA. The use of carbon dioxide snow in the treatment of nevi and other lesions of the skin. JAMA. 1907;49:1354–6.
45. Dr.Herman Allington. http://affiliatesindermatology.com/.
46. Image of Irving Cooper. Private Collection of Family.
47. Cooper I, Lee A. Cryostatic congelation: a system for producing a limited controlled region of cooling of freezing of biological tissue. J Nerv Ment Dis. 1961;133:259–63.
48. Das K, Benzil DL, Rovit RL, Murali R, Couldwell WT. Irving S. Cooper (1922–1985): a pioneer in functional neurosurgery. J Neurosurg. 1998;89(5):865–73.
49. Image of Michael Bryne. Private Family Collection.
50. Brymill Corp. US patent US3534739A. http://www.google.es/patents/US3534739A.
51. Brymill Corp. US patent US3651813A. https://www.google.de/patents/US3651813.
52. Zacarian SA. US patent US3702114. http://www.google.com/patents/US3702114.
53. Tromovitch T. US patent US 3823718A. https://www.google.com/patents/US3823718.
54. Torre D. US patent US4313306 A. http://www.google.com/patents/US4313306.
55. Zacarian SA, editor. Cryosurgery of skin cancer and cryogenic techniques in dermatology. Springfield: Charles C Thomas; 1969.
56. Zacarian SA. Cryosurgery of tumors of the skin and oral cavity. Springfield: Charles C. Thomas; 1973.
57. Zacarian SA. Cryosurgical advances in dermatology and tumors of the head and neck. Springfield: Charles C. Thomas; 1973.
58. Torre D, Lubritz RR, Kuflik EG. Practical cutaneous cryosurgery. Norwalk: Appleton & Lange; 1988.
59. Image of Gilberto Castro-Ron. Private Family Collection.

Cryobiology and Thermodynamics

2

Jānis Ķīsis and Aleksejs Zavorins

Contents

J. Ķīsis, MD, PhD (✉)
Department of Infectology and Dermatology, Riga Stradins University, Riga, Latvia
e-mail: profkisis@inbox.lv

A. Zavorins, MD
Department of Dermatology,
Private Clinic of Prof J. Kīsis,
Brivibas gatve 398-10, Riga, LV 1024, Latvia
e-mail: aleksejs.zavorins@gmail.com

Key Points

- The main mechanisms of tissue damage in cryosurgery include intracellular and extracellular ice formation, solution effects, cold protein denaturation and vascular and inflammatory reactions.
- Four parameters are used to monitor depth, width and circumscription of cryogenic lesion: cooling rate, tissue end temperature, hold time and thawing rate.
- Intracellular ice formation, which is essential for optimal tissue damage, is a result of homogeneous nucleation that can be achieved at rapid cooling rates utilising liquid nitrogen cryosurgical unit.
- Diverse types of tissue have different sensitivity to cryosurgery both in terms of volume of cryogenic lesion and capacity of tissue regeneration.

P. Pasquali (ed.), *Cryosurgery: A Practical Manual*,
DOI 10.1007/978-3-662-43939-5_2, © Springer-Verlag Berlin Heidelberg 2015

2.1 Introduction

Cryobiology is the branch of biology that studies the effects of low temperatures on living tissues. Cryosurgery involves the use of low temperatures in order to induce irreversible damage to the tissue. Cryotherapy is the controlled exposure of living tissues to cold temperatures, usually above freezing point, to induce physiological changes but with no intention to destroy the tissue [1].

With the introduction of advanced/high-tech cryoprobes [2], the opportunity was provided to effectively destroy deeply seated tissues. Study of these effects alongside the achievements in chemistry, physics, thermodynamics and biology provides an opportunity to evaluate changes in the frozen colloid systems. Freezing of water systems involves multiple processes. Complex understanding of these processes both internally and externally opens up a window to accurately plan the effect of cryotherapy on tissues, change parameters of the therapy and accomplish the contemplated therapeutic objective [3].

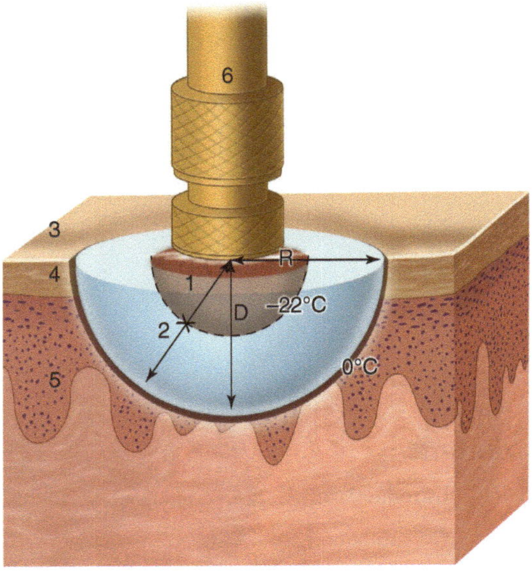

Fig. 2.1 Formation of "ice ball" during application of the timed spot freeze technique [5]. *1* Cryonecrosis area inside isotherm of −22 °C, *2* recovery area between 0° and −22 °C isotherms, *3* cutaneous surface, *4* epidermis, *5* dermis, *6* cryoprobe or cryospray, *R* lateral propagation of "ice ball," and *D* depth of "ice ball." In cryoprobe: $D = 1.3 \times R$; in cryospray: $D = 0.5 \times R$

2.2 Cryoablation

Cryosurgery technique involves performance of one or more freeze-thaw cycles. Thus, heat transfer between the cryogen and tissue occurs followed by tissue damage, vascular stasis and inflammatory response. Upon freezing a certain area with cryospray or cryoprobe, it can be observed how the tissue turns white, extending itself centrifugally as well as turning hard upon palpation; both in depth and surface, the so-called ice ball is formed (Fig. 2.1). Within it, temperature can be measured in isotherms [4].

Visual assessment of the cryogenic lesion (congelation) provides an opportunity to plan and manage the therapy.

Distinction is made between direct and indirect tissue damage mechanisms. Direct mechanisms involve both extracellular and intracellular formation of ice crystals as well as movement of water towards osmotic gradient. Also direct impact of cold on protein structure and enzyme systems is significant.

Indirect tissue damage mechanisms involve vascular stasis, ischaemia in the tissues and inflammatory and immunological responses. A summary of the events that occur during the cryosurgical procedure is given in Table 2.1 [5].

2.3 Types of Heat Transfer

Rate of heat transfer determines the rate of tissue cooling. Rapid heat transfer occurs if there is a high temperature gap between cryogenic agent and tissues. This occurs when the temperature of a cryogen like liquid nitrogen (−196 °C) contacts the skin (36.6 °C).

Heat transfer basically occurs by two manners:

(a) *Boiling heat transfer*: Cryogen comes in direct contact with tissues. Tissues lose their heat, while the cryogen heats up and evaporates. This is the process that occurs when spraying a cryogen on a tissue (as it occurs in cryospray freezing technique).

(b) *Conduction heat transfer*: Through a direct contact (cryoprobe) with tissues, molecules of solid body transfer their kinetic energy to molecules of another body [4].

Table 2.1 The molecular basis of cryosurgical cell destruction

Molecular basis of cryosurgical injury			
Mechanism		Time of cycle	Location
Direct injury	Extra- and intracellular ice crystal formation + coagulation necrosis	Freezing phase	Centre of the cryoinjury
Vascular injury	Microcirculatory failure + ischemic necrosis	Thawing phase	Periphery of the cryoinjury
Apoptosis	Cell death by apoptosis	Up to 8 h after rewarming	Periphery of the cryoinjury
Immnunological	T-cell response mediated by dendritic cells	Late event	Whole body

2.4 Cryogens and Cryosurgical Devices

2.4.1 Cryogens

Once a tissue has been subject to low temperatures, the achieved tissue temperature is the key factor in triggering tissue damage. A temperature of −20 °C in therapy of most neoplasms shall be cautiously evaluated as sufficient. Extensive damage of tissues occurs within the range of −20 and −30 °C, whereas destruction of cancer cells in this range is uncertain and incomplete. In vivo experiments show that vascular stasis after freezing-thawing has changed our understanding of lethal temperature in order to achieve therapeutic objectives. Neel et al. established the temperature necessary for destruction in experiments with animal tumours, *t* −60 °C, as well as argued for the necessity of repeated cooling, this was supported by later findings in studies of the topic [6–12]. In the experiments with diverse animal tissues, the range of lethal temperature is established between −40 and −50 °C [13–15]. Therefore, cryosurgery requires a cryogen capable of freezing at this temperature range. Some common cryogens are given in Table 2.2. Liquid nitrogen (LN) is the cryogen whose boiling point ensures reaching necessary parameters (Fig. 2.2) [3]. Necessary apparatuses are required to manipulate it.

Table 2.2 Temperature of some commonly used cryogens

Temperature of common cryogens	
Liquid nitrogen	−196 °C
Argon gas	−187 °C
Nitrogen gas (N_2O)	−88 °C
Carbon dioxide gas (CO_2)	−78 °C
Organic compressed gases	−55 to −75 °C

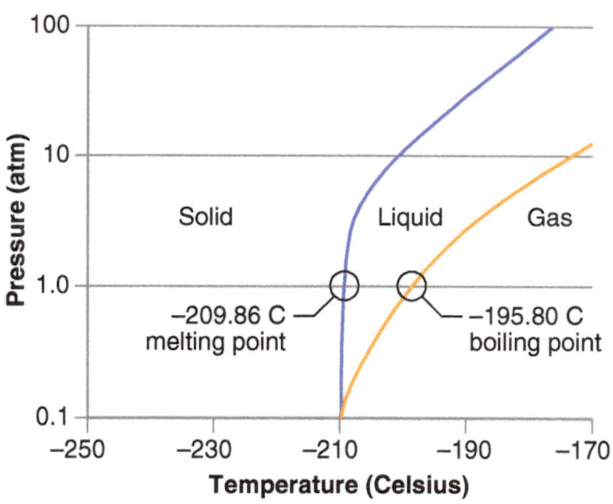

Fig. 2.2 Boiling point of liquid nitrogen

2.4.2 Cryosurgical Devices

LN is commonly delivered to the skin by the following:

Dipstick (cotton swab) permeated with liquid nitrogen: This is a popular method where cotton swabs are dipped into liquid nitrogen and later transferred and contacted to the skin surface. This method prevents from reaching rapid cooling rate of tissues. This is a passive cooling technique in that, once the liquid nitrogen has evaporated, there is no new influx of cryogen, as happens in the case of cryoprobe or cryospray. The result is a non-controlled freezing procedure. In addition, the surrounding liquid nitrogen may block vapour dissipation. It triggers the forming of an insulating layer which protects the site from pronounced cooling. This phenomenon is called the Leidenfrost effect. Therefore, a minimum heat transfer occurs between the dipstick and the skin, and cooling rate is low (<50 °C/min).

Not all cryogens and freezing devices allow achieving a sufficiently rapid cooling rate, whereas units operating without the liquid nitrogen and capable of achieving required cooling rates are too expensive.

Liquid nitrogen cryospray and cryoprobe: Liquid nitrogen comes into contact with the skin or metal of the cryoprobe on the surface of which rapid nitrogen evaporation occurs due to the heat transfer.

Cryospray and cryoprobe of liquid nitrogen allow achieving rapid cooling rate of tissues (>100 °C/min), because they allow for achieving high-temperature rates and because it is an active cooling technique.

Closed devices: A cryoprobe containing nitrous oxide operated based on the *Joule-Thomson* principle; namely, rapid expansion of the nitrous oxide occurs in closed space, which is an adiabatic process, and subsequently a quick drop of temperature of gas occurs. The aforementioned technique allows achieving only moderate cooling rates and is not available in a form of cryospray. Peltier thermoelectric modules (thermoelectric coolers/TEC) have similar deficiencies.

The use of pressurised gases as refrigerants (nitrous oxide, carbon dioxide and argon) spurred development of diverse instruments (thin needle-like probes, clamp devices, catheter probes and balloon structures), which in turn expanded indications of cryoenergy for treatment of a wide spectrum of diseases, including dermatologic, prostatic, hepatic, gynaecologic, ophthalmologic, neurosurgical and oncological disorders [16].

2.5 Monitoring of Cryogenic Lesion

Upon performing cryosurgical treatment of a skin lesion, the volume of frozen tissues can be monitored either visually or upon palpation. Frozen tissues visually become white towards the periphery from the point of cryogen incidence. When the afore-described ice ball is formed, there is interrelation between radius of the frozen region on the surface of the skin and depth of frozen tissues. If the cryoprobe is used, the depth of frozen tissues is 1.3 times greater than the radius on the surface of the skin, whereas in the case of cryospray, the depth is half of the radius [6].

Nowadays, instrumental methods are developed for monitoring freezing and volume of frozen tissues which allows reducing the risk of complications as well as ascertaining if sufficient degree of injury has been achieved. This is of utmost importance when dealing with malignant lesions. These instruments are as follows:

Thermocouple needles: It is possible to monitor tissue temperature using a thermocouple (thermoelectric element); however, in order to evaluate in-depth temperature, the skin has to be penetrated rendering it to be an invasive lesion-monitoring method.

Ultrasound: It allows real-time monitoring of the volume of frozen tissues and is easily available in outpatient practice as well. Cryosurgical equipment has also been developed where ultrasonic probes (transducers) are built in. Efficiency of the technique is limited by occurrence of acoustic shadowing [7].

Other imaging options: These include computerised tomography (CT) scan, magnetic resonance imaging (MRI) [17, 18], electrical impedance tomography [19, 20], optical coherence tomography [21] and confocal microscopy [22].

2.6 Thermal Background of the Cryogenic Lesion and Variables

There are four parameters used to monitor depth, width and circumscription of cryogenic lesion. They are cooling rate, end temperature of tissues, hold time of frozen tissues and thawing rate [23].

2.6.1 Cooling Rate

Freezing rate of tissues may be fast (100–260 °C/min), moderate (10–100 °C/min) and slow (<10 °C/min) [6]. Since the objective is to destroy the tissues, reaching fast cooling rate is essential. In this case, intracellular crystal formation

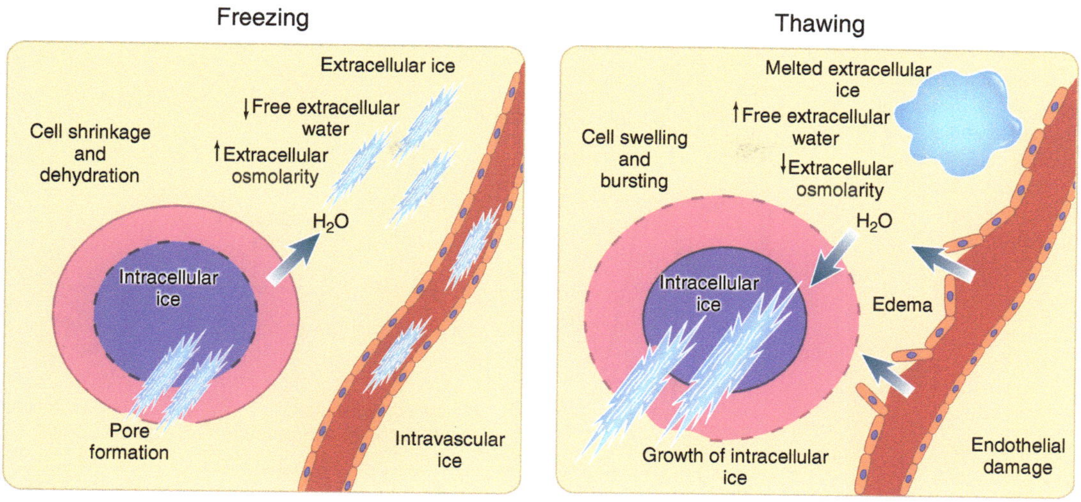

Fig. 2.3 Extracellular ice formation leads to dehydration and shrinkage of the cells due to a high osmolality gradient. Rapid cooling rates allow intracellular ice formation that damages cell membranes. Subsequently, slow thawing leads to rehydration of the cells with their swelling or even bursting (Modified with permission from Erinjeri and Clark [24])

is accomplished inducing irreversible damage to the tissues and necrosis destroying cell organelles and membrane from the inside [23].

Slow and moderate cooling rates cause reversible damage to the tissues forming extracellular crystals, hyperosmolarity in extracellular space and dehydration of cells (Fig. 2.3) [24]. These processes induce programmed death or apoptosis in part of the cells [7]. It is important to note that cooling rates are higher in the center of the lesion, however closer to the periphery cooling rates are low to moderate [23].

Modifications in cell damage according to the cooling rate are not directly proportionate. This is the so-called "inverted U" curve phenomenon (Fig. 2.4) [11]: cell death is marked at low freezing temperatures, when cells are dehydrating, and at high freezing rates, when intracellular crystals form. Between these parameters, high viability of the cells is also observed when cooling rate is sufficiently high to prevent dehydration; however, forming of intracellular crystals does not occur [11].

2.6.2 End Temperature of Tissues

In order to accomplish tissue injury, a sufficiently low tissue temperature has to be reached. Tissue temperature determines the possibility of forming intracellular crystals by homogeneous nucleation, namely, spontaneous crystal nuclei formation inside the cells as long as the temperature is below −40 °C [25]. Furthermore, individual tissues and cells have different susceptibility to cold; thus, it is believed that lethal temperature of keratinocytes is at least −35 °C, while for endothelium it is −15 to −35 °C. On the other hand, upon treatment of benign lesions, the tissue temperature profile of at least −20 to −30 °C has to be reached, whereas in treating malicious lesions – at least −40 to −50°C [7] must be reached.

2.6.3 Hold Time of Frozen Tissues

Hold time of tissues in a frozen state enhances cryogenic injury mechanisms. Once intracellular crystals are achieved, recrystallisation will follow in time. As ice crystal grow in size, the more they will enhance cell injury. On the other hand, upon formation of isolated extracellular crystals, a more marked cell dehydration can be achieved [23]. It is believed that duration of freezing is not of critical importance, as long as the lowest tissue temperature reached is below −50 °C [7].

2.6.4 Thawing Rate (Fig. 2.3)

Slow thawing is the prime destructive factor (<10 °C/min) [6] facilitating recrystallisation

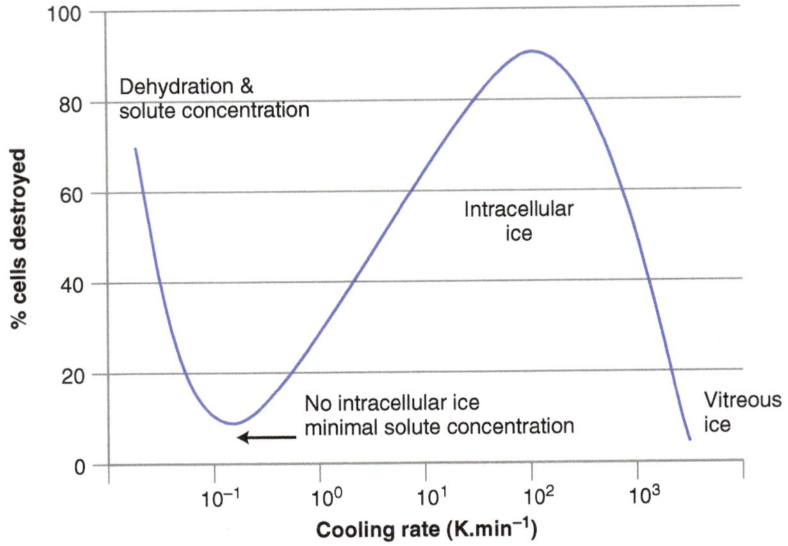

Fig. 2.4 Inverted "U" curve phenomenon: cell death is prominent at rapid cooling rates due to intracellular ice formation and at very slow cooling rates due to prominent solution effects (Used with permission from Takeda et al. [11])

(ice crystal restructuring), namely, crystals growing bigger, and rehydration of cells causing membrane disruption and death of cells [7, 23].

2.7 Vascular Cryogenic Injury

Under the impact of cold, delayed or indirect vasoconstriction of blood vessels occurs which induces occurrence of stasis and tissue ischaemia.

Damage to the endothelium of blood vessels during freezing and thawing is essential for cryolesion formation. Endothelium collapses when tissue temperature is in the range of −15 to −35 °C. The direct cell damage mechanisms described previously are crucial and include forming of crystals and cell dehydration [6, 23]. Nevertheless, it is also important to note that stasis caused by vasoconstriction facilitates hypoxia. Under the impact of hypoxia, cells release vasodilatation cytokines which after thawing enhance refractory vasodilatation and reperfusion injury which, among other, are triggered by excessive oxygen supply to the tissues and forming of free radicals. The free radicals induce lipid peroxidation in the membrane of endothelium cells. Reperfusion also facilitates inflammatory and perivascular oedema of tissues in the first 30 min already [26]. Intensified blood vessel permeability also contributes to occurrence of the oedema because perivascular tissues are dehydrated in the peripheral zone of the ice ball and shrink. That facilitates dilatation, stretching and increase of permeability [6, 23].

These processes create conditions which trigger blood clot formation according to Virchow's triad: stasis caused by vasoconstriction, local thrombophilia triggered by reperfusion and exposing of connective tissue induced by endothelial damage. The first microthrombi appear within 2 h of treatment. Blood vessel clotting leads to ischaemia of tissues and subsequent coagulative necrosis which can be observed after 2 days [6].

2.8 Role of Inflammation and Apoptosis in Cryogenic Lesion

2.8.1 Inflammation

Inflammatory response develops within subsequent 24 h after cryosurgical treatment; it is a response to cellular death, especially in the centre of the lesion, where necrosis forms. Within 30 min of treatment, eosinophilic staining and vacuolisation of cell cytoplasm is observed, as well as nuclei becoming pyknotic, due to irreversible condensation of

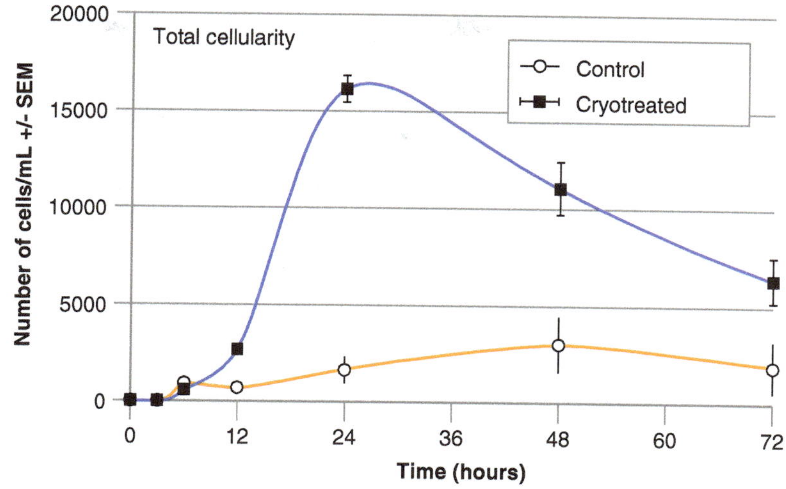

Fig. 2.5 Cellular infiltration of the cryolesion (Used with permission from De Souza et al. [27])

chromatin in the nucleus; epidermal-dermal separation occurs [4]. After vascular dilatation, oedema forms, which is especially marked in locations were the skin is loosely connected to deep tissues, for instance, dorsal surface of hands. Migration of cells to focal point of the lesion occurs, and neutrophils reach it first, whereas after 24 h macrophages and lymphocytes take over – by that time cell count in the lesion zone increases ten times (Fig. 2.5) [27]. In case of inflammation, pain occurs because kinins and substance P stimulates C fibre nociceptors [27]. Production of these agents is secondary to release of inflammatory cytokines in tissues, including TNF-α and IL-1 [27]. These cytokines facilitate production of eicosanoids (icosanoids). It should be noted though that freezing of nervous tissue itself may induce analgesia which will be described next.

2.8.2 Apoptosis and Its Role in Cryosurgery

Apoptosis is a programmed cellular death. During the apoptosis, cell lysis occurs and internal structures and enzymes are not released in the intercellular space. Consequently, there is no immediate inflammatory response and damage to the surrounding tissues.

Apoptosis is observed in peripheral zone of the cryogenic lesion, where the cooling rate is moderate and damage to the tissue is reversible, and it can be established within 8–12 h after the cryosurgical treatment already [7].

Apoptosis is characterised by changes in BAX protein expression which facilitate mitochondrial damage and caspase activation which regulate further process of apoptosis [7]. During apoptosis, phospholipid inversion in the membranes and non-random DNA cleavage occur, and several apoptotic bodies form which can be phagocytised by antigen-presenting cells (APCs), mostly macrophages [28].

2.9 Physical, Chemical and Thermodynamic Processes in Cryosurgery

Arising out of the foregoing, it can be concluded that, upon freezing of tissues, crystals form in the extracellular space. Nevertheless, if the cooling rate is sufficiently fast (>100 °C/min) or if the freezing is sufficiently long, then intracellular crystals begin to form which are the decisive factor in cell death and tissue necrosis. In the present chapter, mechanisms of crystal forming will be described, namely, by way of heterogeneous and homogeneous nucleation; likewise, an explanation will be given of why forming of intracellular crystals is impaired in comparison with forming of extracellular crystals. Furthermore, notion of the osmotic gradient determining movement of water molecules during freezing and thawing will be elaborated upon.

2.9.1 Determinants of Freezing Point of Water

Pure water (with no solutes added) freezes at the temperature 0 °C under pressure of 1 atm. Upon concentration of dissolved substances, freezing point decreases.

According to Raoult's second law, in comparison with pure solvent, the decrease in the freezing point of a solution is directly proportional to the molality of the solute, namely, the temperature decreases by approximately 1.86 °C per unit increase of molar concentration of each solute unit [25].

Theoretically, taking into account the concentration of sodium solution, formation of crystals in the tissue starts from −21.8 °C, although in reality tissue begins to freeze from −0.6 °C [6].

2.9.2 Heterogeneous and Homogeneous Nucleation

Transfer of water into solid phase, namely, formation of ice crystals most commonly occurs through heterogeneous nucleation. In nature, it is virtually impossible to find absolutely clear and homogeneous water in liquid phase. It will always have additions of other substances which are called "impurities." Impurities create favourable conditions for forming crystallisation nucleus on their surface, because they reduce free energy barrier that has to be overcome upon transferring from the liquid water phase to crystal.

Free energy or Gibbs energy (G) defines potential energy of the thermodynamic system. If the Gibbs energy of the system is higher in the initial state compared to the final state, then $\Delta G<0$ and thermodynamic process are possible. The second law of thermodynamics states that the entropy of an isolated system never decreases, because isolated systems spontaneously evolve towards the state of maximum entropy; therefore, the disorder or entropy ($T\Delta S$) (progressing towards thermodynamic equilibrium) has an inherent tendency to grow. $\Delta G=\Delta H-T\Delta S$ (ΔH: changes in thermal capacity of the enthalpy or system characterising overall energy exchange of the system; $T\Delta S$: entropy changes characterising energy dispersed in the system, for example, for movement of molecules; ΔG: Gibbs energy or free energy). Entropy characterises the lack of order in the system. Consequently, thermodynamic processes where increase of entropy (disorder) prevails over heat capacity or enthalpy of the system are potentially possible, and they are characterised by decrease in the Gibbs energy or free energy. There is also overall chemical potential existent. The chemical potential (μ), in essence, is the free energy or Gibbs energy per mole of a substance, namely, if it is lower at the end state than in the initial state, then the process is energetically possible [29].

Heterogeneous nucleation can be reached more easily than the homogeneous one where crystallisation nuclei occur spontaneously in pure water, because less potential or Gibbs free energy is consumed. Heterogeneous nucleation is thermodynamically more beneficial because the surface tension force, which works upon water interfacing with "impurities," reduces necessary Gibbs energy difference. That means that in order to achieve homogeneous nucleation two conditions have to be met. The water has to be without "impurities" that could facilitate heterogeneous nucleation, and its temperature has to be below −40 °C (Fig. 2.6) [29].

It is experimentally proven [25] that intracellular ice crystals may form based on two mechanisms: heterogeneous nucleation at the expense of extracellular ice and spontaneous nucleation inside the cell:

- *Heterogeneous nucleation on the extracellular ice*: In vivo research of mouse oocytes has established that if tissue temperature is above −40 °C, then formation of the intracellular ice is directly dependent on frozen extracellular water fraction. For intracellular crystals to start to form, 94 % or more volume of extracellular water would have to be frozen. Extracellular crystals seem to spread through plasmatic pores of the membrane across to interior of the cells, and on its surface crystallisation nuclei for intracellular ice form on the surface by way of heterogeneous nucleation.Diameter of cellular channels is remarkably small, for example, diameter of aquaporins is 8–10 Å [30, 31]. Consequently, extracellular crystals also have to be sufficiently small to cross them. However, crystals with small radius are less stable, because their surface has high chemical potential. Sufficiently big crystals may be considered flat because their radius gravitates towards infinity. Each water molecule is suspended by hydrogen bonds in the crystal. An individual water molecule has a higher number of surrounding water molecules in a flat crystal which suspend it by hydrogen bonds. On the other hand, a water molecule on the curved interface of the crystal has lower quantity of adjacent molecules. Therefore, small ice crystals may exist in a temperature that is lower than −10 °C, which shall be calculated according to the Kelvin equation. The said condition also explains the recrystallisation phenomenon [32] upon occurrence of prolonged thawing, namely, chemical potential of interface of the big crystals is lower than the chemical potential of the small crystals. Therefore, small crystals shrink in their size, whereas big crystals grow at the expense on these molecules (Fig. 2.7) [32].

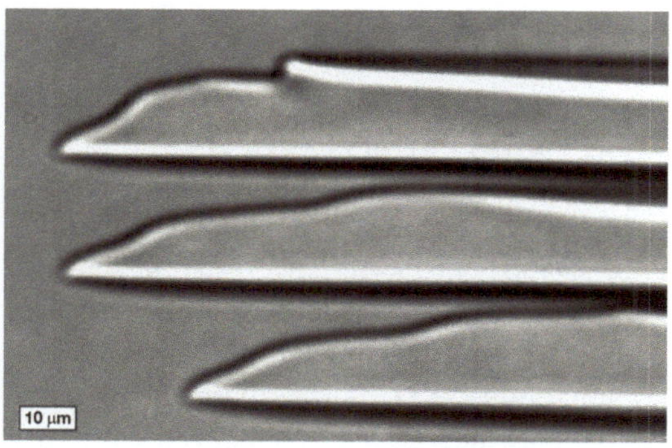

Fig. 2.6 Heterogeneous ice formation (Used with permission from Choi and Bischof [44])

- *Spontaneous intracellular homogeneous nucleation*: It is observed in the experiments that, upon reaching the tissue temperature which is below −40 °C, spontaneous crystallisation nuclei form inside the oocyte even if the frozen water fraction in the extracellular space was below 94 %.

It is not finally established why heterogeneous nucleation and formation of intracellular crystals above −40 °C require extracellular ice crystals. However, one hypothesis links it to an experiment [33] which stipulates that nucleation temperature of water crystals is directly proportional to microscopic volume of water: the lower volume of water, the lower is the nucleation temperature of ice crystals (Fig. 2.8). Therefore, it is possible to speculate that intracellular space

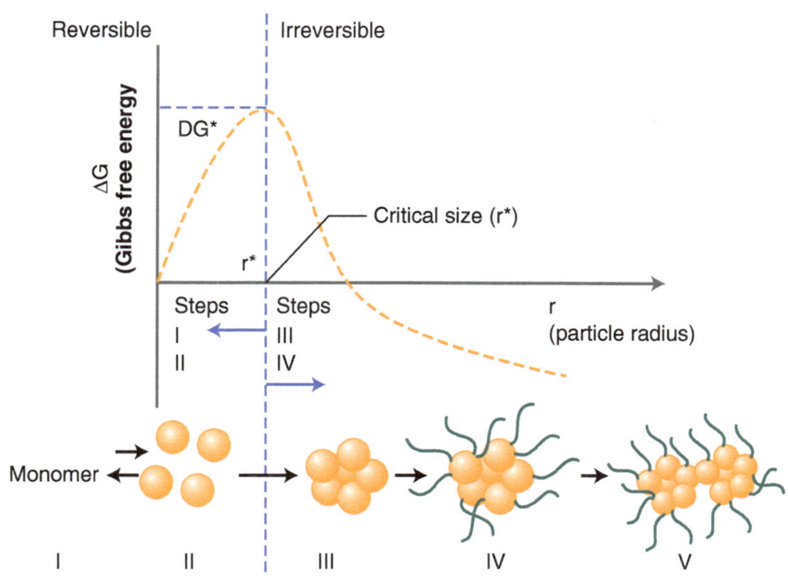

Fig. 2.7 Schematic diagram of the nucleation and growth process showing the five stages and the dependence of the Gibbs free energy (G) on the crystal size. Below a critical radius (r^*), a reversible process occurs; for $r > r^*$, the process becomes irreversible (Modified with permission from Leite and Ribeiro [32])

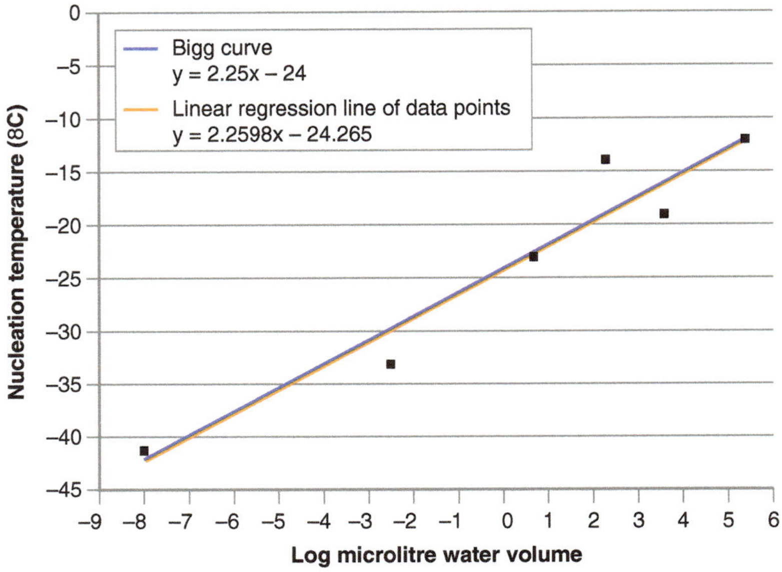

Fig. 2.8 The nucleation temperature of water crystals is directly proportional to microscopic volume of water (Used with permission from Zachariassen et al. [45])

that is divided into small compartments by organelles determines the capability on intracellular ice formation by the means of homogeneous nucleation, namely, at the temperature below −40 °C.

2.9.3 Osmotic Gradient in Cryosurgery

Osmosis is the diffusion of solvents through a semipermeable membrane, namely, a membrane that moves solvent across while retaining dissolved molecules (solutes). Flow of solvent is always directed towards the solution of higher concentration (hypertonic solution). Solvent (water) moves from an environment with a higher chemical potential to an environment with a lower chemical potential. The chemical potential of the solvent is in turn directly proportional to osmolality (M) of the solution or quantity of the solute agent per kilogram of solvent. Osmotic gradient will exist until the chemical potential $\Delta\mu = -vRTM$ – where $\Delta\mu$ is the difference of chemical potential; v, water partial molar volume (0.018 l/mol); R, gas constant; T, absolute temperature; and M, osmolality – on both sides of the plasma membrane of the cells will reach equilibrium as described before in reference to crystal nucleation [29].

2.10 Effect of Cryosurgery on Body Tissues

Diverse types of tissue have different sensitivity to cryosurgery both in terms of volume of cryogenic lesion and capacity of tissue regeneration (Table 2.3). Furthermore, upon tissue temperature decreasing cell enzymes are also inhibited, thus impeding tissue metabolism [34]. Furthermore, organisation of polar water molecules into a clathrate around proteins will facilitate cold denaturation. In these conditions, protein loses its tertiary structure or three-dimensional shape, because non-covalent (hydrophobic) bonds are ruptured. Upon losing its tertiary structure, the protein is no longer able to perform its functions including the enzymatic ones [35].

Factors determining sensitivity of tissue and cells to freezing have been identified mainly by research on reproductive medicine and tissue transplant where it is critically important to prevent possible cryogenic injuries. In vivo studies of freeze-tolerant insects, cell cultures, as well as oocytes and spermatozoids are being carried out.

It is established that permeability of cell membrane plays a significant role in tissue sensitivity to cryosurgery. For example, it has been found that production of aquaporin 3 in prostate cells increases after freezing, while suppressing

Table 2.3 Sensitivity of tissue and cells to cold

Cells/tissues	Lethal temperature
Osteocyte	–2 °C
Melanocyte	–4 °C
Keratinocyte	–35 °C
Adenocarcinoma cells	–40 °C
Sarcoma cells	–60 °C
Endothelium	–15 °C to 40 °C
Fibroblasts	–30 °C to 35 °C

function of aquaporin decreases prostate cells viability [36].

Furthermore, the ratio between surface area of cells and volume of the cell is also relevant. The lower it is, the more pronounced is the cell freezing injury. Thus, for instance, cryopreservation of spermatozoids is easier than cryopreservation of oocytes because the surface-area-to-volume ratio is higher. It is more difficult to prevent formation of intracellular crystals in oocytes. In case of slow and sustained freezing, sufficient dehydration does not occur, and low remaining volumes of water form crystals inside the cells. On the other hand, oocytes are more enduring against fast freezing than spermatozoids because the high surface-area-to-volume ratio of spermatozoids determines exposure to extracellular ice and low water volumes also facilitate intracellular crystallisation [37].

Organisation of tissue is no less important. It is established that tissue where cell density is higher is more sensitive to damage by freezing. Here, both intracellular crystallisation and mechanical destructive impact of extra- and intracellular crystals on cell membranes, organelles and gap junctions (nexus) are enhanced [38].

It is proven that tissue containing more connective tissues is more resistant to freezing [4].

Some of the morphological and pathophysiological changes occurring by freezing on various tissues, including skin, nervous tissue and blood vessels, will be overviewed in the present chapter.

2.10.1 Skin

Skin cryosurgery facilitates forming of marked coagulation necrosis. Derma has high content of collagen, elastin and fibroblasts. These structures have low sensitivity to cryogenic damage; therefore, they form basis for regeneration of tissue. It is observed that, in comparison with burns, collagen is better preserved in case of cryogenic lesion. Gradual degradation by metalloproteinases (metalloproteases) and replacement of new collagen through fibroblasts will result in a more aesthetically cryogenic lesion, unless scar contracture develops [7]. Also, preserved collagen structure facilitates effective re-epithelialisation of the lesion [4]. It should be noted that melanocytes, sudoriferous glands and hair follicles are highly susceptible to cold. Therefore, in deep freezing, hypopigmentation and loss of hair in the frozen region can be expected; however, even in such cases, melanocytes can migrate from peripheral tissues and reduce local hypopigmentation [4].

2.10.2 Blood Vessels

Low temperature initially facilitates vasoconstriction and forming of stasis. If tissue temperature is at least between −15 and –40 °C, then endothelium damage occurs. After freezing, perivascular oedema and tissue hyperaemia occur forming a purple margin around the frozen region followed by microthrombi and tissue necrosis [4].

Under the microscope, one can find oedema, focal capillary damage, haemorrhages and isolated microthrombi formation within 2 h after skin cryosurgery, whereas after 5–8 h avascular segmental necrosis (ASN) is observed [6].

Arteries of bigger size do not lose their thermodynamic functions upon freezing of tissues, although death of smooth muscle cells (SMC) or smooth myocytes and destruction of endothelium are observed. Regeneration of the tissues is achieved through proliferation of the smooth myocytes; myointimal hyperplasia occurs at the expense of growth of collagen and the layer of endothelium is restored with minor disorders of blood flow are observed during this process [7].

In smaller arteries and at the microcirculation level, there is a high risk of thrombosis and subsequent ischemia and necrosis of tissues.

Veins contain less flexible structures and myocytes; they are more resistant to cold than arteries.

At tissue temperatures between 3 and 11 °C, thrombosis in up to 65 % of capillaries and 35–40 % of arterioles and venules is observed, whereas if the tissue temperature is between −15 and −20 °C, then thrombosis is observed in all capillaries, arterioles and venules [6].

Smooth myocytes are more susceptible to cold than endothelium [7, 23].

2.10.3 Nerve Tissue

Damage to nervous tissues and their ability to regenerate after cryosurgery depend on the reached lower temperature of tissues. It is proven in experiments that myelinated nerves suffer most in terms of either electric physiology or morphology. It is established that freezing of nervous tissues induces analgesia [7, 39, 40]. If the lowest temperature in the nervous tissues is −20 °C, then impulse transmission is resumed after several hours, whereas if the lowest temperature is below −60 °C, then impulse transmission resumes after 41 days in average; however, in some cases, it is not restored [39, 41]. It is observed that perineurium and epineurium are less sensitive to cold. The inflammatory response plays a role in regeneration processes [7] which is first observed after 8 days after occurrence of the cryogenic lesion. It occurs in the absence of Schwann cells while as long as the basal membrane is preserved [40]. It is also observed that freezing of nervous tissue down to −140 °C causes complete and irreversible loss of nerve functionality [39].

2.11 Balance Between Cryogenic Lesion and Cryopreservation

Dermatologic cryosurgery aims to selectively destroy skin tumours while preserving surrounding healthy tissue which will give the support for healing by secondary intention.

It is known that cold is used not only in destruction of tissues but also in preservation of ova (egg cells) and spermatozoids. In such cases, tissue freezing is conducted following special protocols. Freezing has to be slow (<10 °C/min) to preclude forming of lethal intracellular ice crystals. On the other hand, in order to mitigate forming of extracellular crystals and osmotic gradient and thus preventing disruption of cells during thawing, it is possible to use cryoprotectors which, for instance, enhance osmolarity inside the cells (dimethyl sulphoxide (DMSO), glycerine) or cover crystallisation centres (HES, antifreeze proteins (AFP) or ice structuring proteins (ISP)) [42, 43].

In the last years, most studies have been focused on immunocryosurgery. It has been observed that immunomodulators can be used as adjuvant therapy to facilitate activation of dendritic cells (accessory cells) and thus also inhibit developing of immune tolerance towards cancer cells (Chap. 3).

The continuous research work done in cryobiology as well as the increased use of cryosurgery for other organ systems will provide further support for this fundamental area of knowledge.

Essential Titbits

- Cryosurgery uses low temperatures to induce irreversible damage. Cryotherapy uses controlled exposure above freezing temperature to induce physiological changes.
- Freezing transfers heat out of the tissue.
- Depth of frozen tissues is greater than the radius for probe freezing than for spray freezing.
- Apoptosis is observed in the peripheral zone of the cryogenic lesion where freezing is not lethal.
- Different tissues have different sensitivity to cold: melanocytes are very sensitive, while fibroblasts are very resistant.

Glossary

ASN	Avascular Segmental Necrosis
Clathrate	Chemical substance consisting of a lattice that traps or contains molecules
Isotherms	A drawn line linking points of equal temperature or constant temperature
LN	Liquid Nitrogen

References

1. Stańczyk M, Telega JJ. Thermal problems in biomechanics – a review. Part III. Cryosurgery, cryopreservation and cryotherapy. Acta Bioeng Biomech. 2003;5(2):3–22.
2. Korpan N. A history of cryosurgery: its development and future. J Am Coll Surg. 2007;204(2):314–24.
3. Rubinsky B. Cryosurgery. Annu Rev Biomed Eng. 2000;2:157–87.
4. Thai KE, Sinclair RD. Cryosurgery of benign skin lesions. Australas J Dermatol. 1999;40(4):175–84, quiz 185–6.
5. Pasquali P. Cryosurgery. In: Rigel DS, Robinson JK, Ross MI, Friedman R, Cockerell CJ, Lim HW, Stockfleth E, Kirkwood JM, editors. Cancer of the skin. 2nd ed. Philadelphia: Elsevier/Saunders; 2011. p. 450–61.
6. Zouboulis CC. Principles of cutaneous cryosurgery: an update. Dermatology. 1999;198(2):111–7.
7. Gage AA, Baust JM, Baust JG. Experimental cryosurgery investigations in vivo. Cryobiology. 2009;59(3):229–43.
8. Zimmerman EE, Crawford P. Cutaneous cryosurgery. Am Fam Physician. 2012;86(12):1118–24.
9. Saliken JC, Donnelly BJ, Rewcastle JC. The evolution and state of modern technology for prostate cryosurgery. Urology. 2002;60(2 Suppl 1):26–33.
10. Swann MH, Taylor TA. Practical cryotherapy for skin disease. Mo Med. 2007;104(6):509–12.
11. Takeda H, Maruyama S, Okajima J, Aiba S, Komiya A. Development and estimation of a novel cryoprobe utilizing the Peltier effect for precise and safe cryosurgery. Cryobiology. 2009;59(3):275–84.
12. Neel 3rd HB, Ketcham AS, Hammond WG. Requisites for successful cryogenic surgery of cancer. Arch Surg. 1971;102(1):45–8.
13. Yiu WK, Cheng SW, Sumpio BE. Synergistic effect of cool/thaw cycles on vascular cells in an in vitro model of cryoplasty. J Vasc Interv Radiol. 2008;19(6):925–30.
14. Seifert JK, France MP, Zhao J, Bolton EJ, Finlay I, Junginger T, Morris DL. Large volume hepatic freezing: association with significant release of the cytokines interleukin-6 and tumor necrosis factor a in a rat model. World J Surg. 2002;26(11):1333–41.
15. Staren ED, Sabel MS, Gianakakis LM, Wiener GA, Hart VM, Gorski M, Dowlatshahi K, Corning BF, Haklin MF, Koukoulis G. Cryosurgery of breast cancer. Arch Surg. 1997;132(1):28–33.
16. Andrade JG, Khairy P, Dubuc M. Catheter cryoablation: biology and clinical uses. Circ Arrhythm Electrophysiol. 2013;6:218–27.
17. Van den Bosch MA, Josan S, Bouley DM, Chen J, Gill H, Rieke V, Butts-Pauly K, Daniel BL. MR imaging-guided percutaneous cryoablation of the prostate in an animal model: in vivo imaging of cryoablation-induced tissue necrosis with immediate histopathologic correlation. J Vasc Interv Radiol. 2009;20(2):252–8.
18. Pease GR, Rubinsky B, Wong ST, Roos MS, Gilbert JC, Arav A. An integrated probe for magnetic resonance imaging monitored skin cryosurgery. J Biomech Eng. 1995;117(1):59–63.
19. Edd JF, Rubinsky B. Detecting cryoablation with EIT and the benefit of including ice front imaging data. Physiol Meas. 2006;27(5):S175–85.
20. Otten DM, Rubinsky B. Front-tracking image reconstruction algorithm for EIT-monitored cryosurgery using the boundary element method. Physiol Meas. 2005;26(4):503–16.
21. Themstrup L, Banzhaf C, Mogensen M, Jemec GB. Cryosurgery treatment of actinic keratoses monitored by optical coherence tomography: a pilot study. Dermatology. 2012;225(3):242–7.
22. Terhorst D, Maltusch A, Stockfleth E, Lange-Asschenfeldt S, Sterry W, Ulrich M, Lange-Asschenfeldt B. Reflectance confocal microscopy for the evaluation of acute epidermal wound healing. Wound Repair Regen. 2011;19(6):671–9.
23. Hoffmann NE, Bischof JC. The cryobiology of cryosurgical injury. Urology. 2002;60(2 Suppl 1):40–9.
24. Erinjeri JP, Clark TW. Cryoablation: mechanism of action and devices. J Vasc Interv Radiol. 2010;21(8 Suppl):S187–91.
25. Mazur P, Pinn IL, Kleinhans FW. The temperature of intracellular ice formation in mouse oocytes vs. the unfrozen fraction at that temperature. Cryobiology. 2007;54(2):223–33.
26. Goel R, Anderson K, Slaton J, Schmidlin F, Vercellotti G, Belcher J, Bischof JC. Adjuvant approaches to enhance cryosurgery. J Biomech Eng. 2009;131(7):074003.
27. De Souza RC, Cunha JM, Ferreira SH, Cunha FQ, Lima HC. Different inflammatory mediators induce inflammation and pain after application of liquid nitrogen to the skin. Cryobiology. 2006;53(3):319–29.
28. Robilotto AT, Baust JM, Van Buskirk RG, Gage AA, Baust JG. Temperature-dependent activation of differential apoptotic pathways during cryoablation

in a human prostate cancer model. Prostate Cancer Prostatic Dis. 2013;16(1):41–9.
29. Mazur P. A biologist's view of the relevance of thermodynamics and physical chemistry to cryobiology. Cryobiology. 2010;60(1):4–10.
30. Day RE, Kitchen P, Owen D, Bland C, Marshall L, Conner AC, Bill RM, Conner MT. Human aquaporins: regulators of transcellular water flow. Biochim Biophys Acta. 2014;1840(5):1492–506.
31. Gonen T, Walz T. The structure of aquaporins. Q Rev Biophys. 2006;39(4):361–96.
32. Leite ER, Ribeiro C. Introduction. In: Crystallization and growth of colloidal nanocrystals. SpringerBriefs in materials. New York: Springer; 2012. p. 1–6.
33. Bigg EK. The formation of ice crystals by the freezing of droplets. London: Imperial College; 1953.
34. Bansal A, Jain S, Gupta S. Cryosurgery in the treatment of oro-facial lesions. Indian J Dent Res. 2012;23(2):297.
35. Dias CL, Ala-Nissila T, Wong-ekkabut J, Vattulainen I, Grant M, Karttunen M. The hydrophobic effect and its role in cold denaturation. Cryobiology. 2010;60(1):91–9.
36. Ismail M, Bokaee S, Morgan R, Davies J, Harrington KJ, Pandha H. Inhibition of the aquaporin 3 water channel increases the sensitivity of prostate cancer cells to cryotherapy. Br J Cancer. 2009;100(12):1889–95.
37. Ledda S, Bogliolo L, Succu S, Ariu F, Bebbere D, Leoni GG, Naitana S. Oocyte cryopreservation: oocyte assessment and strategies for improving survival. Reprod Fertil Dev. 2007;19(1):13–23.
38. Müller-Schweinitzer E. Cryopreservation of vascular tissues. Organogenesis. 2009;5(3):97–104.
39. Zhou L, Kambin P, Casey KF, Bonner FJ, O'Brien E, Shao Z, Ou S. Mechanism research of cryoanalgesia. Neurol Res. 1995;17(4):307–11.
40. Fasano VA, Peirone SM, Zeme S, Filippi M, Broggi G, de Mattei M, Sguazzi A. Cryoanalgesia. Ultrastructural study on cryolytic lesion of sciatic nerve in rat and rabbit. Acta Neurochir Suppl (Wien). 1987;39:177–80.
41. Wagner R, DeLeo JA, Heckman HM, Myers RR. Peripheral nerve pathology following sciatic cryoneurolysis: relationship to neuropathic behaviors in the rat. Exp Neurol. 1995;133(2):256–64.
42. Hovatta O. Methods for cryopreservation of human ovarian tissue. Reprod Biomed Online. 2005;10(6):729–34.
43. Karlsson JO. Effects of solution composition on the theoretical prediction of ice nucleation kinetics and thermodynamics. Cryobiology. 2010;60(1):43–51.
44. Choi J, Bischof JC. Review of biomaterial thermal property measurements in the cryogenic regime and their use for prediction of equilibrium and non-equilibrium freezing applications in cryobiology. Cryobiology. 2010;60(1):52–70.
45. Zachariassen KE, Kristiansen E, Pedersen SA, Hammel HT. Ice nucleation in solutions and freeze-avoiding insects-homogeneous or heterogeneous? Cryobiology. 2004;48(3):309–21.

3 Theoretical Principles of Immunocryosurgery

Aleksandar L. Krunic

Contents

Key Points

- Cryosurgery is well tolerated, is minimally invasive, has low cost, and has good cosmesis.
- Cryosurgery could be capable of destroying not just primary tumors but also distant disease.
- Cryoinjury encompasses cell death by direct and indirect mechanism including necrosis, necroptosis, apoptosis, vascular damage, and inflammation.
- Cryoimmunology characterizes aspects of specific immune response directed towards antigens from the tumor that remains "in situ" upon cryosurgery procedure.
- Initial local inflammation and systemic immune system activation after cryosurgery play key roles in the primary ablation of the tumor and elimination of the distant disease via continued immune surveillance with active cytotoxic cells, Th1 helper cells, and memory immune cells, as well as modification of tumor environment.
- This activity can be further augmented by the addition of cryosurgery adjuvants.
- Future directions include elucidating the importance of specific cytokines and cellular pathways involved in cryodestruction as well as standardization and improvement of techniques available for its various applications.

A.L. Krunic, MD, PhD
Department of Dermatology,
University of Illinois College of Medicine,
502 Park Avenue, River Forest, IL 60305, USA
e-mail: sasakrun@hotmail.com

P. Pasquali (ed.), *Cryosurgery: A Practical Manual*,
DOI 10.1007/978-3-662-43939-5_3, © Springer-Verlag Berlin Heidelberg 2015

3.1 Introduction

Current oncological approach to treating tumors includes surgical removal, chemotherapy, radiation, thermal destruction by heat, or use of superficial/intralesional freezing known as cryodestruction or cryosurgical ablation. Cryosurgery had advantages over other modalities by being minimally invasive and less destructive to surrounding structures as well as having better patient comfort (anesthetic effect), lower cost, and superior cosmetic results. Furthermore, what is unique to cryosurgery is that a frozen tumor remains in the body ("in situ") producing stimulation of immunologic response to tumor-specific antigens released from frozen tissue [1]. The interest in these immunological effects of cryosurgery has risen upon many earlier reports of regressing metastatic foci after cryoablation of primary tumors (prostate cancer, breast cancer, lung metastases). However, it had not been clear whether the immune response was indeed responsible or not for these "distant" effects of freezing. Immunological assays were at the time limited, and rendering the role of responses upon cryoablation as "immunoprotective" or "immunodepressive" was difficult to prove.

Cryoimmunology analyzes a specific immune response that is formed against antigens and debris derived from the cells and tissues after cryodestruction. It comprises all aspects of the innate, humoral, and cytotoxic arms of immunity that may become activated after cryosurgery and contribute further tumor destruction [2]. The strong inflammatory reaction inside the tumor tissue after ablation plays a critical role in the initiation and mediation of the antitumor immune response [3]. For instance, the release of interferon gamma (IFN-γ) and other inflammatory cytokines, upregulated by cryonecrotic tissue, may induce maturation of dendritic cells and other antigen-presenting cells (APCs), leading to immune activation against the cells/tissues damaged by freezing [4]. The key roles in the emerging immunological response upon cryodestruction are performed by macrophages, dendritic cells, neutrophils, and CD4+ and CD8+ cells [5].

The ability of cryoablation to control not just primary tumors but also distant metastases has been described historically, especially in prostate cancer [6, 7]. Some other malignancies have also been shown to regress metastatic foci after cryodestruction, such as breast cancer, myosarcoma, and hepatic rectal tumors [8–12]. Some recent reports have tried to elucidate the mechanisms of cryoablation-induced immune-mediated destruction of tumors and metastases. Interestingly, conflicting results from animal experiments evaluating tumor response to cryoablation have ranged from the desired destruction of the primary tumor and shrinking of distant metastases to the unwarranted growth of tumors and hastened experimental animal death. Earlier studies varied significantly in many factors including but not limited to types of tumors studied, nature of immunological assays used, as well as time frames and techniques of cryoablation, which could have been crucial in the type of immune response generated as we will see in the due course. Modern, controlled cryoimmunology studies have shed more light and suggested better mechanisms of cryo-induced immune response. The current chapter will discuss how the immune system becomes activated after cryoablation, as well as some of the evidence both for and against the use of this approach to treating tumors.

3.2 Mechanisms of Tissue Injury After Cryosurgery

The mechanism of tissue injury and subsequent cell damage after cryosurgery is complex. The nature of cell destruction relies on multiple processes related to the rates of temperature change, target temperature, distance from freezing center, and extracellular/cellular solute concentrations after freezing, among others. Depending on these parameters, either necrosis ("necroptosis") or apoptosis occurs secondary to direct or indirect cellular injury. The direct process occurs due to the sequelae of direct freezing of water. Slow freezing induces ice crystals in the extracellular space, increasing the osmolar concentration,

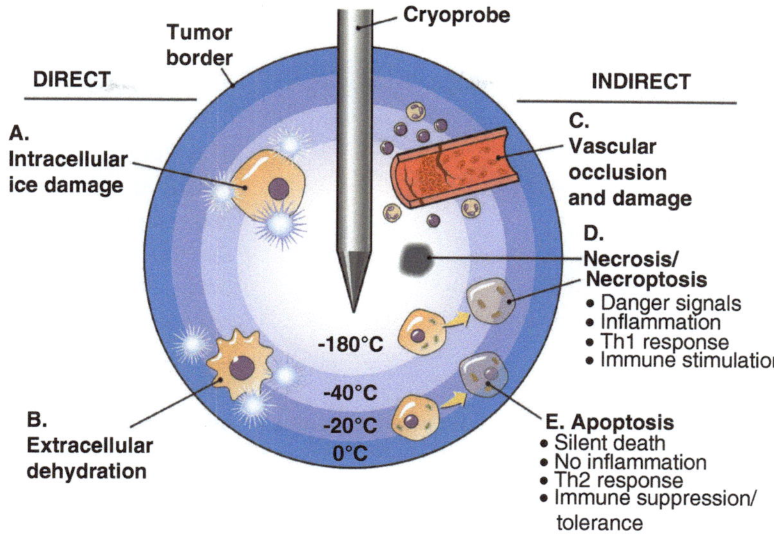

Fig. 3.1 Mechanism of cryodestruction. *A* direct cell damage by intracellular lysis, *B* direct cell destruction by extracellular dehydration, *C* vascular occlusion and damage, *D* inflammatory damage necrosis, necroptosis, *E* silent cell absorption – apoptosis

which results in cell dehydration. The resulting high solute concentration and lower temperatures intracellularly cause reversible conformational change of cytoplasmic enzymes that may lead to direct cell death [13]. However, if freezing rates are rapid, ice crystals form quickly within the cell as well as extracellularly, leading to direct mechanical damage to organelles and cell membranes which cause immediate cell death [14]. This is more commonly observed near the cooling probe (center of cryolesion), where freezing rates are rapid and the temperatures are lowest (Fig. 3.1). Moreover, upon slow thawing of the tissue after freezing, free water rushes into the cells, producing intracellular edema, increasing intracellular ice crystal formation, and producing cell bursting [15].

The direct damage contributes to cell necrosis, release of intracellular contents, and extracellular matrix damage, leading to activation of the short-lived, nonspecific innate immune response and significant inflammation. The direct cell injury resulting necrosis is typical at short distances from the center of the cryogenic lesion where the lower temperatures achieved. Temperatures of approximately −20 °C have been suggested for adequate tissue destruction; however, it is worthwhile to note that malignant cells may be more resistant to cryoinjury and require lower temperatures [16, 17]. Current standards recommend tissue temperatures of 50 °C to −60 °C degrees for effective ablation of malignant tissue [15, 16].

Within higher, sublethal, temperature ranges, cryoablated cells in malignant tissues such as in human colon carcinomas have been shown to undergo apoptosis instead of necrosis [18]. Markers for apoptosis can be observed in cells 4 h after freezing. The percent of apoptotic colon carcinoma cells is maximized at −25 °C with approximately 28 % of cells demonstrating elevated apoptosis markers. Colder temperatures result in lower apoptotic rates likely secondary to a shift towards the mechanism of cell injury described previously, namely, a predominantly cryolytic type of cell death and tissue necrosis (Fig. 3.1). It is important to note that cell death by apoptosis is the primary mechanism of cryoablation in the peripheral zone of the cryogenic lesion (away from the center of cryolesion), given the inherent higher temperatures found away from the source of freezing. Also notable is that apoptotic cell death does not induce an inflammatory response as seen during necrosis. The balance between apoptosis and necrosis may play an important

Table 3.1 Mechanisms of cell death and tissue injury after cryosurgery

Direct injury	Indirect injury
Extracellular matrix ice crystal formation	Thrombus formation
Intracellular osmotic dehydration	Vascular stasis and ischemia
Enzymatic conformational changes	Innate and adaptive immune system-driven injury
Intracellular ice crystal formation and cell bursting	

role in whether a tumor undergoing cryoablation is destroyed or not or whether strong immune response towards the tumor has been induced or not. Furthermore the release of endogenous "danger signals" (fragments of DNA, RNA, hyaluronan products, long CpG sequences, high-mobility group protein B1 (HMGPB1) or amphoterin, TNF-alpha, IFN-alpha, IL-6, IL-1β, heat shock protein (HSP), uric acid, ATP, UTP) has significant proinflammatory properties thus contributing to immune stimulation [19]. Activation of TNF-alpha and binding of FAS-ligand produces necroptosis of the affected cells which is also immune mediated and associated with inflammation in comparison to apoptosis where the death of the cells is silent, with minimal or no inflammation. The apoptotic cell death is main mechanism of tumor-cell turnover to suppress inflammation and avoid protective immune response.

Indirect cell damage also occurs after cryoablation due to the damaging effects of ice crystals on the wall of blood vessels and the lining endothelium. After thawing and reperfusion of affected vessels, platelets become activated causing thrombus formation and subsequent local tissue ischemia. The vascular stasis results in further tissue damage post cryoablation. Furthermore, indirect damage occurs due to immunological response that follows an initial inflammatory response secondary to cryosurgery (Table 3.1). This process of immune system activation is studied by cryoimmunology and is discussed in detail in the following sections along with the development of protective immune response.

3.3 Cryosurgery-Induced Inflammatory Response and Immune Activation

The cornerstones of cryoimmunology can be described as processes involving inflammation and immune attack against damaged target tissue that follow local cryoablation. As described previously, extracellular and intracellular antigens are released after cryosurgery secondary to membrane disruption and cell death. Furthermore, extracellular matrix releases preformed inflammatory cytokines initiating a strong immediate inflammatory response. For instance, studies have demonstrated that levels of IL-1β, IL-6, and TNF-α are elevated after cryoablation of large hepatic metastases [20–22]. IL-12 and IFN-γ have also been detected shortly after freezing [1]. Prostate tumor cell gene expression of several cytokines implicated in stimulating immunity, such as IL-2, IL-15, IL-12p40, IL-18, and TNF-α, was demonstrated to increase after cryoablation. Cells including neutrophils, macrophages, and lymphocytes are recruited by the ongoing inflammatory process and add to the cytokine milieu by secreting other inflammatory mediators marking the activation of the innate immune response [23–25]. Cell infiltration including APCs and T cells may be mediated by the expression of proteins such as heat shock protein-70 (HSP 70) from tumors undergoing cell death [26]. As quickly as within a few hours after cryosurgery, polymorphonuclear (PMN) leukocytes are also recruited to the lesion site and infiltrate the area. Their migration peaks after 3 days and occurs along with an increasing macrophage infiltration that peaks at 7 days [27]. NK cell activity was also shown to increase in a mammary adenocarcinoma mouse model after cryoablation [1].

Following innate immunity activation, the acquired immune response begins with the actions of antigen-presenting cells (APCs). APCs, namely, macrophages and dendritic cells (DCs), engulf the antigens released by cryoablation and present them to T cells via major histocompatibility complex (MHC) Class I and II. A cytotoxic and humoral response follows with APC presentation of antigen to lymphocytic cells. Dendritic cells loaded with antigens now migrate to lymph nodes

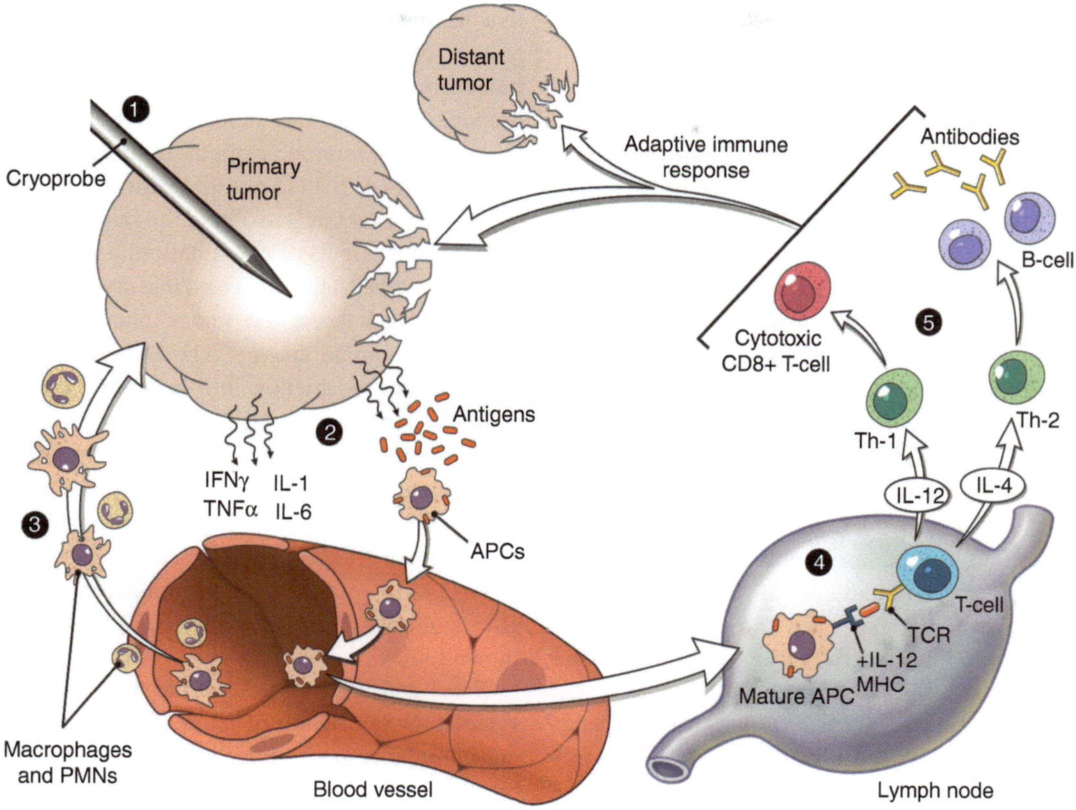

Fig. 3.2 Inflammation and immune activation upon cryoinjury. *1* tumor cryodestruction, *2* antigen and cytokine release, *3* inflammation with polymorphonuclear cells, macrophages, and antigen-presenting cells (*APC*) stimulation, *4* development of the immune response both humoral and cellular in tumor-associated lymph nodes, priming of the cytotoxic T cells, *5* effective immune response – killing of the primary tumor and distant disease

where they undergo maturation, becoming efficient APCs able to prime naïve antigen-specific T cells. They upregulate their maturation gene expression including IL-1, Fas, CDKN1A, ostoprotegrin, and CXCR4, as well as their expression of immunostimulatory cytokines including IL-1β, IL-12p40, IL-15, TNF-α, and IFN-γ. DC maturation estimated by flow cytometric measurement of the surface marker CD86, a ligand that participates in T cell priming, was shown to increase eightfold after freezing prostate cancer cells. Moreover, the expression of class-II MHC, which is a required component of antigen presentation and activation of T cells, was doubled [28].

As APCs present antigens to naïve helper T cells (Th) in the presence of IL-12, T-cell differentiation into Th-1 cells occurs. Th1 cells release IL-2, IL-12, IFN-γ, TNF-α, and GM-CSF, which in turn participate in activating cytotoxic (CD8) T cells. B-cell proliferation and differentiation into antibody-producing cells also occur upon expression of IL-4 by naïve helper T cells, resulting in T-cell differentiation into Th-2 cells. Th-2 cells express IL-4 and IL-5 cytokines promoting B-cell differentiation into antibody producing cells. The afore-described cascade of events marks the initiation of the adaptive arm of the immune response triggered by cryoablation. This response is specific against the antigens derived from cryoablated cells, possibly priming systemic antitumor activity. The specific CD8 T cells now contribute not just to a killing of the primary tumor, but are also carried by circulation to bind to distant foci of metastatic tumor, resulting in antitumor-specific response and killing of tumor cells by necroptosis (Fig. 3.2).

3.4 Cryoablation and Tumor Microenvironment

Tumor survival and progression are partly due to their ability to evade the host immune system. Tumor microenvironments appear to modulate immune response by regulating immune cell phenotype and function both locally and systemically. The knowledge and control of tumor microenvironment are becoming as important as knowledge and control of cancer cells. For instance, patients with progressing hepatocellular carcinoma (HCC) have been demonstrated to have increasing levels of peripheral CD4+CD25+ cells, detected by flow cytometry [29]. CD4+CD25+ cells are some of the best described T-regulatory cells (Treg) that downregulate the immune system. Increases in Treg cell levels have also been shown in other cancers including gastric, lung, pancreatic, and breast cancers [30]. It has been speculated that the response to cryoablation may vary depending on tumor type and the level of Treg cells present. For instance, patients' HCC response after cryoablation with argon-helium cryoprobes to freezing temperatures of −135 °C appeared to be dependent on the quantities of circulating CD4+CD25+ Treg cells prior to treatment. Patients with HCC regression after cryoablation showed significantly decreased Treg frequency by flow cytometry. In contrast, patients with HCC progression and recurrence showed increased Treg cells. Treg frequencies were approximately 6.9 % in early-stage HCC, 8.8 % in intermediate-stage HCC, 10.3 % in advanced-stage HCC, and 13.4 % in terminal-stage HCC. These results indicate the role of immune downregulation in tumor survival, even after therapy. Furthermore, immune-inhibitory cytokines like TGF-β, IL-10, and PG E2 also contribute to suppression of cytotoxic immune response. These data may also help explain why cryoablation is at times ineffective in treating certain tumors, since cytotoxic T-lymphocyte may take at least 6 h to kill one tumor cell in tumor microenvironment (Fig. 3.3a, b), while on the contrary B cell in the healthy lymph node takes less than 60 min to kill the tumor cell [31]. In addition, tumors recruit myeloid-derived suppressor cells (MDSC) from the bone marrow transforming them to tumor-associated macrophages (TAM), thus blocking and suppressing antitumor immune response and enhancing tumor survival. It is likely that adjunctive therapy may be necessary to obtain the full potential of antitumor effects of cryoablation.

Other studies have suggested that cryodestruction may counteract the tumor microenvironment anti-immune activity. The immunological response to cryoablation in a renal cell cancer animal model demonstrated higher IFN-γ to IL-4 levels suggesting an increase in Th-1:Th-2 ratio and demonstrating the interplay between inflammatory cytokines and activation of the immune system after cryosurgery. The increase in Th-1 to Th-2 ratio opposes the anti-immune response effects of renal cell carcinoma (RCC) previously shown [32].

Sabel and colleagues have elegantly demonstrated how rate of freeze could affect the resulting immune response after cryoablation of 4T1 breast carcinoma in balb/C mice [33]. Two weeks after inoculation of mice with the tumor cells, the animals were divided into four groups (control, surgical resection group, and low- and high-freeze group). High-freeze technique used argon cryoprobe for 30 s and duty cycle of 100 %, while low-freeze technique used the same probe, but with duty cycle of 10 % for several minutes. One week later, high-freeze group demonstrated significant reduction in CD4+CD25+ T-regulatory cells in examined tumor lymph nodes, while the number of cytotoxic CD8+ cells was not significantly affected. Both, low-freeze group and surgery group had dramatically higher Treg levels, producing more immunosuppression and increased levels of lung metastases in the latter. Furthermore, the cytotoxic CD8 T-cell responses to exposure to tumor cells in vitro were almost tripled in the high-freeze group in comparison to low freeze, surgery, and control. Specific evidence of antitumor activity following cryoablation is discussed in more detail in the following section. We can now emphasize that cryoablation apart from direct and indirect tumor cell damage may also contribute significantly to a change

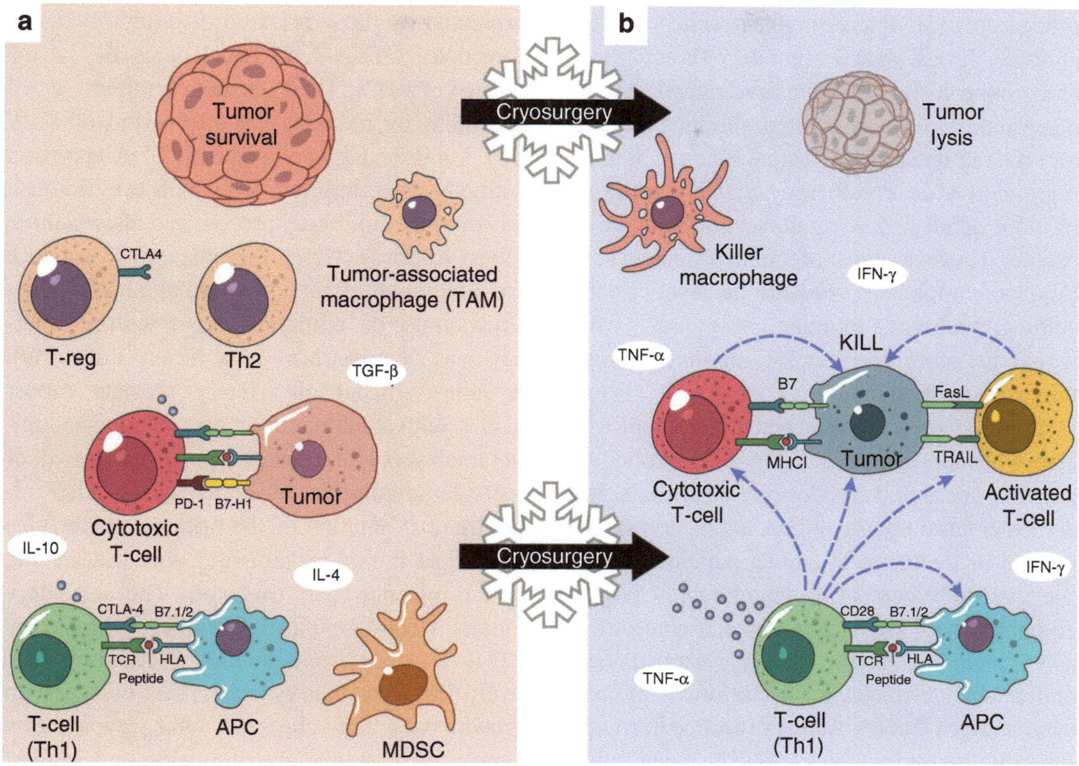

Fig. 3.3 (**a**, **b**) Tumor microenvironment switch induced by cryosurgery. (**a**) Tumor survival. Th-2 – immune-inhibitory microenvironment. (**b**) Tumor lysis. Th-1 immunostimulatory microenvironment. *Abbreviations*: *MDSC* myeloid-derived suppressive cells, *APC* antigen-presenting cells, *CTLA-4* cytotoxic T-lymphocyte antigen 4, *PD1* programmed cell death receptor 1, *TCR* T-cell receptor, *HLA* major histocompatibility complex

from tumor-supportive (Th-2) tumor microenvironment to tumor-suppressive one with Th-1 predominance (Fig. 3.2).

3.5 Cryosurgery-Induced Primary and Metastatic Antitumor Activity

The formation of specific antibodies against cryoablated tissue antigens was demonstrated many decades ago. Early experiments with cryoablation of the rabbit benign prostate, seminal vesicle, and bulbourethral glands showed that autoantibodies specific to these tissues could be isolated from the serum of respective animals. These antibodies did not react with other autologous tissues such as the kidney, liver, or thyroid and did not recognize human-derived tissues, demonstrating the specificity of the antibodies for the cryoablated tissue [34]. Autoantibody formation was detected as early as within 7–10 days of cryoablation, suggesting that at least period of 2 weeks should be allowed for the first attempts to detect the immune response. The same study also explains the lack of the immune response detection in sera analyses performed earlier in the immediate post-freezing period [1]. These data inspired more research exploring the generation of immune system-targeted therapy against malignant tissues with cryosurgery. Cryoablation of prostate cancer has become increasingly popular in urological oncology and has shed light into the widespread potential applications of cryoimmunology as primary or adjuvant therapy for cancer. The reports of cryosurgery of prostate tumor demonstrated that antibodies specific to prostate cancer antigens were found in the serum after the procedure [35]. Interestingly, despite increased antibody levels, actual secondary tumor growth and tumor histology were unchanged. Several other reports have suggested similar contradictory data in regard to the actual efficacy of tumor regression after cryotherapy and are discussed in more detail in a separate section later in this chapter. However, most of the investigators at the time were not able to measure the level of actual cellular/cytotoxic immune response, which would be more specific for immune-mediated tumor destruction.

Later studies, where better immunological assays became available and more controlled and precisely measured cryodestruction feasible, have demonstrated impressive benefits of cryosurgery for cancer treatment in human patients. A retrospective study comparing the effects of targeted cryoablation of prostate cancer and control therapies including brachytherapy, external beam radiation, or 3-dimensional conformal radiation demonstrated that cryosurgery resulted in equal or superior disease free rates [36]. The mean follow-up time was 5.3 years, and the outcome measures were prostate-specific antigen (PSA)-based cut-offs. No serious complications were reported and only minimal morbidity was observed.

Patients with nonmetastatic prostate cancer have also been treated using a percutaneous approach to cryoablation [37]. Biopsy of treated tissue after percutaneous cryotherapy showed elevated levels of TNF-α and IFN-γ as well as increased Th-1:Th-2 ratio. A significant increase in peripheral blood mononuclear cells was also shown along with increased cytolytic activity of cytotoxic T-lymphocytes against autologous prostate cancer cells. This activity was specific to prostate tissue. It is prudent to note, however, that despite evidence of immune system activation, this approach was not sufficient to prevent cancer relapse. Moreover, the level of differentiation of the prostate tumor cells also plays a role in the effectiveness of cryosurgery. More differentiated tissue proved to be associated with advantageous survival in patients [38], since the capacity for proliferation decreases in cells as they mature and differentiate.

Some of the rationale for the limited effectiveness of cryosurgery in eradicating tumors may be explained by the expression of inhibitory T-cell coreceptor CTLA-4. CTLA-4 binds B-7 at the surface of APCs. Their interaction inhibits T-cell activation by reducing the expression of IL-2. CTLA-4 is the target of a recently FDA-approved antibody drug, ipilimumab, which can diminish this immune-inhibitory process and allow a more robust response. Given the potential to enhance the antitumor effects of thermal ablation, the adjuvant use of ipilimumab along with cryotherapy was demonstrated in a recent study [39]. A mouse model of primary prostate cancer treated with combination of cryoablation and ipilimumab was utilized showing that the growth of secondary tumors seeded at distant sites after initial thermal ablation of the primary tumor (also known as tumor rechallenge) was slowed and tumor rejection was triggered. The secondary tumors were found to be highly infiltrated by CD4+ T cells as well as CD8+ T cells and relatively less T-regulatory cells. This cessation in growth was not observed after cryoablation alone. These results are promising and suggest augmentation of antitumor immunity with combination therapy. Another possible mechanism of tumor survival is activation PD-1 (programmed cell death) receptor on active T and B cells which blocks their activity when stimulated by tumor cells produced ligands PD-L1/PD-L2. Thus, the binding of PD-1 receptor has profound immunosuppressive properties and is crucial for tumor survival [40]. Promising new studies are now on the way in metastatic melanoma with new PD-1 inhibitor lambrolizumab [41], which could also serve as a potential adjuvant to cryodestruction in selected cases.

Many other types of cancers have been targeted using cryoimmunology. For instance, tumors created by human melanoma cell lines that were xenografted in mice and treated with cryoablation were evaluated for necrosis-induced recruitment of inflammatory cells and induction of immune-mediated activity [27]. After freezing, congestion, edema, and endothelial cell activation were detected, as well as a polymorphonuclear leukocytes infiltration into the tumor. Antibodies against the tumor cells were also detected.

In mammary adenocarcinoma, a striking reduction in the development of tumors was demonstrated in mice after treatment with cryoablation [1]. Mice were first treated with either surgical resection or cryoablation of the primary mammary adenocarcinomas. Later, the same two groups of mice were subjected to rechallenge with the same tumor type and while the group that had been treated with surgical resection alone developed new tumors 86 % of the time, only 16 % of the group previously treated by cryoablation had recurrence. These data exemplify that cryoablation of the primary tumors likely resulted in an adaptive immune response with memory specific to the tumor type, reducing the development of new tumors/recurrences. The investigators also noted that natural killer (NK) cell activity was increased.

Zeelenberg et al., in her study of suspension of fibrosarcoma cells, compared the ability of different antigen presentation to induce sustained cytotoxic immune response and decrease in Treg cells upon cryoablation. The most efficient form of antigen was vesicle bound (exosomal) which was superior to intact cell or antigen molecule per se [42]. Exosomes can also be tumor-derived (breast, colon, pancreas, lung, and head and neck melanomas) as 50–100 nm membrane bound vesicles containing among others the following components: RNA, microRNA, receptors, ligands, cytokines, tumor markers, adhesion molecules, enzymes, and HLA/peptide complexes. They present hallmark of tumor survival promoting tumor growth, carcinogenesis, angiogenesis, and herald metastases and modifying and preparing tumor microenvironment for survival and also have strong immunosuppressive activity [43]. Considering effects that cryodestruction has on cell membrane, it is plausible to deduct that one of the mechanisms of tumor suppression could also be freezing-induced modification of the tumor-derived exosomes, making them instead more immunogenic and less capable of tumor promotion. Curcumin, a very well-known supplement with antioxidant properties, was also found to be able to produce membrane alteration of tumor-derived exosomes and as such exhibiting anticancer properties [43]. Another membrane system possibly targeted by cryodestruction could also be mitochondrial membrane where sudden release of enzymes could evolve in generation of "signals of danger" switching the response from immunosuppressive to immunostimulating upon cryoablation, contributing as such to cryonecrosis already produced by direct damage of the tumor cells by freezing [44]. Baust et al. showed in his analysis of caspase-inhibition assays that cryodamage of mitochondrial membrane in prostate cancer cells is responsible for >30 % cryonecrosis upon temperature decrease to −15 °C and below [45]. The effect gets enhanced further if cryosensitization was performed with pretreatment with vitamin D as an adjuvant.

In human studies involving patients with rectal carcinoma, 13 patients with inoperable cases were subjected to cryosurgery [46]. The investigators reported raised concentrations of IgG and IgA in biopsies of the tumors, detected by direct immunofluorescence. Although no prognostic factors were evaluated, the authors proposed that the immunoglobulin increase would likely result in antitumor properties, similar to previous studies in other organ systems. Patients with colon cancers were also treated with cryoablation of their metastatic liver masses [47]. The levels of serum total gangliosides (STGs) and antibody titers against these STGs were measured as an indicator of cryoablative-related necrosis and induction of humoral immunity against colon cancer-specific gangliosides. IgM titers were increased significantly after cryoablation, correlating to the increase in serum ganglioside levels. No increase in IgM was observed against normal tissue gangliosides, again, illustrating the tissue-specific immunity.

Nishida et al. studied a group of 24 patients with different primary (chondrosarcomas, osteosarcomas) and metastatic bone tumors using tumor curettage and treatment of affected bone with cryosurgery. Frozen bone was then replanted back to the patient using "free-freezing technique" for flat bones like pelvis or "pedicle-freezing technique" for long bones. The authors reported disease-free survival in more than half of the group that correlated with posttreatment elevation of IFN gamma and IL-12 levels which doubled, even tripled, in patients with disease-free survival during the 6–12-month follow-up period [48].

Given that the immune response against malignant cells is specific and systemic, activity against metastatic cancers has also been shown. It has been proposed that cryoablation of breast cancer prior to surgical resection can be an effective adjuvant therapy in preventing recurrence and reducing metastases in mice [49]. These investigations led to the illustration of increased fraction of tumor-specific T cells as shown by IFN-γ release assay. Strikingly, the number of pulmonary metastases was reduced after cryoablation when compared to surgery alone or controls. The progression of metastasizing comedo-type breast adenocarcinoma in rats was also evaluated after cryotherapy in comparison to surgical resection alone [50]. Ten weeks after local cryotherapy of tumors, rats were rechallenged with breast adenocarcinoma cells. The investigators reported an increased rejection rate of secondary tumors in the cryoablation group compared to surgery alone. Moreover, the number of lymph node metastases and tumor weight was also lower.

Splenic and lymph node reaction to cryotherapy of metastasizing mammary tumor cells was studied in a rat model [2]. It was shown that the spleen increased in weight by 1 week post treatment and regressed to preoperative values by 6 weeks. Lymph nodes draining the site of tumor implantation and treatment showed paracortical hyperplasia, histiocytosis, and germinal center hyperplasia, indicating T-cell activation and increased B-cell and macrophage activity. Furthermore, tumor rechallenge after cryosurgery resulted in increased resistance rate that peaked at 10 weeks post cryoablation.

3.6 Conflicting Data

The size and amount of tissue that is cryoablated may play a significant role in whether the immune response is stimulated or actually suppressed. For instance, when myosarcoma and carcinosarcoma tumors were treated with cryosurgery, regression of secondary tumors was observed if a large portion of the cryoablated tumor was also concomitantly removed surgically during therapy. Interestingly, the antitumor immune response was suppressed if most of the cryoablated tissue was not removed [19]. Perhaps the anti-immunity properties of the tumor microenvironment involving CD25+ Treg cells, even after cryoablation as discussed previously, may overcome immune activation and protect against immune attack locally. Surviving malignant cells may then repopulate the area and reform tumors resulting in cancer recurrence. Furthermore, soft-tissue sarcomas are in general more resistant to freezing and are probably not as feasible for studies as epithelial tumors, more dependent on the proper stromal response for their survival.

Similarly, liver metastases appear to respond in the same fashion [51]. When only a single colon cancer-derived metastatic liver nodule was treated with cryoablation in a mouse model, the overall number of metastatic liver nodules and size of primary tumor was reduced. However, if multiple nodules were treated, an actual increase in the number of lesions was found, although this difference was not statistically significant.

It is important to mention that many of the studies reporting conflicting results (including actual tumor progression upon cryodestruction) did not standardize their methodology entirely, which has varied significantly from the type of the tumor studied, presence or absence of preexisting immune recognition of the tumor by the host, method and volume of tissue frozen, as well as timing of the monitoring and detection of immune response.

3.7 Augmentation of the Effects of Cryodestruction: The Use of Cryosurgery Adjuvants

Molecular adjuvants can be used to enhance cryodestruction within frozen tumors. The use of adjuvants is bifactorial: first, it could increase control of local disease in the area of cryoinjury reducing risk for local recurrence; second, it could decrease complications due to over freezing into adjacent healthy tissues near the treatment site, enhancing the wound healing and postsurgical recovery. The adjuvants [52] can be broadly categorized into three groups: (a) thermophysical adjuvants, which enhance the injury caused by ice formation, (b) chemotherapeutic approaches that act at a molecular level to induce apoptosis, and (c) cytokines or vascular-based agents that modulate the inflammatory response or stimulate immune cells to enhance tissue destruction. The most common thermophysical adjuvants are glycine and eutectic salts, studied in human breast and rat prostate tumors, respectively. Chemotherapy agents, like 5-FU and doxorubicin, have been used systemically 1–4 days before cryoablation of prostate or hepatoma, respectively. The potential for tumor necrosis factor alpha (TNF-α) and imiquimod in enhancing vasodilatation, apoptosis, and immune response upon cryoablation has been analyzed in prostate and breast cancers as well. Combined use of podophyllotoxin immediately after cryoablation may contribute significantly to control of genital HPV infections, especially when combined with Bowenoid papulosis [53] (Fig. 3.4a, b). Other adjuvants to cryosurgery which possibly are to be considered are lambrolizumab (PD-1 inhibitor) [41] or cyclophosphamide (Treg suppressor) [54].

Some common factors to be considered once cryosurgery adjuvants are selected include: (a) the sensitivity of the tumor to the adjuvant, (b) the selectivity of the adjuvant towards the tissue, (c) the dose of the adjuvant needed to enhance injury in the temperature range (up to −0.5 °C), (d) side effects associated with the adjuvant, (e) the mode of delivery of the adjuvant, and (f) the time of application of the adjuvant relative to cryosurgery procedure [52]. A summary of some of the mechanisms involved in the immunology of cryoinjury is shown in Fig. 3.5.

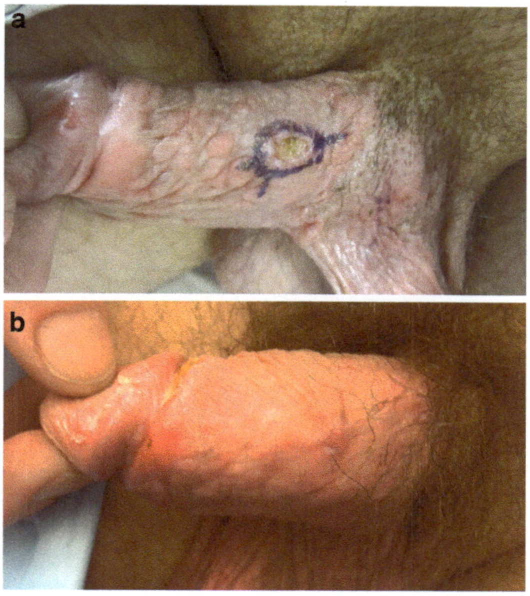

Fig. 3.4 (**a**, **b**) The use of podophyllin as cryosurgery adjuvant. (**a**) A 45-year-old male with advanced HPV disease and bowenoid papulosis on the penile shaft. (**b**) Successful ablation after single session of cryodestruction with podophyllin applied immediately on treated lesions, enhancing the effect of freezing

Essential Tidbits

- During a cryosurgery procedure, a tumor remains "in situ" and induces an antitumoral response triggered by natural absorption of malignant tissue. This should be an advantage over surgical removal of a tumor.
- Necrosis or apoptosis induced by cryosurgery will be secondary to direct or indirect cellular injury. The first is typical at short distance from the center (lower temperatures); the latter at the periphery (higher temperatures).
- Molecular adjuvants can be used to enhance cryodestruction within frozen tumors. They can be categorized into: (a) thermophysical adjuvants (glycine and eutectic salts), (b) chemotherapeutic (5 FU), and (c) cytokines or vascular-based agents.

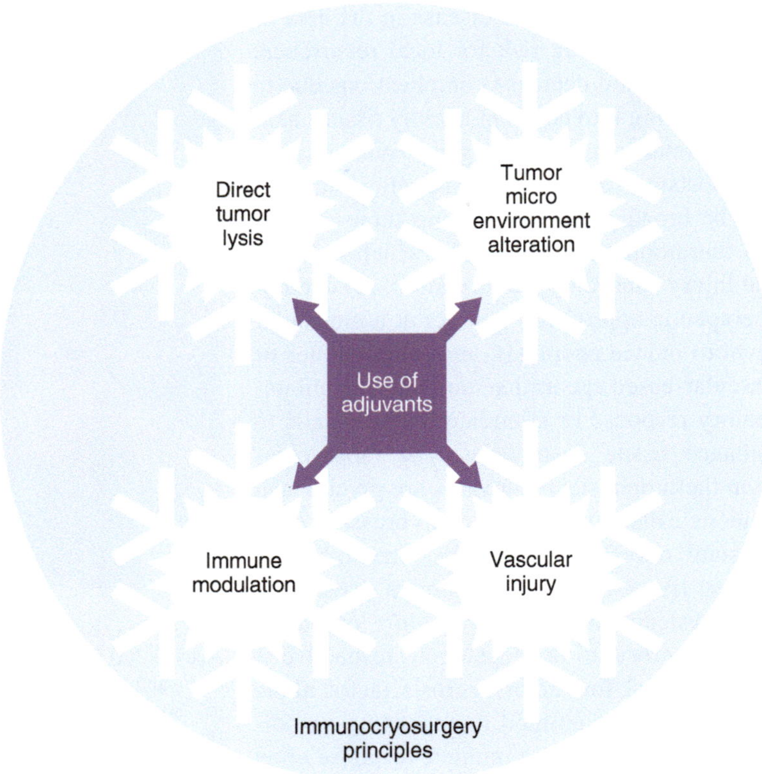

Fig. 3.5 Summary of basic principles of immunocryosurgery

Conclusions

Immunological effects of cryosurgery continue to attract substantial interest not just in oncological therapy but also in understanding of the human immune response to tumor growth and progression. Furthermore, cryoablation has the potential for both local and systemic therapy, i.e., direct ablation of the tumor and eradication of micrometastases through the immune system with minimal systemic toxicity. However, the specifics of generated antitumor immune response are very complex and dependent on many factors capable of inducing not only immune stimulation but also immune suppression. Further directions would possibly include clarification of (1) cytokine profile triggered by cryoablation; (2) the availability of the antigens and the forms of their presentation to be processed by antigen-presenting cells; (3) the timing of the immune response post cryoinjury; (4) ideal ratio of apoptosis vs. necrosis/necroptosis for induction of immunoprotective and not immunosuppressive response; (5) the type and subsets of phagocytic cells responsible for clearing of tumor debris (dendritic cells vs. macrophages); (6) the effects of freezing on tumor microenvironment, vascularity, and suppressive T-regulatory cells; (7) the discovery of adjuvants capable of tilting/switching the immune balance towards stimulation – augmentation and as such enhancing the therapeutic effects of cryodestruction.

As the field of cryosurgery continues to expand, extensive research in the mechanism of the immunomodulatory effects of cryoinjury is necessary. The induction or augmentation of protective and effective antitumor immune response, triggered by use of proper and controlled cryosurgery technique, especially when used with adjuvants, could make this approach very attractive to cancer therapy. The ultimate goal of modern oncology where the single modality is capable of the destruction of primary tumor and its micro- and macrometastatic disease with minimal toxicity to the patient may not be that far off.

Glossary

Apoptosis	Silent cell death, with cell absorption and no inflammation
Cryoablation	Removal of tumor tissue by freezing
Cryoadjuvants	Compounds use to augment destructive or immunostimulatory effects of cryosurgery
Cryosurgery	Destruction of diseased tissue by freezing
Cryotherapy	Therapeutic application of cold in medicine
Necroptosis	Cell death caused by immunological process with cytotoxic T cells and inflammation
Necrosis	Cell death produced by inflammation, chemical or physical destruction of the cell membrane and subcellular structures
Th-1 tumor microenvironment	Immune response-modified stromal tissue that destructs a tumor and blocks its survival, immunostimulatory
Th-2 tumor microenvironment	Tumor-induced stroma that helps a tumor to survive, immunosuppressive
Treg	T-regulatory cells, induced by the tumor tissue to suppress immune response

References

1. Sabel MS, Nehs MA, Su G, Lowler KP, Ferrara JL, Chang AE. Immunologic response to cryoablation of breast cancer. Breast Cancer Res Treat. 2005; 90:97–104.
2. Miya K, Saji S, Morita T, Niwa H, Takao H, Kida H, et al. Immunological response of regional lymph nodes after tumor cryosurgery: experimental study in rats. Cryobiology. 1986;23:290–5.
3. Osada S, Imai H, Tomita H, Tokuyama Y, Okumura N, Matsuhashi N, et al. Serum cytokine levels in response to hepatic cryoablation. J Surg Oncol. 2007; 95:491–8.
4. He T, Tang C, Xu S, Moyana T, Xiang J. Interferon gamma stimulates cellular maturation of dendritic cell line DC2.4 leading to induction of efficient cytotoxic T cell responses and antitumor immunity. Cell Mol Immunol. 2007;4:105–11.
5. Matin SF, Sharma P, Gill IS, Tannenbaum C, Hobart MG, Novick AC, et al. Immunological response to renal cryoablation in an in vivo orthotopic renal cell carcinoma murine model. J Urol. 2010;183:333–8.
6. Gursel E, Roberts M, Veenema RJ. Regression of prostatic cancer following sequential cryotherapy to the prostate. J Urol. 1972;108:928–32.
7. Ablin RJ, Soanes WA, Gonder MJ. Immuno-cryourogenital treatment of benign and malignant diseases of the prostate. Gerontol Clin. 1970;12:302–13.
8. Staren ED, Sabel MS, Gianakakis LM, Wiener GA, Hart VM, Gorski M, et al. Cryosurgery of breast cancer. Arch Surg. 1997;132:28–33; discussion 4.
9. Wong LL, Limm WM, Cheung AH, Fan FL, Wong LM. Hepatic cryosurgery: early experience in Hawaii. Hawaii Med J. 1995;54:811–3.
10. Crews KA, Kuhn JA, McCarty TM, Fisher TL, Goldstein RM, Preskitt JT. Cryosurgical ablation of hepatic tumors. Am J Surg. 1997;174:614–7; discussion 7–8.
11. Wang ZS. Cryosurgery in rectal carcinoma – report of 41 cases. Zhonghua Zhong Liu Za Zhi. 1989;11: 226–7.
12. Blackwood CE, Cooper IS. Response of experimental tumor systems to cryosurgery. Cryobiology. 1972;9: 508–15.
13. Privalov PL. Cold denaturation of proteins. Crit Rev Biochem Mol Biol. 1990;25:281–305.
14. Mazur P, Rall WF, Leibo SP. Kinetics of water loss and the likelihood of intracellular freezing in mouse ova. Influence of the method of calculating the temperature dependence of water permeability. Cell Biophys. 1984;6:197–213.
15. Baust JG, Gage AA. The molecular basis of cryosurgery. BJU Int. 2005;95:1187–91.
16. Yang G, Zhang A, Xu LX. Intracellular ice formation and growth in MCF-7 cancer cells. Cryobiology. 2011;63:38–45.
17. Tatsutani K, Rubinsky B, Onik G, Dahiya R. Effect of thermal variables on frozen human primary prostatic adenocarcinoma cells. Urology. 1996;48: 441–7.
18. Hanai A, Yang WL, Ravikumar TS. Induction of apoptosis in human colon carcinoma cells HT29 by sublethal cryo-injury: mediation by cytochrome c release. Int J Cancer. 2001;93:526–33.
19. Sabel MS. Cryo-immunology: a review of the literature and proposed mechanisms for stimulatory versus suppressive immune responses. Cryobiology. 2009; 58:1–11.
20. Weber SM, Lee Jr FT, Chinn DO, Warner T, Chosy SG, Mahvi DM. Perivascular and intralesional tissue necrosis after hepatic cryoablation: results in a porcine model. Surgery. 1997;122:742–7.
21. Glasgow SC, Ramachandran S, Csontos KA, Jia J, Mohanakumar T, Chapman WC. Interleukin-1beta is prominent in the early pulmonary inflammatory response after hepatic injury. Surgery. 2005;138: 64–70.

22. Seifert JK, Junginger T. Cryotherapy for liver tumors: current status, perspectives, clinical results, and review of literature. Technol Cancer Res Treat. 2004;3:151–63.
23. Bishoff JT, Chen RB, Lee BR, Chan DY, Huso D, Rodriguez R, et al. Laparoscopic renal cryoablation: acute and long-term clinical, radiographic, and pathologic effects in an animal model and application in a clinical trial. J Endourol. 1999;13:233–9.
24. Chosy SG, Nakada SY, Lee Jr FT, Warner TF. Monitoring renal cryosurgery: predictors of tissue necrosis in swine. J Urol. 1998;159:1370–4.
25. Campbell SC, Krishnamurthi V, Chow G, Hale J, Myles J, Novick AC. Renal cryosurgery: experimental evaluation of treatment parameters. Urology. 1998;52:29–33; discussion –4.
26. Todryk S, Melcher AA, Hardwick N, Linardakis E, Bateman A, Colombo MP, et al. Heat shock protein 70 induced during tumor cell killing induces Th1 cytokines and targets immature dendritic cell precursors to enhance antigen uptake. J Immunol. 1999;163: 1398–408.
27. Gazzaniga S, Bravo A, Goldszmid SR, Maschi F, Martinelli J, Mordoh J, et al. Inflammatory changes after cryosurgery-induced necrosis in human melanoma xenografted in nude mice. J Invest Dermatol. 2001;116:664–71.
28. Ismail M, Morgan R, Harrington K, Davies J, Pandha H. Immunoregulatory effects of freeze injured whole tumour cells on human dendritic cells using an in vitro cryotherapy model. Cryobiology. 2010;61: 268–74.
29. Zhou L, Fu JL, Lu YY, Fu BY, Wang CP, An LJ, et al. Regulatory T cells are associated with post-cryoablation prognosis in patients with hepatitis B virus-related hepatocellular carcinoma. J Gastroenterol. 2010;45: 968–78.
30. Baecher-Allan C, Anderson DE. Regulatory cells and human cancer. Semin Cancer Biol. 2006;16:98–105.
31. Vasievich E, Huang L. The suppressive tumor microenvironment: a challenge in cancer immunotherapy. Mol Pharm. 2011;8:635–41.
32. Rayman P, Wesa AK, Richmond AL, Das T, Biswas K, Raval G, et al. Effect of renal cell carcinomas on the development of type 1 T-cell responses. Clin Cancer Res. 2004;10:6360S–6.
33. Sabel MS, Su G, Griffith KA, Chang AE. Rate of freeze alters the immunologic response after cryoablation of breast cancer. Ann Surg Oncol. 2010;17:1187–93.
34. Shulman S, Brandt EJ, Yantorno C. Studies in cryo-immunology. II. Tissue and species specificity of the autoantibody response and comparison with iso-immunization. Immunology. 1968;14:149–58.
35. Hoffmann NE, Coad JE, Huot CS, Swanlund DJ, Bischof JC. Investigation of the mechanism and the effect of cryoimmunology in the Copenhagen rat. Cryobiology. 2001;42:59–68.
36. Bahn DK, Lee F, Badalament R, Kumar A, Greski J, Chernick M. Targeted cryoablation of the prostate: 7-year outcomes in the primary treatment of prostate cancer. Urology. 2002;60:3–11.
37. Si TG, Guo Z, Wang HT, Han YP, Hao XS. Cryoablation for prostate cancer induces tumor-specific immune response. Zhonghua Nan Ke Xue. 2009;15:350–3.
38. Petersen DS, Milleman LA, Rose EF, Bonney WW, Schmidt JD, Hawtrey CE, et al. Biopsy and clinical course after cryosurgery for prostatic cancer. J Urol. 1978;120:308–11.
39. Waitz R, Solomon SB, Petre EN, Trumble AE, Fasso M, Norton L, et al. Potent induction of tumor immunity by combining tumor cryoablation with anti-CTLA-4 therapy. Cancer Res. 2012;72:430–9.
40. Francisco LM, Sage PT, Sharpe AH. The PD-1 pathway in tolerance and immunity. Immunol Rev. 2010;236:219–42.
41. Robert C, Soria J-C, Eggermont AMM. Drug of the year: programmed death-1 receptor/programmed death-1 ligand-1 receptor monoclonal antibodies. Eur J Cancer. 2013;49:2968–71.
42. Zeelenberg IS, van Maren WWC, Boissonnas A, et al. Antigen localization controls T-cell mediated tumor immunity. J Immunol. 2011;187:1281–8.
43. Kharziha P, Ceder S, Qiao L, Panaretakis T. Tumor-cell derived exosomes: a message in a bottle. Biochim Biophys Acta. 1826;2012:103–11.
44. Thicr J, Acker JP. Mitochondria and membrane cryoinjury in micropatterned cells: effects of cell-cell interactions. Cryobiology. 2010;61:100–7.
45. Baust MJ, Klossner DP, Robilotto A, et al. Vitamin D3 cryosensitization increases prostate cancer susceptibility to cryoablation via mitochondrial mediated apoptosis and necrosis. BJU Int. 2011;109: 949–58.
46. Kogel HGR, Fohlmeister I, Pichlmaier H. Cryotherapy of rectal cancer. Immunologic results. Zentralbl Chir. 1985;110:147–54.
47. Ravindranath MH, Wood TF, Soh D, Gonzales A, Muthugounder S, Perez C, et al. Cryosurgical ablation of liver tumors in colon cancer patients increases the serum total ganglioside level and then selectively augments antiganglioside IgM. Cryobiology. 2002;45: 10–21.
48. Nishida H, Yamamoto N. Cryoimmunology for malignant bone and soft-tissue tumors. Int J Clin Oncol. 2011;16:109–17.
49. Sabel MS, Arora A, Su G, Chang AE. Adoptive immunotherapy of breast cancer with lymph node cells primed by cryoablation of the primary tumor. Cryobiology. 2006;53:360–6.
50. Misao A, Sakata K, Saji S, Kunieda T. Late appearance of resistance to tumor rechallenge following cryosurgery. A study in an experimental mammary tumor of the rat. Cryobiology. 1981;18:386–9.

51. Urano M, Tanaka C, Sugiyama Y, Miya K, Saji S. Antitumor effects of residual tumor after cryoablation: the combined effect of residual tumor and a protein-bound polysaccharide on multiple liver metastases in a murine model. Cryobiology. 2003;46:238–45.
52. Goel R, Anderson K, Slaton J, Schmidlin F, Vercellotti G, Belcher J, et al. Adjuvant approaches to enhance cryosurgery. J Biomech Eng. 2009;131:074003.
53. Aleksandar L. Krunic, personal communication
54. Levy MY, Sidana A, Chowdhury WH, et al. Cryoimmunology for malignant bone and soft-tissue tumors. J Pharmacol Exp Ther. 2009;330(2):596–601.

Basic Equipment for Cryosurgery

4

Paola Pasquali

Contents

Key Points

- Dermatological cryosurgery utilizes specialized equipment.
- An overview of the different accessories necessary to perform the most common procedures will be shared.
- The most relevant features of each instrument will be discussed.

4.1 Introduction

Dermatologic cryosurgery requires its own set of equipment. When compared to other subspecialties in the field, cryosurgical equipment is relatively inexpensive. A basic starter kit for most dermatologists includes a unit, a set of spraying tips, and a cryogenic storage Dewar [1].

However, for those surgeons that want to do something more than a wart removal and an occasional seborrheic keratosis, the tool box will necessarily have to expand. One will need to have a whole set of gadgets in order to solve a difficult case, besides using all your cryosurgical wit. As in anything in life, once one becomes passionate about a technique, more equipment will be needed.

This chapter will take you step by step through the different equipment used in basic dermatologic cryosurgery using liquid nitrogen (LN) as the cryogen.

P. Pasquali, MD
Department of Dermatology, Pius Hospital de Valls, 43800 Tarragona, Spain
e-mail: pasqualipaola@gmail.com

P. Pasquali (ed.), *Cryosurgery: A Practical Manual*,
DOI 10.1007/978-3-662-43939-5_4, © Springer-Verlag Berlin Heidelberg 2015

The equipment and needed materials include:

1. Liquid nitrogen (LN), LN producers, storage Dewars, and other useful gadgets regarding manipulation of LN (gloves, withdrawn tubes)
2. Cryosurgical unit
3. Attachments for units:
   - Spraying tips
   - Probes
   - Chambers
4. Rubber cones, plastic plates, and other restrainers
5. Tweezers
6. Other equipment

4.2 Liquid Nitrogen (LN), LN Producers, Storage Dewars, and Other Useful Gadgets

4.2.1 Liquid Nitrogen and Storage Dewars

LN is readily available and purchased through specialized dealers. It is relatively easy to manipulate and fairly safe. Since it is used by other professions (veterinary, laboratory, engineering, computer, food industry), finding a dealer is not difficult. This is true for many countries, though each place has regulations that differ from one place to another, and in certain parts of the world finding an LN dealer is almost impossible. When available, most LN distributors will come to your office, pick up your storage Dewar (vacuum flask), and return it full (with the accompanying bill).

LN has to be maintained in special flasks. Throughout history, these vacuum flasks have received many names. Although first introduced in 1881 by Adolf Ferdinand Weinhold, it was Sir James Dewar who in 1892 invented and developed the first insulated flasks [2]. A researcher in the field of cryogenics, Dewars developed a double flask system (1892) (one flask inside another joined at the neck) separated by partially evacuated air that creates a semi-vacuum area which prevents heat transfer (Fig. 4.1).

It took two German glassblowers (1904) [3] to visualize the potential commercial use of the vacuumed flask for keeping drinks hot or cold. They rebaptized the flask into the "thermos," which 60 years later became a metonym for such containers.

Modern day Dewars are structurally the same: they are still one big container contained in another with a vacuum in between. However, they have been improved in many ways:

- They are available in different sizes. This gives you a whole range from which to choose, adapting it to different needs.
- They have improved insulating systems that make LN last longer.
- They are lighter because they are aluminum. This weight reduction has made Dewar handling simpler and more practical.
- They are safer thanks to improvements in the cap/neck system.

Size is an important issue when it comes to choosing a storage Dewar. The most commonly

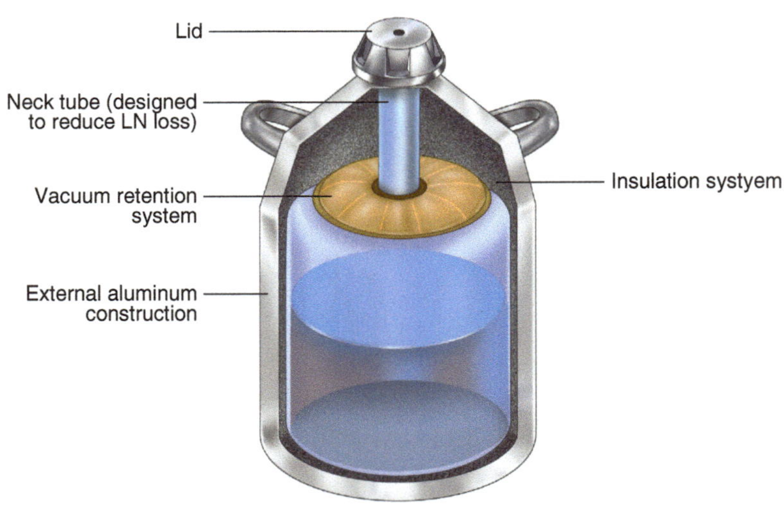

Fig. 4.1 Anatomy of a Dewar (taken from MVE): (**a**) lid, (**b**) neck tube (designed to reduce LN loss), (**c**) vacuum retention system, (**d**) external aluminum construction, (**e**) insulation system

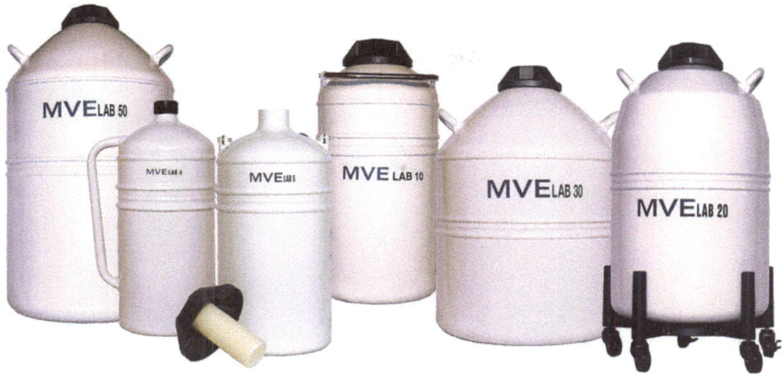

Fig. 4.2 Dewars from MVE (Courtesy of Chart Biomedical)

Table 4.1 MVE Dewars: size, static holding time, empty weight, and full weight

Size (liters, l)	Static holding time	Static evaporation rate (liters/day)	Weight empty (lb)	Weight full (lb)
5 l	4–5 weeks	0.15	8	17
10 l	6–8 weeks	0.18	13	30
20 l	8–12 weeks	0.18	19	53.
Long last 20 l	220 days	0.095	19	53.
30 l	14–16 weeks	0.22	26	77.
50 l	14–17 weeks	0.49	34	123

Data courtesy of MVE Biomedical

used Dewars in dermatology range from 5 up to 50 liters (l). (Fig. 4.2). One commercial manufacturer is MVE [4], and the holding time and weights (empty and full) can be seen in Table 4.1. Small Dewars are easier to handle with the disadvantage that LN lasts a shorter period of time (they contain less), making continuous recharge necessary. They are useful in order to drain off the remaining LN from a larger Dewar that needs to be sent for refill. Larger ones (50 l) are more cumbersome but last longer. They are ideal for daily and continuous use (such as in a large dermatology department), weight being their sole drawback.

An excellent alternative is to have an intermediate-sized Dewar (20–30 l) and a small one (5 l), used to hold the little amount left in a larger Dewar that needs to be sent for refill. It might sound as an unnecessary precaution but one needs to take into account that most retails need at least 24 hours for picking up, refill and bringing back a Dewar. This spared LN in a small Dewar will allow doing cryosurgeries for a day, while waiting for LN delivery.

Dewars can be placed on a roller base, a necessary item for flasks larger than 20 l. This simplifies transferring from one place to another (for instance, for cleaning the floor) or for taking it away for refill.

LN can be withdrawn from the storage Dewar by:

1. Simple pouring. Pouring using a funnel is the standard procedure for small Dewars (5 l). It is not recommended for large Dewars: one might end up hurting ones back or accidentally pouring LN all over the floor. Another inconvenience with single pouring is pouring residues that are sitting at the bottom of the Dewar. This increases the risk of clogging the equipment.
2. Fixed device affix (Fig. 4.3): This is screwed at the top of the Dewar and left in place until refill is required. The fixed affix has its own pressure control and it works like a faucet. Once the LN is reduced inside the flask, so does the internal pressure, making refill necessary. This affix includes a filter that keeps the LN poured from inside the unit clean.

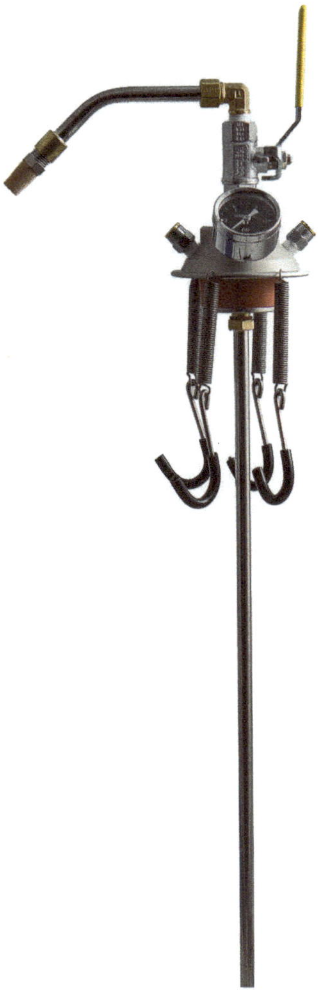

Fig. 4.3 Fixed device affix to leave on Dewar to withdraw liquid nitrogen (LN) (Courtesy of Brymill Cryogenic Systems)

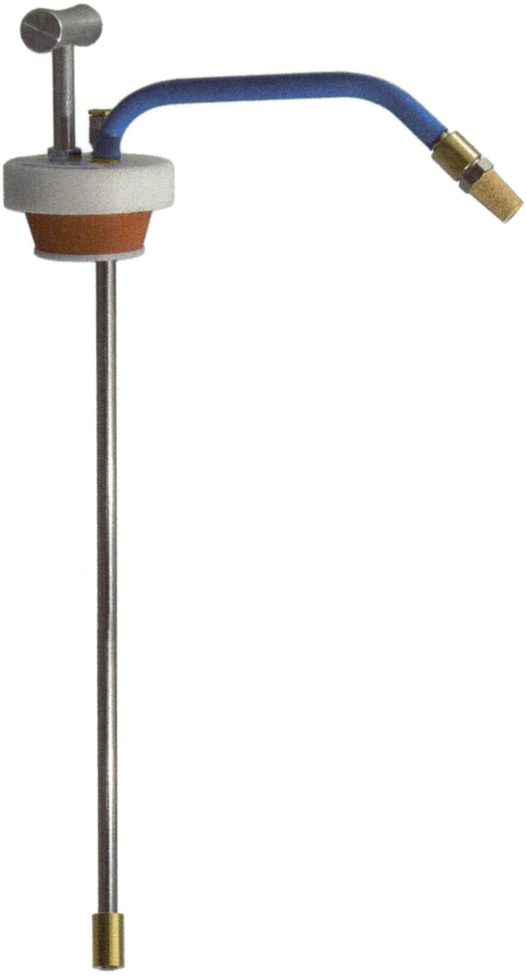

Fig. 4.4 Removable device left on Dewar to withdraw liquid nitrogen (LN). It is placed with slight pressure once the cap is removed. It is meant to be taken out of the Dewar once LN is withdrawn (Courtesy of Brymill Cryogenic Systems)

3. Removable affix (Fig. 4.4). This is placed into the opening of the Dewar once the cap is removed. Once firmly placed, instant pressurization is obtained and unit refill can be done. It must be removed after each refill, and one must remember to place the Dewar cap right back in place to avoid evaporation. If the withdrawal procedure is to be done for several units one after another, the affix can occasionally get clogged due to freezing. If this happens, one must let it thaw for several minutes and restart the charging procedure of the units.

4.2.2 Other Cryogens

There are other cryogens available on the market and used for cryosurgery. Among them are argon gas (Ar, boiling point −187 °C), nitrous oxide (N_2O, −88 °C) [5, 8], carbon dioxide gas (CO_2, −78 °C), and other compressed gases that boil on the order of −55 to −75 °C.

Argon is mostly used in visceral cryosurgery (prostate [9], lung, bone [10, 11]). N_2O and CO_2 are used in dermatologic situations but should be reserved for benign lesions. Wallach [12, 13], Cryo S classic and mini by Metrum CryoFlex [14], Cryosucess by Schuco [15] and CryOmega by Premier Medical [16] are some of the options availble for carbon dioxide and nitrous oxide cryosurgery.

4.2.3 Dewar's Maintenance

Modern Dewars need little maintenance; however, they still need to be kept clean since there is a tendency for detritus accumulation at the bottom of the flask. With sufficient time, a dusty residue accumulates at the bottom and gets sucked into the unit during the LN withdrawal. This detritus will cause malfunction in the unit. The first "symptom" of an unclean Dewar is the darkening of the central pick up tube of the cryosurgical unit. It will start losing its brightness and begins to turn grayish. Once this process begins, the LN will start getting clogged, making maintenance necessary.

Cleaning Dewars is a usually a forgotten but necessary procedure both for the maintenance of the flask and cryosurgical unit. Cleaning the Dewar is a good idea to assure its long life. The best time to do this is right before you send it for refill. Just turn the Dewar upside down and let all the residues pour out. If one thinks that it needs extra cleaning, one can proceed to wash it. MVE suggests using any household detergent or mild soap solutions for sanitizing and decontaminating their Dewars (Table 4.2). They suggest spraying the solution into the inner vessel, although agitation of the solution inside the inner vessel will suffice. Rinsing is important, and the flask has to be thoroughly dry before use; accomplish this by setting the Dewar inverted to drain and dry. If cleaning a Dewar seems a difficult chore, have the technical support from your suppliers take care of this. Basically, cryosurgeons use Dewars to store LN and not as containers for specimens (semen, embryos, bone marrow). Therefore, cleaning is simplified since there is no need to use disinfectants for maintenance.

Another aspect to take into account is that Dewars can lose their vacuum if they are accidentally hit. Care should be taken when handling. Unfortunately, some LN dealers treat empty Dewars like suitcases. When dealing with careless LN dealers, it might be a good idea to put some external protection around the Dewar or change dealer.

Table 4.2 Dewar filling instructions, measuring and withdrawal of LN

Dewar filling instructions
To avoid damage to the aluminum cryogenic vessel which may result in premature vacuum loss, it is important to follow this procedure during the addition of liquid nitrogen to a warm vessel and on subsequent additions
1. Slowly pour liquid nitrogen into new or warm vessels with a funnel or transfer line when possible
2. Allow liquid nitrogen to settle in vessel for 2 h to completely cool
3. Fill the vessel to the desired level after the 2 h settling (cool down) time
4. If filling the Dewar from a pressurized source, make sure that the source tank is at a low pressure (1.52 bar or below)
5. If transfer hose is used for extracting liquid nitrogen from a pressurized liquid source, always use a phase separator on the end of the hose
6. Remember to always wear proper safety attire over clothing; also use face shield, cryogenic gloves, and apron
7. Never overfill your Dewar with liquid nitrogen. Overfilling the tank may cause pumped out components to leak, leading to immediate or premature vacuum failure to occur
How to measure liquid nitrogen quantity
1. Use wooden or plastic dipstick. Never use a hollow tube to measure liquid nitrogen
2. Level will be indicated by frost line, which develops when dipstick is removed
Liquid nitrogen withdrawal
1. Liquid withdrawal from Dewars must be accomplished by pouring or utilizing a withdrawal device. Withdrawal device pressurizes to approximately 0.35 bar and the pressure forces liquid up the withdrawal tube out the valve
2. Always wear proper safety attire: shield, gloves, and apron

Data courtesy of MVE Biomedical

4.2.4 Gloves and Apron (Fig. 4.5)

Proper safety attire is recommended when manipulating LN. A set of cryogenic gloves is a useful item to have, especially if filling is done by somebody not familiar with LN. Occasionally, LN can spatter on the dorsum of the hand and cause burning, particularly on fair skin. Glove use gives confidence. They are a good investment to maintain happy personnel and avoid lawsuits.

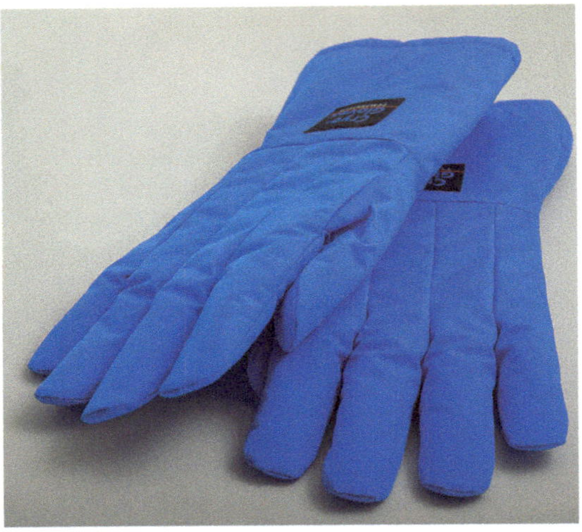

Fig. 4.5 Cryogenic gloves (Courtesy of Brymill Cryogenic Systems)

4.2.5 LN Producers (Fig. 4.6)

For those who have difficulty in accessing a reliable source of LN or live far away from the circuits of delivery, an LN generator can be the solution. This equipment looks like a water dispenser and works by taking nitrogen from the air and turning it into liquid nitrogen. Air is extracted through a particle filter and then compressed to a moderate pressure of 6–8 atmospheres. The compressed air is fed to a membrane that separates the nitrogen portion (78 %) from the air and liberates oxygen, carbon dioxide, and water vapor back into the atmosphere.

This nitrogen is later liquefied through a cryogenic system. Once full, the unit stops, and the LN is transferred by pressure into a liquefier and later forced out a transfer siphon into the Dewar or unit.

This equipment is called elan2™ Liquid Nitrogen Generators [17] and is based on MMR Technologies patented refrigeration technology. They are safe and allow for the production of liquid nitrogen in the office every time it is needed. These units are left powered on all the time. When full, they go into standby mode waiting to power back on as soon as the unit is less than full.

There are two types of units:

- The office unit: it comes with an internal storage container of 0.75 L. Once full (it takes roughly 4 h to produce this amount of LN), a button is pushed and it takes roughly 60 s to transfer it to the external container.
- The auto transfer unit automatically transfers from the internal Dewar to the external Dewar. It takes roughly 4 days to fill the 20 L Dewar, but you can use and take liquid nitrogen from it at any time using a provided transfer tube. Transfer from the 20 L Dewar to a handheld can take approximately 60 s.

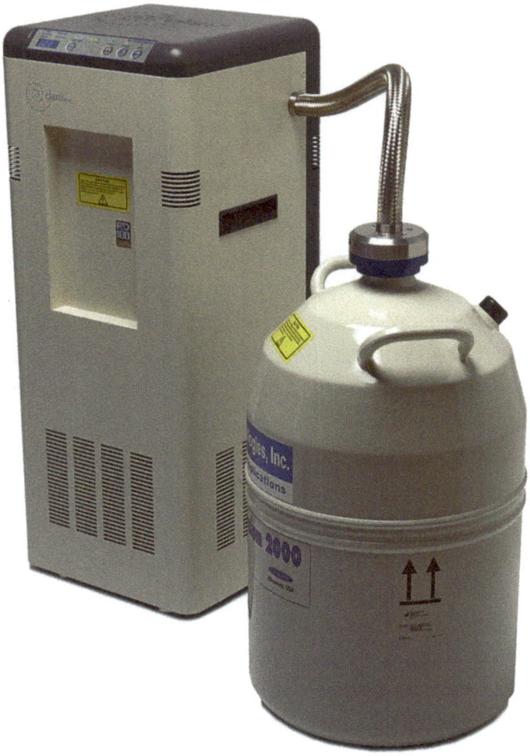

Fig. 4.6 elan2 Liquid Nitrogen Generators (Courtesy of MMR Technologies)

4.3 Cryosurgical Units

Cryosurgery requires cryosurgical units. From the times when Zacarian and Adham (1960) immersed copper disks in LN, many advances have been made in this field. In 1966, Michael Bryne (Brymill Co.) developed the first commercially available handheld cryosurgical device which has been the prototype that has inspired all the equipment available in the market today.

With the existence of these units, the use of cotton swabs is long gone. Cotton swabs for cryosurgical purposes should be avoided for the following reasons:

- They do not allow a controlled application of LN. There is no temperature control whatsoever.
- Commonly used in benign lesions, they do not permit a precise application of cold, therefore destroying areas of healthy skin that should not have to be treated. One ends up with all the undesired secondary effects of cold with little of the expected results.
- Verrucous lesions have large amounts of keratin, a bad cold conductant. If a continuous spraying with margins included using a unit does not eliminate the lesion, needless to say a cotton swab will not either.
- Vascular tumors are nests of vessels with hot blood circulating through them. The destruction of such vessels requires previous pressure and a controlled application of cold via previously frozen copper probes. The use of cotton swabs for this purpose should be avoided.
- There is the bad habit of refreezing the cotton swab by plunging it back into the open unit after contacting the skin. This might cause contamination of the unit. If a cotton swab is reused, this should be immersed in LN placed in a Styrofoam cup which should later be discarded.

Therefore, a cryosurgical unit is a *must have* in order to perform cryosurgery correctly. The common characteristic of this device is that it delivers LN through different tips or probes in a safe, precise, and controlled manner.

The first units were cumbersome and heavy. Nowadays, they are light, easy to handle, and contain sufficient LN to treat several patients, without requiring continuous refills. The most common models come with 300, 350, or 500 cc bottles. The main manufacturer who developed the original units is Brymill [18]. Some other well known trademarks have followed and include Wallach [19], Delasco [20], Cortex [21] (Fig. 4.7a–d), Schuco [22], Premier Medical [23] and KS-2 by Kriosystem [24].

The main breakthrough of the past years has come with the new Cry-Ac® TrackerCam (Fig. 4.8), the new unit by Brymill which measures skin temperature and records the settings and procedures. It does so through infrared technology. Up to now, cryosurgeons used freezing time as a main parameter. However, this could be imprecise because it depended on the distance from the skin and the diameter of the spraying

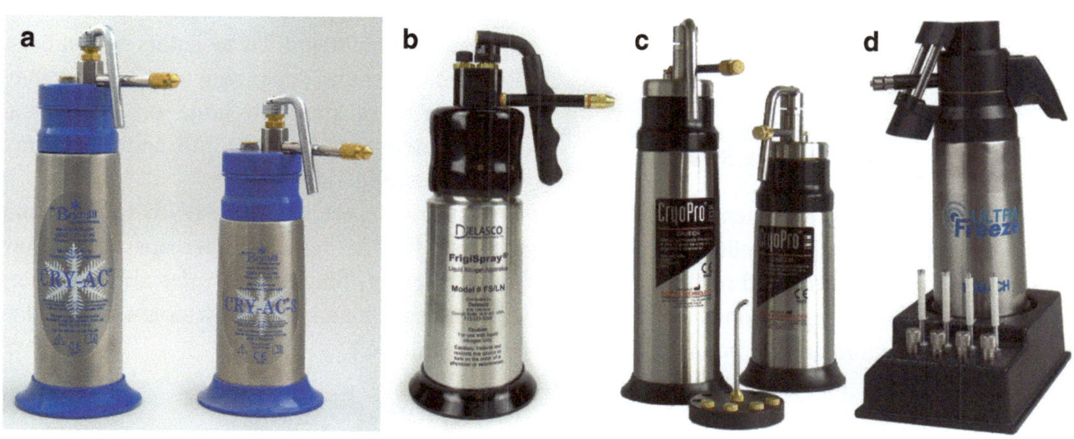

Fig. 4.7 (**a–d**) Cryosurgical units. (**a**) Brymill's Cry-Ac (500 cc capacity) and Cry-Ac 3 (300 cc) (Courtesy of Brymill Cryogenic Systems); (**b**) Delasco's FrigiSpray (350 cc) (Courtesy of Delasco); (**c**) Cortex's CryoPro (500 and 350 cc) (Courtesy of CortexTechnology, Denmark); (**d**) Wallach's UltraFreeze (350 cc; also available in 500 cc) (Courtesy of Cooper Surgical, Inc.)

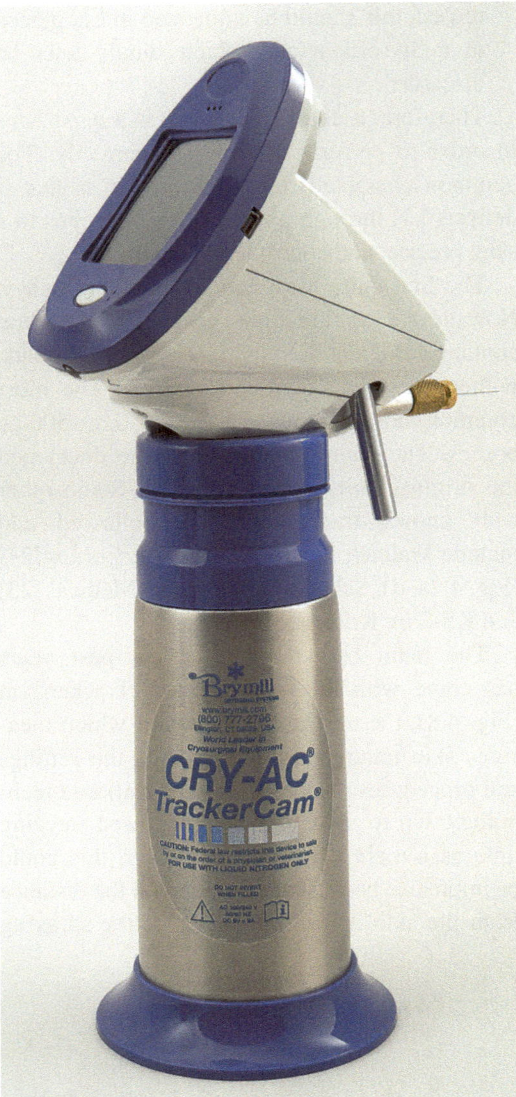

Fig. 4.8 The Cry-Ac® TrackerCam (Brymill) which measures skin temperature and records the settings and procedure (Courtesy of Brymill Cryogenic Systems)

tip, among other issues. Experience was determinant in assuring a correct procedure.

Temperature measuring and recording can be justified for the following reasons:

- It allows for a more precise freezing. One will freeze just until the desired temperature is reached: −10 to −20 °C for benign lesions and −50 °C for malignant lesions.
- It allows standardization of procedures.
- Help in training inexperienced cryosurgeons. For most benign lesions, an experienced cryosurgeon will probably not need to measure surface temperature. However, inexperienced cryosurgeons or doctors in training can certainly benefit from this information.
- By previously setting the temperatures parameters, the cryosurgeon will avoid over or under freezing.
- It allows you to keep a record of the procedure for the patient's chart and for future reference.

Freezing of the skin will turn it white; however, freezing time, distance from the skin, size of the spraying tip, anatomical area, and underlying vascularization are variables that can result in −10, −20, or −25 ° C temperature differences in local freezing. Whiteness of the skin should not then be the sole feature to determine correct freezing.

In the subsequent chapters, the advantages of measuring temperature will be discussed.

4.4 Attachments for Cryosurgical Units

4.4.1 Spraying Tips or Apertures

The spraying tips are probably the most commonly used attachments in cryosurgery. They are tips (mostly built in brass) with openings of different diameters that allow LN release from the unit. Some have a flat surface, and some are conical.

Depending on the manufacturer, the different tip apertures are identified by letters or numbers. Be careful because, depending on the brand, they can start from small to large or vice versa. A comparison between Brymill and FrigiSpray tips is shown in Table 4.3.

For larger apertures, more LN is released and freezing will be faster. Larger apertures allow faster freezing. Smaller apertures allow a better control of the margins of the lesions (since LN is released slower).

4.4.1.1 Other Options

Luer Lock Adapter (LLA)

You can attach an LLA at the end of the release. (Some units, like Wallach's, already have it incorporated.) This allows you to use disposable

Table 4.3 Comparison between Brymill and FrigiSpray (Delasco) apertures

Brymill 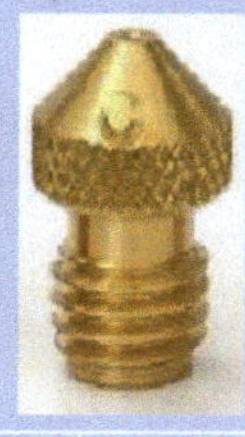		Delasco 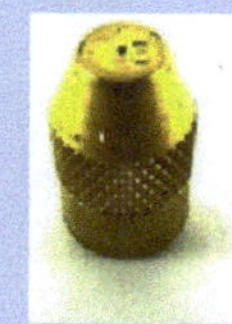		
Tip aperture		Tip aperture	Tip aperture	
A	.040 in. (1.0 mm)	1	Extra small	0.4 mm (0.016 in.)
B	0.031 in (0.79 mm)	2	Small	0.5 mm (0.020 in.)
C	0.022 in. (0.56 mm)	3	Medium	0.6 mm (0.024 in.)
D	0.016 in. (0.41 mm)	4	Large	0.8 mm (0.031 in.)
SuperSpray E	0.013 in. with back vent (0.33 mm)			

Images courtesy of Brymill Cryogenic Systems and Delasco

needles of different diameters, previously prepared for the purpose: make sure the cutting edges are sanded down in order to avoid accidental pinching of the patient. By using needles, the options of tip diameters will be extended. Long needles work as extensions, allowing for hidden areas to be reached, such as the external ear canal or inside the mouth.

Extensions

These are used to reach difficult to reach areas such as lesions in the ear canal or inside the mouth. Some are bendable.

The Advanced Acne Aperture (Brymill) (Fig. 4.9)

This is useful for peelings. It gives a soft, vaporized spray for superficial desquamation.

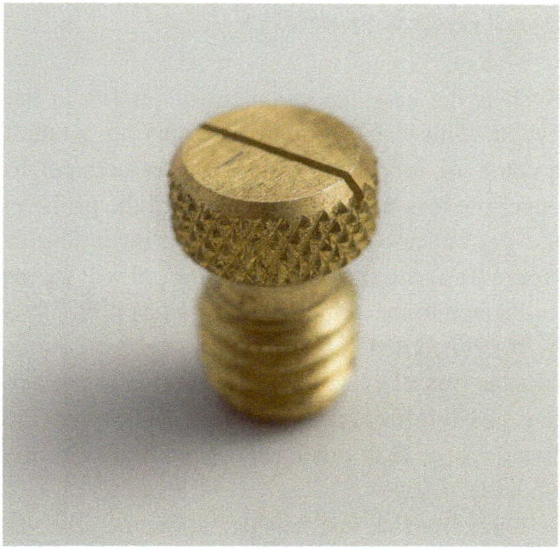

Fig. 4.9 Acne aperture spraying tip (Courtesy of Brymill Cryogenic Systems)

SuperSpray E (Brymill) (Fig. 4.10)

This is a tip that delivers a stronger, more concentrated and streamlined spray. It treats lesions faster and clogs less.

4.4.2 Probes

Probes are close LN circuits. They are built with metal (an excellent cold-conducting material), and once LN starts circulating, the outer metal gets frozen and stays at a constant temperature as long as the LN goes through it. If properly applied, the temperature of the skin lesion will drop very fast in a continuous manner and in a circumscribed place.

Some probes are Teflon-coated in order to reduce the risk of sticking to the surface. This outer cover makes them ideal for treating lesions in the mucosa. Another way to reduce the risk of getting stuck to the surface is by previously freezing the probe before applying to the skin.

One might want to fix the probe to the lesion before the start of freezing for better accuracy.

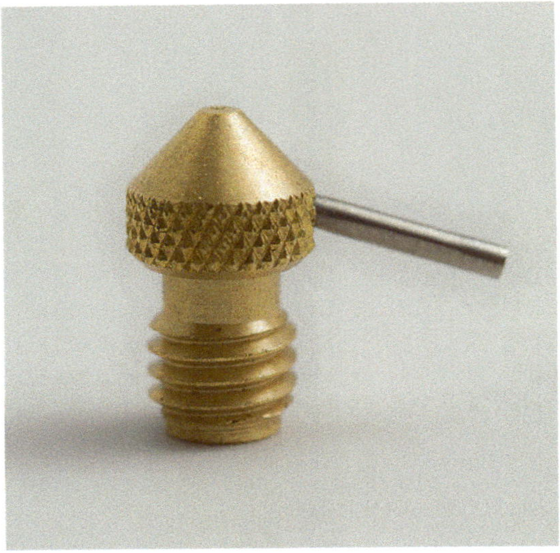

Fig. 4.10 SuperSpray E Tip with back vent (Courtesy of Brymill Cryogenic Systems)

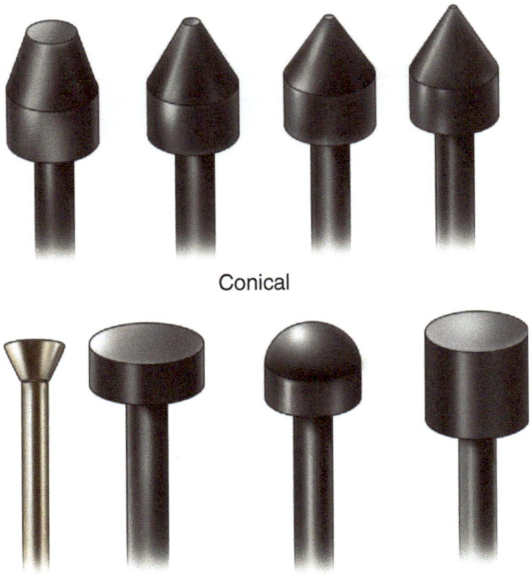

Fig. 4.11 Set of probes by Brymill, Delasco, Cortex, and Wallach

Such is the case for treatment of tumors in the eyelid. This can be done by applying a small amount of lubricant jelly or ultrasound gel to cover the lesion, touching the end of the probe to the gel but not the skin, and then beginning to freeze. In approximately 5–7 s, the gel will freeze and attach to the skin (cryo-adhesion) [25].

If concerned about underlying structures (nerves, vessels, tendons) and wanting to prevent any possible freezing, pull back slightly on the fixed probe, thus raising the skin, and continue freezing.

Once freezing has finished, allow the probe to thaw before trying to separate it from the skin/mucosa/gel. If the probe is stuck to the skin and one tries to force it off, the tissue may tear. The area has to thaw before the probe can be detached. To avoid excess freezing, pour warm water over it. A slight gentle twisting motion of the unit may expedite the release of the probe even when thawing is not complete.

Probes have to fit the lesion. They should be approximately of the same size. If such a probe is not available, then choose a smaller probe rather than a larger one. An oversized probe (larger than the lesion to be treated) will cover its margins and prevent visualization of the procedure. A much smaller one will cause excess freezing at the center before the freezing front reaches the margin. Instead, if the probe is just slightly smaller than the lesion, the outer margin of the lesion will be visible and the freezing front will be seen as it advances.

Probes come in various shapes and are commercially available through different manufacturers. The ideal situation is to have a set of different sizes and shapes (Fig. 4.11).

Probes have a silicone vent tube attached to the base from which LN is liberated once it has circulated through the conduit line. Care should be taken to point the hose away from anyone (patient, nurse, or even the operator) in order to avoid burns. Since LN comes out of a flexible hose, the initial released LN might cause a whiplash, a situation that can startle the patient. Holding the hose in the correct direction until frozen will maintain the position and avoid accidents. Once the tube freezes, it can be released. The tube will harden after approximately 5 s and remain in a predetermined fixed position.

Probes can also be custom made in order to satisfy various demands of cryosurgeons, as is the case with the half moon shape for the base of the mouth (Fig. 4.12), custom designed Teflon-coated tweezers for vascular lesions that need to

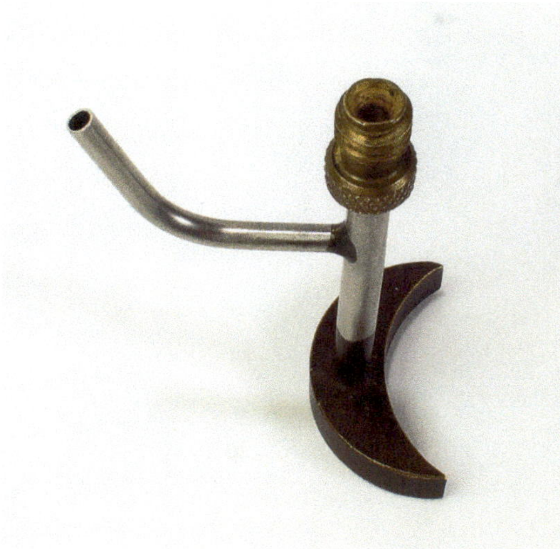

Fig. 4.12 Custom-made half moon probe for vascular lesion under the tongue

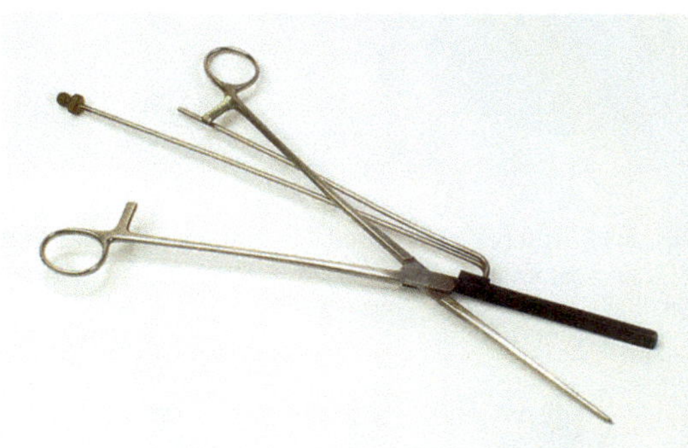

Fig. 4.13 Custom-made Teflon-coated tweezers for vascular lesions, placed in the posterior part of the tongue (custom made)

be "grasped" when placed in difficult to reach areas (like the base of the tongue) (Fig. 4.13), and the knob probe for "ironing" the surface of hypertrophic capillary malformations to reduce thickness (Fig. 4.14).

Depending on the type of procedure, probes will need to be cleaned and sometimes sterilized. For low-risk procedures (probes in contact with bloodless areas or with ultrasound probe cover), cleaning is sufficient. No immersion is necessary. Wipe with alcohol and properly dry with an absorbent cloth.

For intermediate- and high-risk procedures (contact to curettage lesion, blood, breaks in the skin, mucous membranes, genital and anal regions), clean the probe and then sterilize it. Remove the silicone vent tube before sterilization.

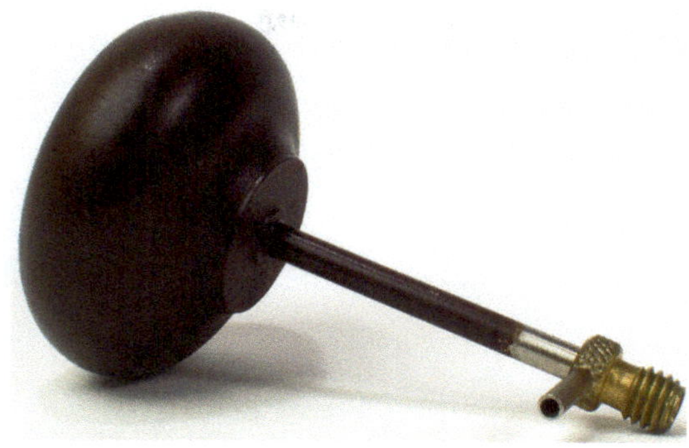

Fig. 4.14 Custom-made door knob probe for flattening hypertrophic capillary malformations

In immunocompromised patients, sterilize the probe before and after the procedure.

Remember to replace the silicone vent tube prior to use.

If one wants to avoid contact with the skin (as in a Kaposi's sarcoma lesion), cover the probe with a latex or rubber protector (ultrasound transducer cover, vaginal probe cover, latex finger cover, finger glove, or simply cut off one "finger" out of a medical glove).

4.4.3 Chambers

Chambers are cylinders totally open at the distal end (the part that will touch the skin) and closed at the proximal end, with the exception of the opening through which LN will flow from the unit. The border of the cylinder that will be in touch with the skin is covered with a rubber band to prevent damaging and sticking to the skin.

This semi closed system confines LN and allows for a potent and precise freezing. They come in different sizes: 6, 10, 15, 18, and 31 mm (Fig. 4.15).

Chambers also have a silicone vent tube attached to the base as in probes. The tube will harden after approximately 5 s and remain in a predetermined fixed position. This position is determined by the operator. By doing so, the tube is pointed away from the patient, assistant, or user at the onset of the procedure.

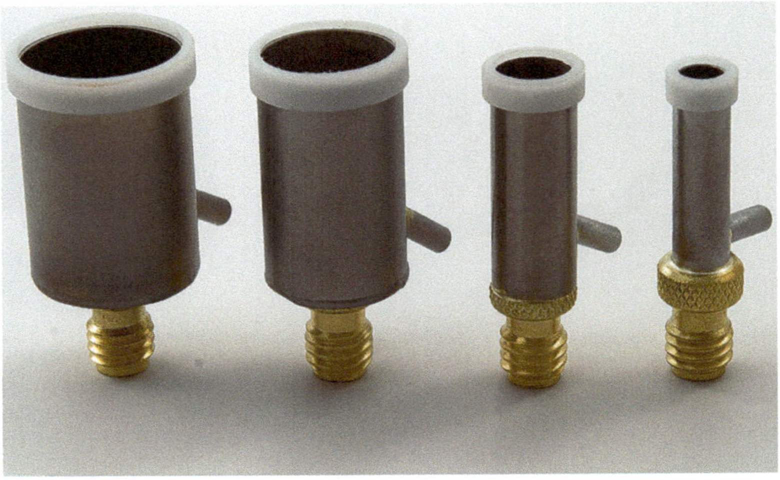

Fig. 4.15 Set of chambers

4.5 Rubber Cones, Lexan Plates, and Otoscope Disposable Specula Tips

In order to restrain sprayed LN, cones can be fitted to the lesion. They have to be made either of plastic, neoprene, or rubber. They cannot be made of metal; otherwise they will freeze as well (due to the high conductivity of metal) and damage the healthy skin.

The use of these "restrainers" allows a more precise and localized freezing, limiting the sprayed LN just to the selected area and reducing spattering, a common cause of local discomfort; it also spares the perilesional healthy skin. Furthermore, freezing is more potent because LN remains in one spot instead of vaporing on the sides, concentrating all the cold in the limited area. Limiting the LN allows selective tissue destruction.

There are sets of neoprene cones commercially available that come in 6, 11, 16, 25, 30, and 38 mm (Fig. 4.16). There are also transparent Lexan plates with conical openings (4, 7, 9, and 12 mm). Otoscope disposable specula tips, which come in different diameters, work also very well for this purpose (Fig. 4.17).

Essentially, these attachments have to be made of nonconductant material, and the edge applied to the skin should not be sharp. Never use metal, and never use blunt edges.

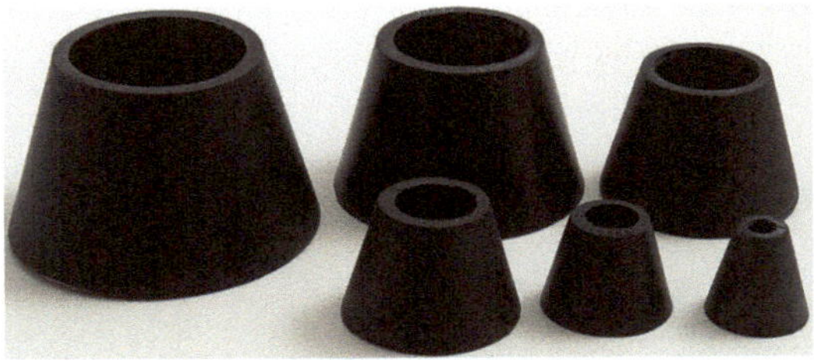

Fig. 4.16 Rubber cones used for limiting spraying to a defined anatomical area

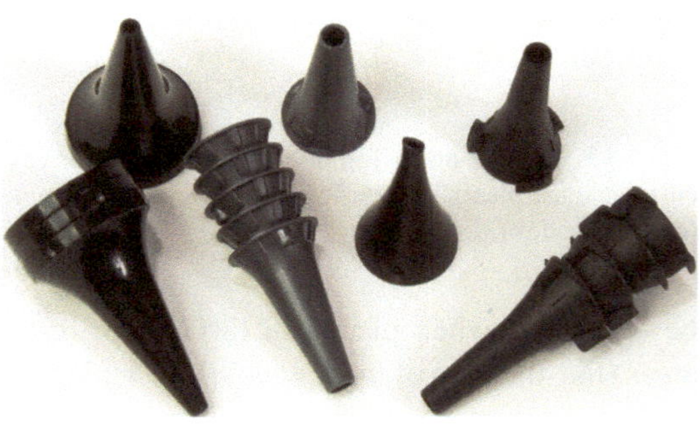

Fig. 4.17 Otoscope tips used for limiting spray to a defined anatomical area (Courtesy of Brymill Cryogenic Systems)

4.6 Tweezers

Teflon-coated tweezers (Fig. 4.18) are used to grab lesions. They allow treatment of small- and medium-sized protruding tumors. They are meant to be dipped in a styrofoam cup filled with LN

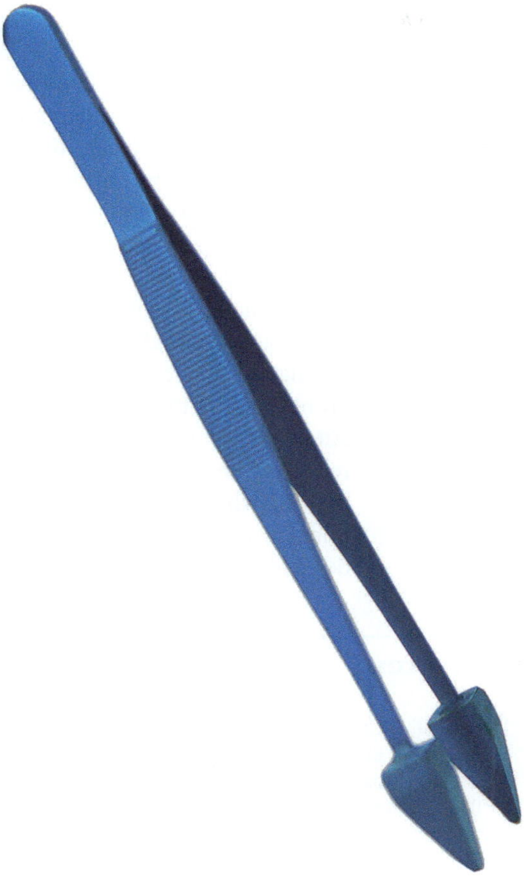

Fig. 4.18 Teflon-coated tweezers (Courtesy of Brymill Cryogenic Systems)

and left immersed for around 30 s until LN stops boiling. Lesions are then grasped, and the freezing front is allowed to advance just to the base of the lesion.

4.7 Other Equipment

There is equipment that is not specific to cryosurgery but indispensable. Since cryosurgery is a surgical procedure, one needs to have minor surgical equipment such as sterile gloves, syringes, local anesthesia, gauze, disinfectants, sutures, biopsy jars, curettes, and hemostatic solutions. One has to be ready for any situation: sticking the skin, stopping excess bleeding, curettaging, and so on.

Since cryosurgery has to be performed on bloodless skin, hemostatic solutions are frequently used, especially after curetting a lesion. If the chosen solution is trichloroacetic acid, keep in mind that it will leave a white spot. Care should be taken not to confuse it with the freezing front.

Keep a record of all your procedures. Part of this record includes an excellent picture of the lesion one plans to treat and a postoperative control picture. This is the best way to remember what has been done. A good before and after sequence will become the best teacher; it will also help in teaching others, and it allows both patient and operator to remember what was done. Believe it or not, the operator's memory is short and so is the patient's.

No freezing should ever be done unless there is certainty of the nature of the tumor. If in doubt, a biopsy is mandatory. Wait for the results before freezing a tumor of uncertain nature. With surgery, there is no place for rushing: things should be done correctly from the beginning. Do not freeze a pigmented lesion without previously confirming its diagnosis. Freezing a melanoma thinking that it is a seborrheic keratosis can be a fatal error no one should ever make.

This is why dermoscopy has become an indispensable tool for surgeons. Since many consultations have to do with benign lesions (solar lentigos, SK, warts, skin tags, etc.), a dermoscopic confirmation of benignity reassures the surgeon and allows correct decision making.

For tumors, it is important to know the depth of the lesion, and a high-frequency ultrasound is becoming indispensable for such purpose (Chap. 13). HFUS with Doppler will help identify the presence of a large feeding vessel. The presence of medium or large vessels is a common cause of recurrence of vascular tumors. If a nest of small vessels is destroyed using cryosurgery but a medium feeding vessel is left untouched, the tumor will recur.

When working with large vascular tumors, nuclear magnetic resonance with contrast is indispensable to visualize the extent of the tumor and the feeding vessels.

Confocal microcopy can be crucial to determine with certainty a diagnosis before freezing, especially if in doubt. It is particularly useful in pigmented lesions.

Essential Tidbits

- Standard equipment includes a Dewar and a handheld unit with different apertures and probes. It is essential to have a reliable LN delivery system.
- Maintenance is minimal, a trifle compared to other procedural alternatives.
- Rubber cones, Lexan disk, otoscope tips, extensions for apertures, and a reliable, simple LN delivery system are essential.
- The larger your toolbox, the better. The more probes, apertures, and attachments available, the more possibilities you will have to treat diverse conditions.

Conclusions

Cryosurgery requires a whole set of equipment, most of which is specific to this technique. Many manufacturers have products available, and one can find a vast selection of attachments to suit most needs.

Remember that cryosurgery is a surgical procedure: it is cryosurgery and not cryotherapy. Therefore, all precautions need to be taken.

Never freeze a lesion without being certain of the diagnosis, and keep a record of the whole procedure, starting with the consent form, clinical pictures, and a detailed description of the procedure including technique and temperature.

As in other surgical specialties, cryosurgery has improved its outcomes by actively incorporating diagnostic tools and procedures such as dermoscopy, high-frequency ultrasound, confocal microscopy, and optical coherence tomography, among others.

Glossary

Dewar Vacuum flask

Luer Lock A standardized system used for making leak-free connections between a male taper fitting (made in brass and screwed to the cryosurgical unit) and a mating female part (a disposable hypodermic syringe)

Probe Close conduit system made of metal and through which LN circulates. The end part of the probe contacts the skin

Spraying tip Attachment screwed at the releasing end of the cryosurgical unit through which LN is released through an orifice of a determined size

References

1. Pasquali P. Cryosurgery. In: Robinson J et al., editors. Surgery of the skin: procedural dermatology. 2nd ed. London: Mosby-Elsevier; 2010.
2. "Dewar, James." Complete dictionary of scientific biography. 2008. Encyclopedia.com. Weblog. [Online]. Available from: http://www.encyclopedia.com/topic/James_Dewar.aspx. [Accessed 4th Dec 2013].
3. Cryogenic Society of America, Inc. 1984–2013. History of cryogenics April 2008. Weblog. [Online]. Available from: http://www.cryogenicsociety.org/resources/cryo_central/history_of_cryogenics/ [Accessed 4th Dec 2013].
4. MVE Biomedical. Aluminum specimen Dewars. 2013. Weblog. [Online]. Available from: http://www.chartbiomed.com/Cryopreservation_Products/Aluminum_Specimen_Dewars.aspx. [Accessed 4th Dec 2013].
5. Peksayar G, Altan-Yaycioglu R, Onal S. Excision and cryosurgery in the treatment of conjunctival malignant epithelial tumours. Eye (Lond). 2003; 17(2):228–32.
6. Wang H, Zhang N, Tao M, Li D, Zhou Y, Zou H, Liang S, Li J. Application of interventional bronchoscopic therapy in eight pediatric patients with malignant airway tumors. Tumori. 2012;98(5):581–7. doi:10.1700/1190.13198.
7. Mariategui J, Santos C, Taxa L, Jeronimo J, Castle PE. Comparison of depth of necrosis achieved by CO_2- and N_2O-cryotherapy. Int J Gynaecol Obstet. 2008;100(1):24–6.
8. Winkler JL, Jeronimo J, Singleton J, Janmohamed A, Santos C. Performance of cryotherapy devices using

nitrous oxide and carbon dioxide. Int J Gynaecol Obstet. 2010;111(1):73–7.
9. Theodorescu D. Cancer cryotherapy: evolution and biology. Rev Urol. 2004;6 Suppl 4:S9–S19.
10. Meller I, Weinbroum A, Bickels J, Dadia S, Nirkin A, Merimsky O, Issakov J, Flusser G, Marouani N, Cohen N, Kollender Y. Fifteen years of bone tumor cryosurgery: a single-center experience of 440 procedures and long-term follow-up. Eur J Surg Oncol. 2008;34(8):921–7. Epub 2007 Dec 26.
11. Robinson D, Halperin N, Nevo Z. Two freezing cycles ensure interface sterilization by cryosurgery during bone tumor resection. Cryobiology. 2001;43(1):4–10.
12. Wallach Surgical Devices. Cryosurgical systems. Weblog. [Online]. Available from http://www.wallachsurgical.com/Products/LLCO2?ApplicationId=4
13. Wallach Surgical Devices. Cryosurgical systems. Weblog. [Online]. Available from: http://www.wallachsurgical.com/Products/LL100-Cryosurgical-System?ApplicationId=4
14. Metrum CryoFlex. Cryo-S mini devices for dermatosurgery. Weblog. [Online]. Available from: http://www.metrum.com.pl/en/products/cryosurgery-devices/cryo-s-mini. [Accessed 4th Dec 2013].
15. Cryosuccess by Schuco. Weblog. [Online]. Available from: http://www.schuco.co.uk/cryosurgery/cryosuccess.html. [Accessed 4th Dec 2013].
16. CryOmega by Premier Medical. Weblog. [Online]. Available from: http://www.premusa.com/medical/dermatology.asp. [Accessed 4th June 2014].
17. MMR Tecnologies, Inc. Introducing the Elan2 liquid nitrogen generator. 2013. Weblog. [Online]. Available from: http://www.elan2.com/. [Accessed 4th Dec 2013].
18. Brymill Cryogenics Systems. Introducing the new Brymill Cry-Ac® TrackerCam™. 9 octubre 2013. Weblog. [Online]. Available from: http://www.brymill.com/. [Accessed 4th Dec 2013].
19. UltraFreeze Liquid Nitrogen Cryosurgical Sprayer. Weblog. [Online]. Available from: http://www.wallachsurgical.com/Products/UltraFreeze-Liquid-Nitrogen-Cryosurgical-Sprayer?ApplicationId=4. [Accessed 4th Dec 2013].
20. Delasco. Dermatology Labs&Supply Inc. 1995–2013. Cryosurgery. Weblog. [Online] Available from: http://www.delasco.com/pcat/1/Cryosurgery/. [Accessed 4th Dec 2013].
21. Cortex Technology. CryoPro® Cryosurgical equipment. Weblog. [Online]. Available from: http://www.cortex.dk/cryosurgical-equipment.html. [Accessed 4th Dec 2013].
22. Schuco cryospray 350 ml sch-cry-350. Weblog. [Online] Available from: http://www.schuco.co.uk/cryosurgery/schuco-cryospray-350ml.html. [Accessed 4th Dec 2013].
23. Nitrospray Plus. Weblog. [Online]. Available from: http://www.premusa.com/medical/dermatology.asp. [Accessed 4th Dec 2013].
24. K2-Device. Weblog. [Online]. Available from: http://www.kriosystem.com.pl/en/offer/cryosurgery.html. [Accessed 4th Dec 2013].
25. Colver GB, Jackson A, Dawber RPR. Cutaneous cryosurgery: principles and clinical practice. London: CRC Press, Taylor & Francis Group; 2005.

5 Cryosurgical Techniques

Paola Pasquali

Contents

Key Points

- There are six common cryosurgical techniques: open, semi-open, close, semi-close, tweezers, and intralesional.
- Each one uses different equipment. Each technique tends to be used for different types of lesions (open technique in benign, close technique in malignant), but there are special uses that will improve the cryosurgical outcome.

5.1 Introduction

Once the correct equipment is available, mastering certain techniques is the focus. For each technique, there is specific equipment, and there are some common indications. First, one has to feel confident and master the common techniques; after this occurs, one can begin to apply techniques in nonconventional manners.

For the sake of clarity, techniques have been named as follows:

1. Open or spraying technique
2. Semi-open technique
3. Close or probe technique
4. Semi-close or chamber technique
5. Tweezers technique
6. Intralesional technique

P. Pasquali, MD
Department of Dermatology, Pius Hospital de Valls, 43800 Tarragona, Spain
e-mail: pasqualipaola@gmail.com

P. Pasquali (ed.), *Cryosurgery: A Practical Manual*,
DOI 10.1007/978-3-662-43939-5_5, © Springer-Verlag Berlin Heidelberg 2015

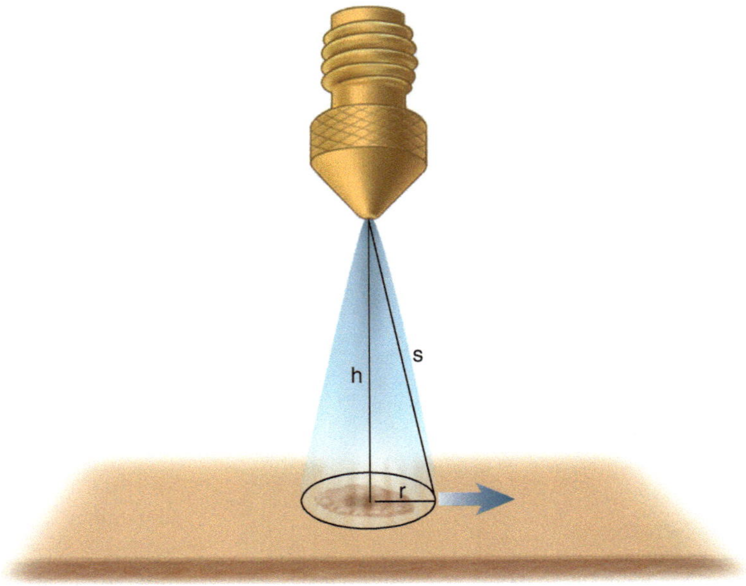

Fig. 5.1 Sprayed LN exits, forming a conical pattern. This cone will have a height (*h*) which corresponds to the distance from the tip opening to the skin, a radius (*r*) which is the distance from the center of the freezing area towards the periphery, and a side length (*s*)

5.2 Common Cryosurgical Techniques [1]

5.2.1 Open or Spray Technique

This is probably the most utilized cryosurgical technique. The cryogen (LN) is sprayed out from the unit through nozzles (tips or terminals) of different apertures (Chap. 4) directly on the skin surface [1].

As LN exits through a standard aperture, it forms a conical pattern and cools upon expansion (Joule-Thomson process). With the unit kept perpendicular to the skin, this cone will cool in a uniform manner and have a height (*h*) which corresponds to the distance of the nozzle opening to the skin, a radius (*r*) which is the distance from the center of the freezing area towards the periphery, and a side length (*s*) (Fig. 5.1).

Once LN reaches the skin surface, the freezing front advances horizontally on the skin surface as well as vertically (in depth) following an isotherm pattern (Fig. 5.2). Isotherms are temperature zones of equal temperature; the isotherm pattern in skin freezing will have a center where the temperature is the lowest, and the temperature at the periphery where it will be the highest.

There are three important points to keep in mind when using the spray technique:

1. *Tip diameter.* The amount of released LN will depend on the diameter of the tip opening. Larger openings release more LN. Choose small openings for delicate, superficial freezing and whenever you need to be sure to freeze a small and well-defined lesion (like a lentigo). Large openings are used to freeze large tumoral masses or extended large lesions. A small opening will result in a slower freezing. It will take longer to freeze a lesion (Fig. 5.3).
2. *Distance.* The distance between the releasing tip and the lesion is very important. Since air is a bad conductor, the farther away you spray, the less freezing you will achieve. Furthermore, the spray angle is not constant for larger h (distance to the skin). Since spray coverage will depend on the spray angle, the distance has to be maintained constant. Keep this in mind and always work at the same distance from the subject (Fig. 5.4).
3. *Inclination.* The cone of LN released from a unit parallel to the skin will be spherical. Instead, if the unit is not kept parallel to the skin, it will be an oblique cone. A tilted spraying will result in an irregular freezing: the side closer to the skin will have a lower temperature

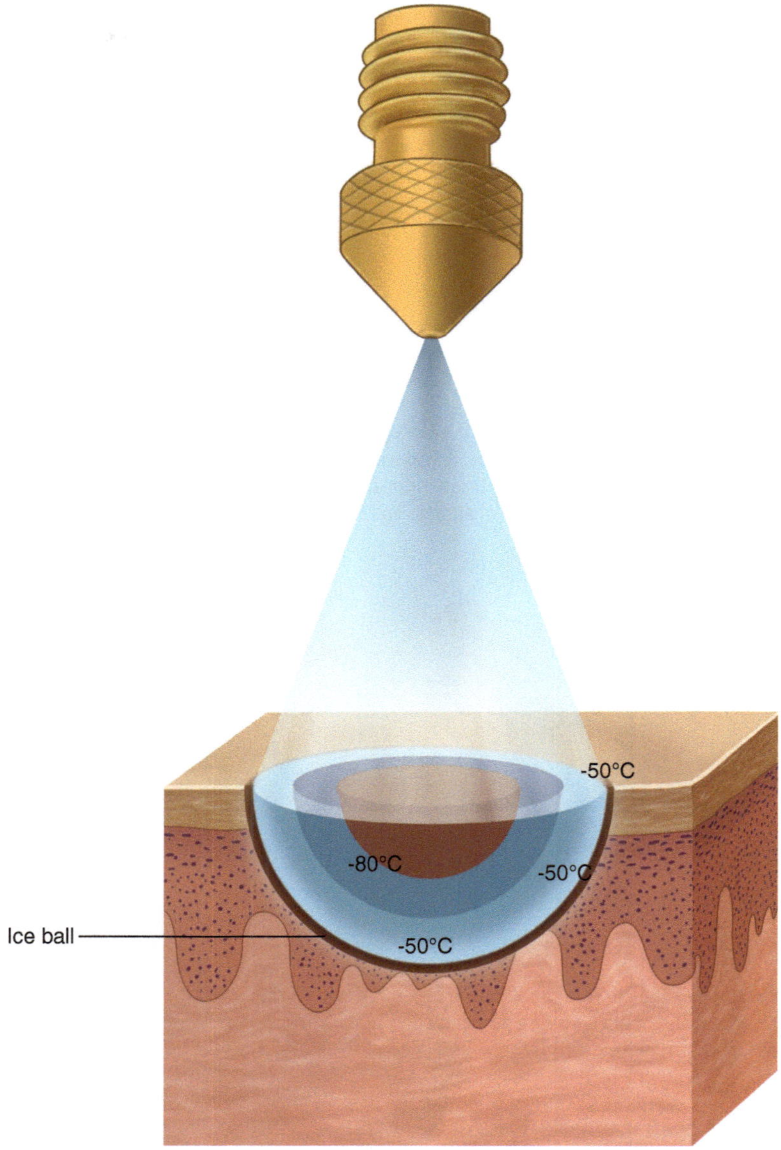

Fig. 5.2 Superficial freezing front extends radially. In depth, it does so in approximately a half sphere with concentric isothermal rings

and therefore experience larger destruction, while the other end will have a higher temperature (less destruction) (Fig. 5.5).

As LN hits the skin and freezing begins, the skin turns white. With pendular movements (Fig. 5.6), whiteness appears in every area the LN has reached, giving a false freezing front. Pendular movements are used for very superficial freezing, as is the case in cryopeelings. It is a good idea to delineate in advance with a marker the lesion and the margins because freezing (ice whiteness and the edema) can blur the margins.

For spray freezing where one needs to guarantee a regular freezing front, it is necessary to maintain a stable freezing at the center and allow it to expand towards the periphery. Maintain the same distance and the same position. This technique has also been called the time spot freeze [2].

Having more than one nozzle helps adjust to different needs. For instance, there is a spray nozzle called advance acne aperture (Brymill®). It produces a spray pattern which appears flat and elongated. It is used for acne lesions, and it is particularly useful for cryopeelings.

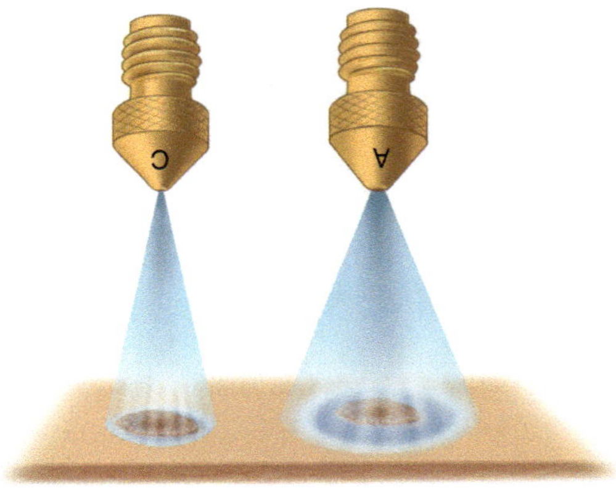

Fig. 5.3 Diameter of aperture. For nozzles placed at the same distance, perpendicular to the skin and different apertures, the larger aperture will release more LN. Freezing will be faster, larger in superficial surface and deeper

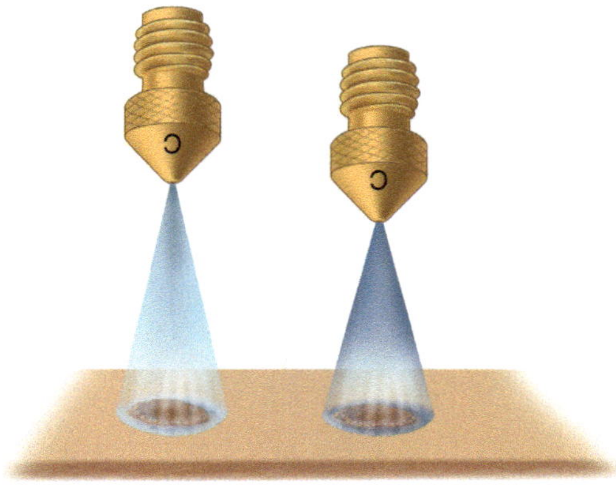

Fig. 5.4 Distance from the skin. For two nozzles with the same aperture, both spraying perpendicular to the surface, the more distant one will freeze less

The open technique is ideal in:

- Superficial flat lesions, like lentigos solaris
- Dome-shaped or thick lesions, such as seborrheic keratosis or small keloids
- Superficial freezing for cryobiopsy (Chap. 7)
- Irregular tumoral masses where the irregularity of the surface would not enable probe use

The open technique should be avoided in:

- Protruding skin lesions (like skin tags). Freezing elongated lesions with the open technique will cause an unnecessary rim of healthy skin to freeze, with a resulting hypo- or hyperpigmented spot.
- In orifices (nose, mouth).
- In vascular lesions unless you freeze in an intermittent manner and allow the freezing

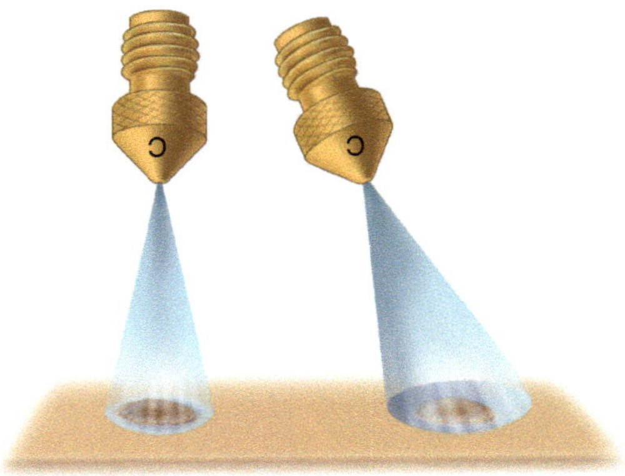

Fig. 5.5 For two nozzles that share the same size of aperture and distance but different positions (one perpendicular to the skin surface and the other tilted), freezing of the tilted spray will cause irregular freezing (colder in the area close to the opening and warmer at the distal extreme)

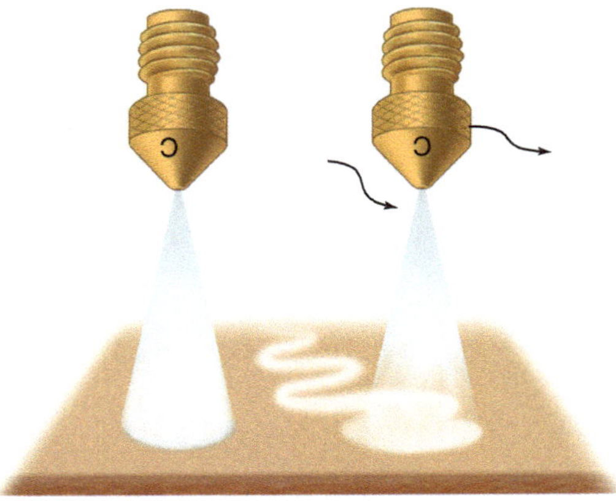

Fig. 5.6 Spraying turns the surface skin white. By freezing without moving the unit, freezing will spread from the center outward. With swinging or brush movements, the skin turns white but for a shorter period since freezing is very superficial

front to advance slowly until it reaches the bottom (see the discussion of the pyogenic granuloma technique in Chap. 12).

5.2.1.1 Advantages

- It tends to be quicker and less laborious than other techniques.
- It is especially convenient in multiple lesions, such as seborrheic keratosis.
- Since there is no contact, there is no risk of sticking on the surface and over-freezing. Once the spraying stops, thawing begins.
- It is ideal when treating irregular bulky tumors that cannot be curetted.

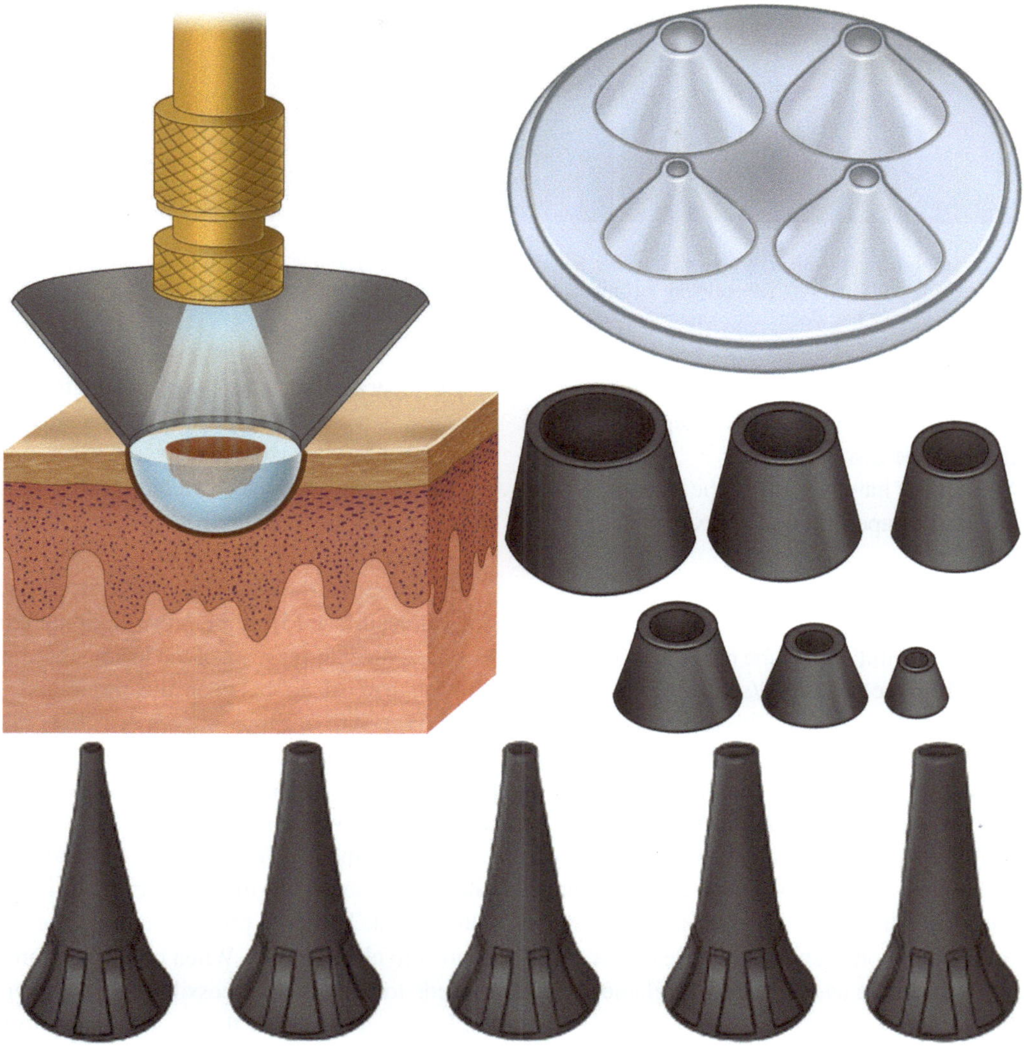

Fig. 5.7 Sprayed LN can be confined with lexan plastic plates, rubber cones, or otoscopes

- Since there is no contact, it is the safest technique. There is no contact with blood or other secretions.

5.2.1.2 Disadvantages

- Swinging the unit as you freeze can cause false freezing fronts and yield the wrong impression of having frozen the whole lesion at the expected temperature.
- Distance and tilting is operator dependent and will change the outcome of a procedure.
- Its initial impact on the skin, once freezing starts, can startle the patient.
- Peri lesional LN spattering is possible which might cause discomfort.

5.2.2 Semi-open Technique

It is as a variation of the spraying technique [3] in which the released spray is constrained into one area. The limits are set by a rubber cone, the opening on a lexan plate, or an otoscope disposable specula tip (Fig. 5.7). Metal cones should never be used because they are excellent conductors of cold and they will get stuck to the surface, causing addition destruction.

Concentrating LN in a limited area will cause faster and deeper freezing.

The opening of the attachment has to fit the lesion. If it is too large, you will be freezing unnecessary healthy skin. If it is too small, the entire lesion will not be included.

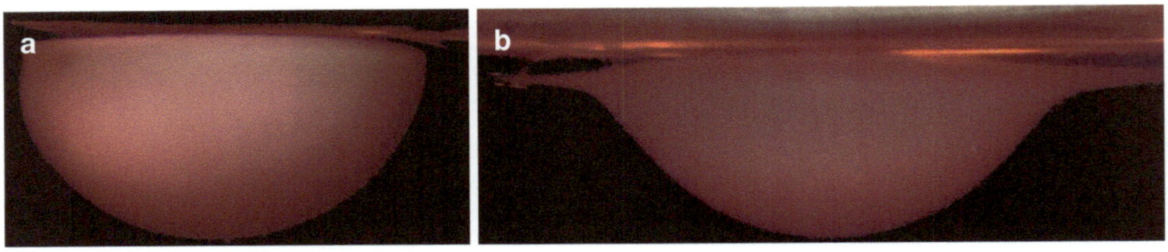

Fig. 5.8 (**a**) Freezing with a probe will cause a half sphere freezing ball. (**b**) With the spraying technique, the shape is more like a hat: deep in the center and thinner at the periphery. The final depth in probe freezing is deeper (4×2) than in spray freezing (4×1.5)

It is the ideal for:

- Small warts or molluscum contagiosum

It should be disregarded if:

- You do not have a cone of the correct size or the cone or aperture on the lexan plate.

5.2.2.1 Advantages

- Freezing is faster.

It is less painful. Part of the pain sensation might be caused by the splashing (spattering) of the LN drops over the healthy skin. This problem is reduced by having the lesion restrained within the cone. Part of the pain is also believed to be due to sputtering caused by LN "boiling" from liquid to gas [3].

- Children are distracted by the presence of the lexan plate or specula. They seem to tolerate the procedure better. It sometimes gets stuck for a few seconds and that amuses them.
- Costrainers are usually easily available.

5.2.2.2 Disadvantages

- Need to have the proper constrainer that adjust to the size of the lesion.
- It is limited in use to lesions of up to 6–8 mm.
- There is no visibility of the superficial freezing front.

5.2.3 Close or Probe Technique

This technique is performed by using probes, which are closed-circuit systems into which LN travels from the unit and finally exits through a rubber hose [4].

They are built with metal and some are Teflon-coated to reduce the risk of sticking to the surface of the lesion. Freezing is constant, not dependent on the operator because they contact the skin. Distance is not an issue because it is also a constant given by the size of the probe. Since metal is an excellent conductor of cold, probes freeze very fast, and the freezing front is deeper than the one obtained by spray freezing (Fig. 5.8a, b).

A requirement when using probes is to have a flat lesion surface [5]. If the probe does not completely contact the surface of the lesion, there will be "pockets" of air between the probe and the lesion. The sum of theses spaces is called "interphase," and these are air spaces. Since air is a poor conductor of cold, the larger the interphase, the less effective the freezing (Fig. 5.9).

Probes come in different forms and diameters. The ideal probe is one that best fits the lesion you plan to treat. The more probes available, the more options to choose from. When choosing a probe, it needs to fit as best as possible the diameter of the lesion. As a rule of thumb, it is better to use a slightly smaller probe than a larger one. The latter will not allow visualization of the freezing front and thus tend to over-freeze. If it is too small, the center of the lesion will be destroyed very deeply (more than needed) before the freezing front reaches the periphery (Fig. 5.10a–c).

Care should be taken when working in humid areas like the oral mucosa or previously curettaged tumors. Even Teflon-coated probes can get stuck to the surface. One trick is to previously freeze the probe. This will reduce the chances of it sticking to a wet surface. If in spite of the precautions the probe gets stuck to the surface, do not try to detach it. Avoid maneuvers aiming at forcing the probe off of the site. Pulling out the probe can cause breakage of the tissue, unnecessary damage, and profuse bleeding. Always allow thawing. To avoid

Fig. 5.9 Probes need to be applied to a flat surface. If the probe does not completely contact the surface of the lesion, air "pockets" between the probe and the lesion ("interphase") will raise the final freezing temperature

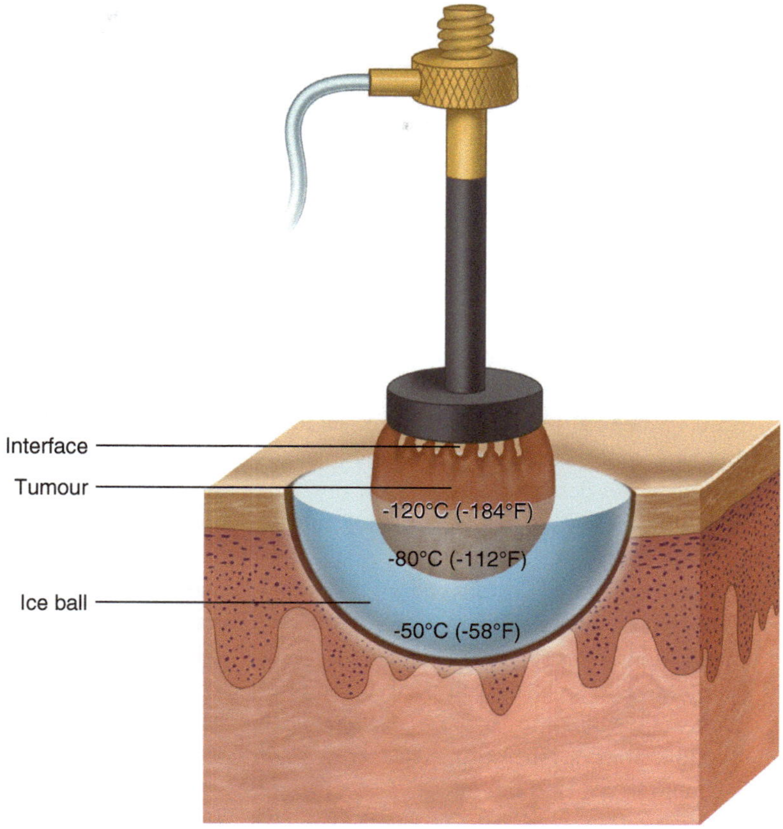

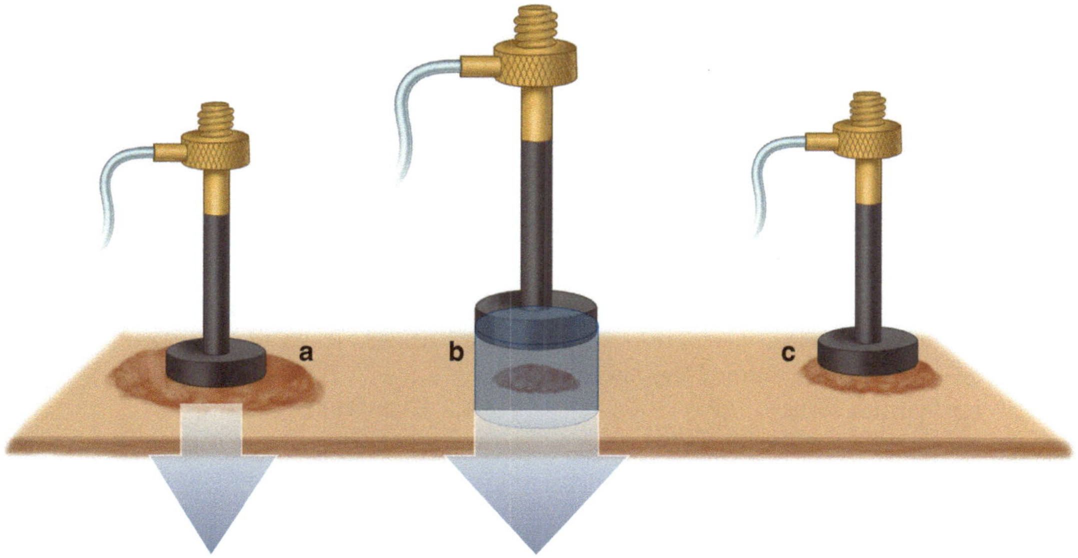

Fig. 5.10 (**a–c**) In relation to the lesion: A probe that is too small will freeze the center of the lesion in excess (**a**). If the probe is larger than the lesion (**b**), it will not allow visualization of the freezing front and there will be tissue destruction of perilesional normal skin. Therefore, if a probe of the exact size (**c**) is not available, it is better to use a slightly smaller one than a larger one

excess freezing, let some warm water run over it: As a precaution, always keep some warm water at hand when using a probe. By using this approach, the probe will immediately separate. On the other hand, if one wants the probe adhered to the surface (as for eyelid tumors) pre wetting or applying some ultrasound gel will do the job.

Care should also be taken with the releasing hose. Since LN comes out of the hose under pressure, one can inadvertently burn the patient, nurse, or even oneself. A free hose can whiplash and startle the patient.

Before freezing, the hose has a free end that moves back and forth. Grab it with your hands and set it in the desired position. In a few seconds, it will freeze (due to the continuous release of LN) and stay in place.

The probe technique is ideal for:

- Skin cancer. It is the ideal technique for skin destruction of deeply seated lesions.
- Vascular tumors, where you need to use pressure over the tumor to "squeeze" the blood out.
- Eyelid lesions or other lesions near orifices.

It should be avoided in:

- Irregular surface tumors where there will not be proper contact of the probe with the surface.
- Extra care should be taken in wet mucous areas. Water will form ice and keep the probe stuck for a longer period after releasing the unit trigger.

5.2.3.1 Advantages

- Fast and deep freezing
- Allows pressure over vascular lesion, emptying it of its warm content

5.2.3.2 Disadvantages

- It requires having a complete set of probes.
- Needs the correct surface.
- Risk of sticking to the surface and involuntarily breaking the surface.

5.2.4 Semi-close or Chamber Technique

Chambers are metal cones with a rubber safety ring at one end (in order to avoid cutting or damaging the skin) and a small aperture from which LN exits. These need to be firmly planted onto the skin in order to keep the liberated LN inside the cone. They have a blowoff (or release) hose to liberate LN just as in probes.

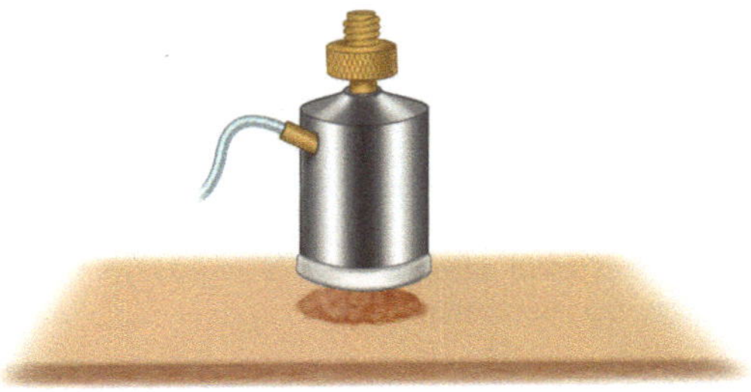

Fig. 5.11 Chambers are metal cones with a rubber safety ring at one end that needs to be firmly placed in order to keep LN inside the cone. They generate a very potent freezing

The turbulence generated inside the cone makes this freezing very potent, and it is usually reserved for skin cancer, particularly metastatic skin disease.

These come in different diameters and need to be matched as close as possible to the lesion (Fig. 5.11).

When first applied to the skin, LN pressure might kick back the whole unit. Start releasing very slowly until you get the feeling that it is held in place.

As with probes, care should be taken with the release hose in order to avoid accidental burns to the patient, nurse, or even oneself.

This technique is ideal for:

- Skin cancer [5]
- Skin metastasis

It should not be used in:

- Benign lesions

5.2.4.1 Advantages

- Potent, fast, and very deep freezing
- Less risk of sticking to the surface

5.2.4.2 Disadvantages

- It causes an extremely fast freezing, and there is a risk for over-freezing. Use only if experienced.

5.2.5 Tweezers Technique

Teflon-coated tweezers [6] are a very simple and useful means of treating filiform or protruding

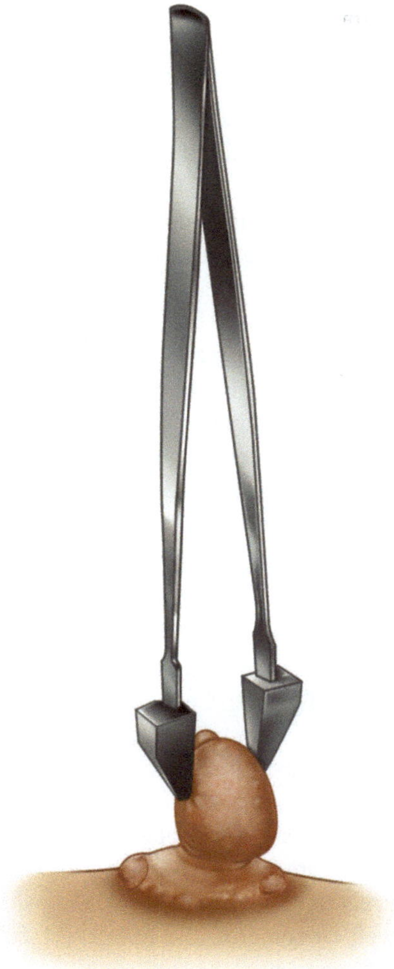

Fig. 5.12 Cryotweezers are ideal for protruding lesions where no deep freezing is required

small lesions (Fig. 5.12). They are commercially available through Brymill®, and the instructions for their use are in Table 5.1. Regular tweezers can also be used, but care should be taken that they are grabbed in the correct place to avoid accidental burns to the operator.

Basically, they are meant to be placed into a Styrofoam cup full of LN just to the narrow neck point. They are left there until LN stops bubbling.

They should be wiped with alcohol after each use.

This technique is ideal for:

- Protruding lesions such as skin tags or molluscum
- Cryobiopsy of a protruded lesion (Chap. 7)

It should be avoided in:

- Skin cancer
- Deeply seated lesions

5.2.5.1 Advantages

- No anesthesia is required.
- Fast and comfortable for the patient.
- Can treat many lesions at once.
- Low risk of hyper- or hypopigmentation.

5.2.5.2 Disadvantages

- Care should be taken not to burn one hand. This can happen when the tweezers are left for too long in the LN, or placed in a cup with excess LN, or grabbed too distally.

Table 5.1 Basic operating principles for tweezers

1. Decant a small quality of liquid nitrogen into the tweezer cup (Styrofoam cup)
2. Insert the tweezers into the liquid nitrogen only as far as the narrow neck point indicates. This point is located approximately ½″ (12 mm) behind the tweezer head
3. Keep the tweezer head immersed in liquid nitrogen until the rapid boiling has stopped. This may take approximately 30 s
4. Remove the cryotweezers from the liquid nitrogen and wait approximately 30 s until the tweezer heads turn frosty white
5. Carefully grasp the end of the skin tag between the tweezer heads
6. With the tweezer holding the skin tag, pull the tweezers away slightly to extend the skin tag
7. Continue holding the skin tag for 5–10 s or until the frosting has extended to the base of the skin tag
8. Release the skin tag and allow it to thaw
9. At the end of the procedure, simply allow any remaining liquid nitrogen in the tweezer cup to evaporate
Decontamination
Thorough cleaning and then disinfection of the cryotweezers and cup using an alcohol wipe prior to use is recommended between patient episodes

Recommended by Brymill®

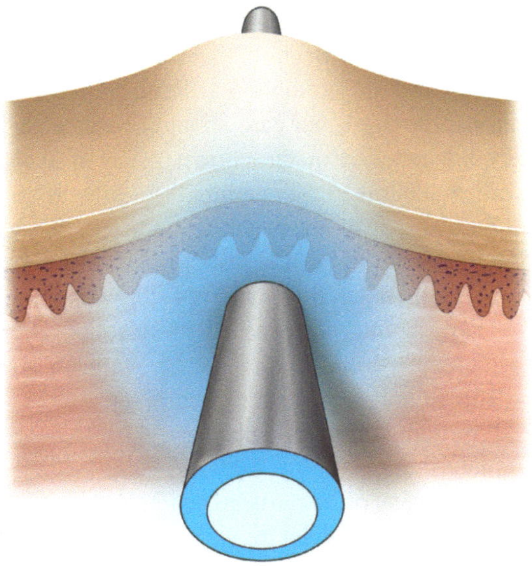

Fig. 5.13 In the intralesional technique, a thick needle is introduced into the mass in its longest axis. The needle needs to stick out from the other end of the tumor to liberate LN

5.2.6 Intralesional Technique [7]

The intralesional technique consists of passing a thick needle longitudinally through the center of a tumor. It has been mostly proposed for keloids but can also be used for skin metastasis or large malignant tumors. Keloids are deeply seated lesions with a large amount of fibrous tissue (bad conductor of cold). By treating them with the intralesional technique, one preserves the surface skin.

The needle needs to be attached to the unit through a Luer-Lock adapter and then introduced through the tumor by its longer axis until it reappears at the other end. Once the LN is allowed to go through the needle, freezing will occur from the center out (Fig. 5.13). For this technique, one can use regular needle or preferably Teflon-coated ones. There are disposable needles commercially available through Cryoshape® [8, 9] specially designed for keloid treatment.

It is a technique developed for keloids but can also be used for skin metastasis or large malignant deeply seated tumors. It should be avoided for superficial treatment or in vascular lesions.

5.2.6.1 Advantages

- When used in keloids, it spares the superficial skin.
- In deeply seated metastasis, it is an option of treatment although superficial skin sparing is not an issue.

5.2.6.2 Disadvantages

- Not simple to do. Requires experience.
- It is time consuming.
- Requires special equipment.
- With freezing, the needle can get stuck in the center of the lesion. Complete thawing is required before attempting to remove the needle.

Essential Tidbits

- Intermittent spraying allows for a more precise freezing. Continuous spraying is faster.
- Smaller apertures release less LN and are very useful for small lesions. Large apertures are best for large tumors.
- Probes are best used on surfaces with no irregularities (like crusts); also works well on compressible lesions (vascular, sebaceous hyperplasias).
- Prefrozen probes tend to stick less to the skin surface.
- Running some warm water helps detach stuck probes.

Conclusions

This chapter has presented the most common cryosurgical techniques. They have been summarized in Table 5.2. As one proceeds though the subsequent chapters, one can find nonconventional uses tailored to the patient's needs.

For the sake of clarity, the names of each technique as indicated in this chapter will be maintained throughout the subsequent chapters.

Table 5.2 Summary of the most common cryosurgical techniques

Technique	Equipment required	Recommended	Not recommended	Advantages	Disadvantages
Open or spray	Tips or apertures	Superficial lesions	Peduncular	Fast and less laborious; convenient in multiple lesions	Distance and inclination are operator dependent
	Needles adjusted to Luer-Lock	Dome shaped	Skin tags	No risk of contamination	
		Irregular surface	Orifices	No risk of sticking to the skin and over-freezing	
		Cryobiopsy	Vascular lesions		
Semi-open	Same as in spray + lexan plate or rubber cones or otoscope tips	Small dome shaped	Same as in open spray	Best in small lesions (under 6)	Requires restrainer of the appropriate size
				Fast freezing	
				Less painful	
				Children seem to tolerate it better	
Close or probe	Probes	Skin cancer	Irregular surface tumors	Fast and deep freezing	Requires availability of set of probes to adapt to lesion
		Vascular lesions		Empties content of vascular tumors when applied with pressure	Need to curettage if surface is irregular
		Eyelid lesions and other lesions close to orifices			Contact to surface
					Maintenance/cleaning of probes
					Risk of breaking tissue if incorrectly removed
Semi-close	Cryochambers	Skin cancer	Benign lesions	Potent, deep freezing	Requires availability of a set of chambers to adapt to lesion
		Metastasis		No need to curettage to adapt to surface irregularities	Contact to surface
					Maintenance/cleaning of probes
					Risk of breaking tissue if incorrectly removed
Tweezers	Cryotweezers	Peduncular	Flat lesions	Multiple lesions	Delicate and can be time consuming with multiple lesion treatment
	Teflon tweezers	Dome shaped (small lesions)	Skin cancer	Fast	
			Deeply seated lesions	Painless	
Intralesional	Specially adapted	Keloids	Vascular or vascularized tumors	Superficial skin sparing	Post op can be very prolonged
	Needles	Skin metastasis	Operator inexperience		
	Cryoshape™ probe				

References

1. Andrews MD. Cryosurgery for common skin conditions. Am Fam Physician. 2004;69(10):2365–72.
2. Zimmerman EE, Crawford P. Cutaneous cryosurgery. Am Fam Physician. 2012;86(12):1118–24.
3. Andrews MD. Letters to the editor. Adapter provides constant spray of liquid nitrogen. Am Fam Physician. 2005;72(4):573–4.
4. Zouboulis C. Principles of cutaneous cryosurgery. An update. Dermatology. 1999;198(2):111–7.
5. Gage AA. Cryosurgery of advanced tumors. Clin Dermatol. 1990;8(1):86–95.
6. Delasco Dermatology Lab & Supply Inc 1995–2013. Brymill Cryo Tweezers. Weblog. [Online]. Available from: https://www.delasco.com/pcat/1/Cryosurgery/BCT/BCT/. Accessed 4 Dec 2013.
7. Goldenberg G, AJ Luber AJ. Use of Intralesional Cryosurgery as an Innovative Therapy for Keloid Scars and a Review of Current Treatments. J Clin Aesthet Dermatol. Jul 2013;6(7):23–26.
8. Har-Shai Y, Amar M, Sabo E. Intralesional cryotherapy for enhancing the involution of hypertrophic scars and keloids. Plast Reconstr Surg. 2003;111(6):1841–52.
9. Cryoshape™. Weblog. [Online]. Available from: http://cryoshape.com/patients/. Accessed 4 Dec 2013.

Preoperative Care for Cryosurgery

6

Paola Pasquali

Contents

Key Points

- Cryosurgery requires minimal previous preparation.
- Some preoperative procedures are common to all surgical procedures, such as having the patient complete a consent form, obtaining correct diagnosis before surgery, and choosing the best technique that suits the patient's needs.
- A careful explanation of the procedure and the expected results as well as the time required to obtain such results is mandatory. Many patients are not familiar with cryosurgery and will need to be given thorough explanations.

6.1 Introduction

Many common benign and malignant lesions are amenable to be treated with cryosurgery. As in any other type of intervention, patients need to receive a thorough explanation on the procedure and give their consent. Once decided that a lesion can be treated with cryosurgery, explain to the patient all the treatment options as well as the expected secondary effects, the possible complications, the postoperative care, and the time expected for final healing. Questions about pain are frequent. Let the patient know what to expect in order to reduce anxiety. Cryosurgery tends to be a quick procedure with a long postoperative

P. Pasquali, MD
Department of Dermatology, Pius Hospital de Valls, 43800 Tarragona, Spain
e-mail: pasqualipaola@gmail.com

P. Pasquali (ed.), *Cryosurgery: A Practical Manual*,
DOI 10.1007/978-3-662-43939-5_6, © Springer-Verlag Berlin Heidelberg 2015

period. The more explanations are given to patients on all the possible side effects, the better the compliance.

While some cryosurgical procedures can be performed without any previous preparation, in some cases better results can be obtained if the patient follows some simple instructions prior to the procedure.

The first questions must be asked by the physician himself/herself. Then, the physician will need to attend to queries from the patient or his/her family.

6.2 Doctor's Queries

1. *Has the correct diagnosis been made?*

   Before attempting to freeze a lesion, be completely sure of the diagnosis. If in doubt, it becomes mandatory to biopsy. Never freeze if not completely certain what is about to be eliminated by the cold.
2. *Is the patient's type of lesion amenable to cryosurgical treatment?*

   Once a diagnosis is made, one should stop and consider all of the options available for the removal of a lesion. For instance, pigmented lesions are very sensitive to cold. A lentigo solaris responds very well, while melasma treated with cryosurgery can be a disaster. It is therefore important to know where to freeze and where not to freeze.
3. *Is the patient's skin type adequate to ensure the expected result?*

   Skin types I and II tend to have excellent cosmetic results with cryosurgery. In darker skin types, one can expect hyperpigmentation with light freezing or hypopigmentation with deep freezing. If one is doing a cosmetic procedure on someone having darker skin, it is recommended to treat a small lesion in a not visible area and observe the results before attempting to do all the lesions at once.
4. *Location, location, location.*

   Even when a lesion can be treated with cryosurgery, its anatomical location will help decide whether one surgical technique should be used over another. For instance, doing cryosurgery on a nodular basal cell carcinoma (BCC) on the earlobe or on the eyelids will give an excellent cosmetic result, while a BCC on the leg will take forever to heal and leave an anesthetic scar.
5. *Is there one lesion or are there several lesions?*

   If the patient has a single, small, actinic keratosis, probably cryosurgery is the faster and cheaper curative treatment. The same is true for single or multiple seborrheic keratoses. Instead, a patient with numerous warts might benefit from a previous treatment before attempting to freeze many lesions.
6. *Will the patient benefit from a prior preparation?*

   Preparing the skin for a cryosurgical procedure can reduce the time required to perform the procedure, reduce pain experienced by the patient, and produce better curative and cosmetic results. If one thinks that the patient will benefit from a prior preparation, explain this in detail to the patient in order to increase compliance, and postpone the procedure until the lesion/area has been properly prepared. Some suggested presurgical preparations are summarized in Table 6.1.
7. *What is the best technique?*

   Choose carefully the technique and ensure that you have all the necessary instruments to carry out the procedure. Do not treat some skin tags in the neck with the open (spraying) technique when the tweezer technique will work better, even if it is more time-consuming.
8. *Will someone be available to attend to the patient if needed in case of an unexpected occurrence?*

   With any surgical procedure, doctors have a responsibility to ensure that the patient can be attended to in case of an unexpected event. In cryosurgery, the postoperative time can be of long duration; therefore, one has to mentally "draw" a timeline of the expected occurrences and the final healing time in order to make the necessary arrangements. The patient needs to have at hand the adequate staff to meet any eventuality. This is an important consideration to keep in mind: avoid extensive cryosurgical procedures (such as for large

Table 6.1 Some of the pretreatments suggested for the most frequent skin conditions amenable to cryosurgical treatment

Skin condition	Pretreatment
Macular (lentigines, lentigo simplex, lentigo solaris)	Retinoic acid/glycolic acid
Papular (molluscum)	In children with molluscum: Hydrate skin Indicate topical antibiotic in infected lesions Topical anesthesia before procedure
Dermatofibroma	None
Verrucous warts	Immunomodulators/salicylic acid solution or patches with daily shaving Shaving/wet before freeze Topical anesthesia especially in younger patients
Condilomas	Immunomodulators
Seborrheic keratosis	Glycolic acid gel or cream
Keloids	None
Skin cancerization	Topical fluorouracil, tretinoin, isotretinoin, tazarotene, ingenol mebutate, diclofenac sodium, salycilic acid
Basal cell carcinomas	See Immunocryosurgery (Chap. 20)

tumors) right before anticipated absences (physician, nurses, caretakers).

6.3 Patient's Queries

1. *Preoperative preparation*

   Make sure the patient understands the need for preoperative preparation in order to guarantee compliance. An example of such preparations can be the simple topical application of local anesthesia. However, others involve using immunomodulators for a long period, which in themselves have side effects.

2. *Pain*

   Patients are usually concerned about the possibility of having to suffer through a surgical procedure, and this is quite normal. Reassure the patient about this. Pain threshold is different from one patient to another. Individuals vary in their sensitivity to cold. A single superficial freezing is usually well tolerated. However, multiple superficial freezings increase responsiveness to further freezing and make the patient reach his/her maximum level of tolerable pain.

   Deep freezing is more painful than a superficial one. Once freezing begins, there is a cold sensation. When continuing to freeze, the sensation turns into a "burning" one. It improves when the procedure stops and then suddenly there is a new peak of pain which corresponds to the beginning of the thawing period. Explain this to patients from the beginning.

3. *Location*

   In cryosurgery, wounds heal by second intention. Daily cleaning and sometimes ointment application are necessary. The patient will need to let the surgeon know if he/she will be able to take care of the wound either on his/her own or with the help of someone else. Otherwise, one should wait to do the procedure. For example, in lesions of the back or those in anatomical locations not reachable by the patient, a patient will need help with postoperative care.

4. *Healing time*

   Once the patient knows how long the healing process will take, he/she will be able to decide the correct timing for the surgery. Sometimes it is best to wait until after a patient returns from a vacation or until after a special family event. The patient will also need to have at their disposition someone who will assist with the postoperative care.

6.4 Preoperative Considerations

Once the patient has agreed to have a cryosurgical procedure, the doctor will need to:

- Obtain a signed consent form to include in the patient's chart (Fig. 6.1). This consent form should include the operative and postoperative course of action. Every country/hospital/private clinic has different forms. Some are available online and can be adapted to your practice needs [1]. Ensure that the consent form is signed before doing a procedure. This is very

CONSENT FORM

CRYOSURGICAL PROCEDURE CONSENT FORM

I, ..., have been informed by Dr................. of my diagnosis of.....................

After having the different modalities of treatment explained to me, I have accepted treatment with cryosurgery with/without local/infiltrative anesthesia.

Skin cryosurgery is a procedure to treat a skin lesion by freezing. It uses Liquid Nitrogen as a freezing substance (-196°). The treated area will be replaced by healthy tissue in a few weeks. I might need cryosurgery more than once.

I have been informed of the alternative treatments available for this condition.

The purpose and reasonable expected benefits of this specific procedure have been explained to me. The immediate effects (some discomfort, sometimes pain, inflammation, redness) as well as later effects (oozing, blister and crust formation), hypo- (loss of skin pigment) or hyper-pigmentation (more pigment than originally present) that can be transitory and sometimes permanent have also been explained to me.

Swelling can be notorious if freezing has been performed around the eye (s). Blisters can be removed or left to heal spontaneously. Cryosurgery in the legs heals more slowly than in the face.

Healing will be by granulation. I understand that healing might take..........days. I am aware that I am responsible for caring for the treated area according to instructions that will be handed to me right after the procedure. I need to wash the treated area daily and apply..

Some of the unexpected complications include allergic reaction to cold, to the local anesthesia; others are: pain, infection, hematoma, and bleeding as well as an anesthetic scar.

I am aware that in the practice of medicine other unexpected risks and complications not discussed may occur. If any complication might occur, the surgeon might require a change in the surgical technique, in which case I will be informed.

The information given has been discussed with me, and I have been given time to ask questions and receive specific answers.

I certify that I have read and fully understand the content of this form. The disclosures referred to above were made to me and all blanks filled in before I signed my name below.

Patient Name.................................... Date.....................................

Id #

If patient is minor or unable to give consent,

Signature of person authorized to consent for the patient (Relationship)...

Name..

Signature.. .

ID #...

Fig. 6.1 A proposed consent form

important because it guarantees that the patient has all the necessary information, and it prevents legal issues for the physician. Dr Suhonen R. has suggested that it is best to have two different consent forms: a "small" consent form for small procedures and a "large" consent form in big procedures. An example of a "small" procedure could be freezing a seborrheic keratosis. An example of a "large" procedure could be the deep freezing of a skin cancer.

- Reduce expected pain. In most procedures, no anesthesia is required. In some procedures, topical anesthesia can be helpful such as: (a) superficial treatment in children (warts, molluscum) and (b) cryopeeling for sun-damaged skin. For procedures where one can expect pain, infiltrate local anesthetics will be required (deep freezing as in skin cancer treatment).
- Reduce hyper-/hypopigmentation. For skin types III and darker, perform a test in a not-too-visible area and have the patient return later to the office so that the results can be observed.
- Control for excessive edematous or allergic reaction. If the patient's skin is very lax and the procedure is in the face and/or around the eyes, perform a test or do just a few lesions at a time in order to avoid excessive edema. If the doctor suspects that the patient might have an allergic reaction to cold, a small test on the inner side of the arm (with a few seconds of spraying) should be performed before the cryosurgical procedure.
- Ask the patient face to face before a procedure if he/she has a trip, a party, or any important event coming up. The patient may not remember at first, but double-checking will be worth the time: the patient will be very upset if the procedure takes place and then he/she realizes that they had forgotten about such an event and now have a crust on the face due to the procedure, for example. This is something to be very aware of especially in those cases in which an in-office procedure is performed during a medical visit and has not required any preparation (like freezing one seborrheic keratosis in the face). It is best to postpone the procedure to another time when there are no special events planned in the patient's life after a procedure.
- Confirm that the presurgical procedure has been done properly. Some of the most common presurgical treatments are:
  (a) Warts: one small wart can be shaved and wet before freezing. Multiple lesions might be reduced in size and number by a previous 15–21-day shaving treatment and/or immunomodulator treatment.
  (b) Multiple molluscum in an atopic child: send the patient home for a few weeks of intensive skin hydration. Some of the lesions will simply fall off. The child will be very grateful to have less cryosurgery done on him/her.
- Ensure that, for single recurrent lesions, a previous biopsy has been obtained. This is mandatory.
- Last but not least, make sure to have enough LN before starting a procedure. One can have a waiting room full of patients and suddenly realize the Dewar is empty.

Essential Tidbits

- In many instances, preparing the skin for cryosurgical treatment will yield better results.
- Keratin removal will allow for a better penetration of the freezing front.
- In skin cancerization, a previous removal of small subclinical lesions will leave only larger, hyperkeratotic lesions (additive effect).
- Previous treatment can have an enhancing effect. The end result will be better than either cryosurgery or topical treatment used alone.

Conclusions

Patients need to be previously prepared for a cryosurgical procedure. Consent forms need to be signed. In addition, clear explanations of all surgical options, expected end results, required postoperative care, and possible complications are part of the information that should be made available to the patient.

Some procedures will have better cosmetic and curative results if a prior preparation of the lesion or the whole area is performed. Some of these are very simple and others are more time-consuming and have side effects of their own. Explaining them to the patient will help achieve better compliance.

Reference

1. Surgical consent forms. Weblog. [Online] Available from http://www.docstoc.com/docs/84831222/Procedure-Consent-Form-Template. Accessed 19 Feb 2014.

Part II

Benign Conditions

Cryobiopsy, Cryoanesthesia, and Cryoanalgesia

7

Angeles Fortuño-Mar and Paola Pasquali

Contents

Key Points

- Sub-zero temperatures can be used to anesthetize a small area of tissue. The transient numbness is sufficient for shaving biopsy or needle sticking without generating any major discomfort.
- No cellular changes or artifacts are generated on the specimen.
- Freezing nerve endings has also been used in neuralgic pain.

7.1 Introduction

Skin biopsy is a common dermatologic procedure performed to confirm or rule out a disease or diagnosis. It can be performed by removal of the outer layers (shave biopsy) or by taking superficial or deep layers (as in punch biopsy), either excisionally (the whole lesion) or incisionally (part of the lesion). Local infiltrating anesthesia is required even in superficial procedures. Needle injection and the stinging sensation caused by the acidic pH of the anesthesia are both causes of discomfort [1].

Cryoanesthesia offers the possibility of performing a superficial procedure without having to apply anesthesia. Cold acts as an anesthetic, and a superficial freezing of a few seconds will give the operator sufficient time to take a shave biopsy. This procedure is particularly useful in sensitive areas, such as the nipple, genitals, ear, or nose (Fig. 7.1a, b).

A. Fortuño-Mar, MD, PhD, MBA (✉)
Eldine Patologia Laboratory, Avenida Roma, 7-A, 8° 4°, 43005 Tarragona, Spain
e-mail: afortunyo@eldinepatologia.com

P. Pasquali, MD
Department of Dermatology, Pius Hospital de Valls, 43800 Tarragona, Spain
e-mail: pasqualipaola@gmail.com

P. Pasquali (ed.), *Cryosurgery: A Practical Manual*,
DOI 10.1007/978-3-662-43939-5_7, © Springer-Verlag Berlin Heidelberg 2015

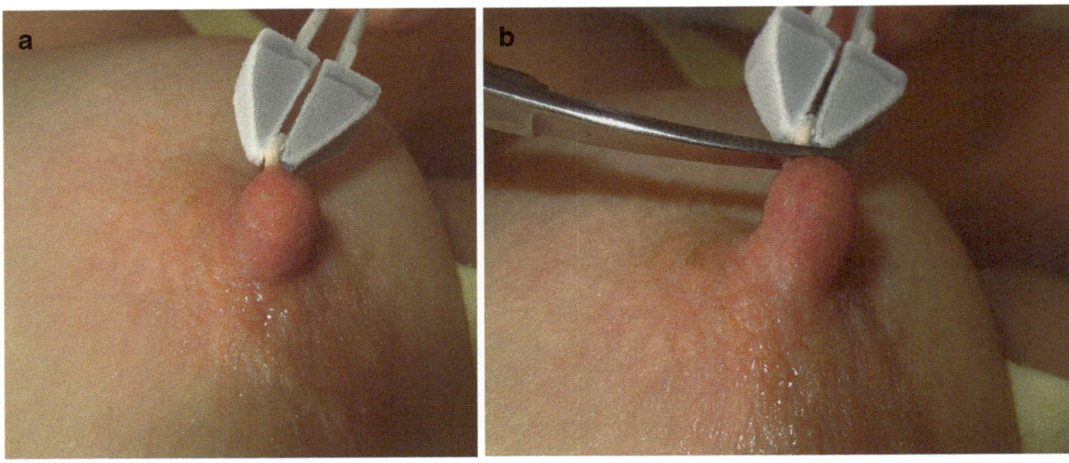

Fig. 7.1 (**a**, **b**) Cryoshaving of a lesion in the nipple done with cryotweezers. (**a**) The area was cleaned, and the lesion grabbed with frozen cryotweezers. The freezing front was left to advance just to the surface of the skin. (**b**) Cutting was performed with scissors right at the base at the beginning of the thawing. The patient felt no discomfort

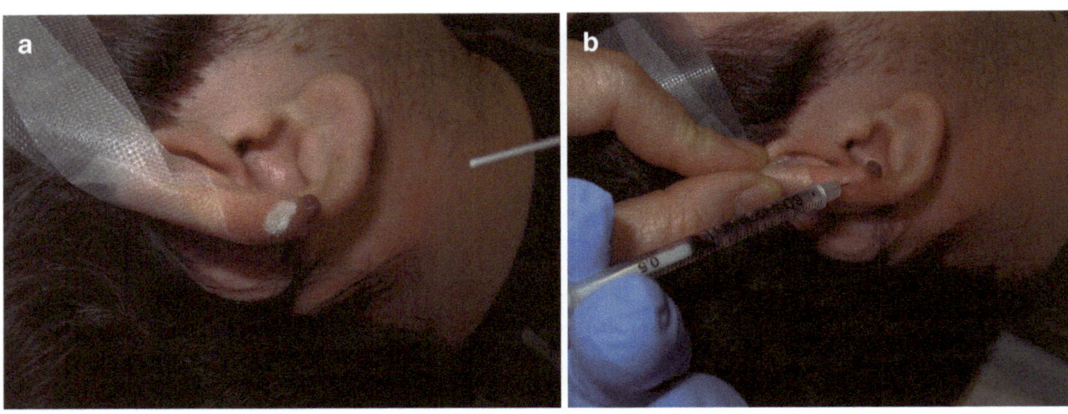

Fig. 7.2 (**a**) Superficial spray freezing where the needle will prick. (**b**) Immediate pricking at frozen site

The use of cold to reduce pain or swelling is called cryotherapy. Instead, when low temperatures induce irreversible damage to a tissue, it is called cryosurgery [2]. In cryobiopsy, the freezing is fast and superficial. No tissue destruction occurs.

Another use of cold as analgesia is spot spraying an area where a needle needs to be introduced. By freezing the surface, the patient will not feel the prick of the needle (Fig. 7.2a, b), therefore reducing discomfort and fear; this procedure is especially useful in children and in delicate areas such as the genitals where a needle prick generates a lot of anxiety.

7.2 Histopathologic Evaluation of Cryobiopsy Specimens

The preservation of original components in cells and tissues is necessary for the study and correct interpretation of histopathology changes. Therefore, a correct tissue fixation consists of interrupting degradation processes which appear after cellular death, trying to preserve both tissue structure and composition.

There are two concepts in histopathology that deserve mention: real and equivalent image. A real image of a tissue is the one which shows this tissue when it is still alive. This is an image that

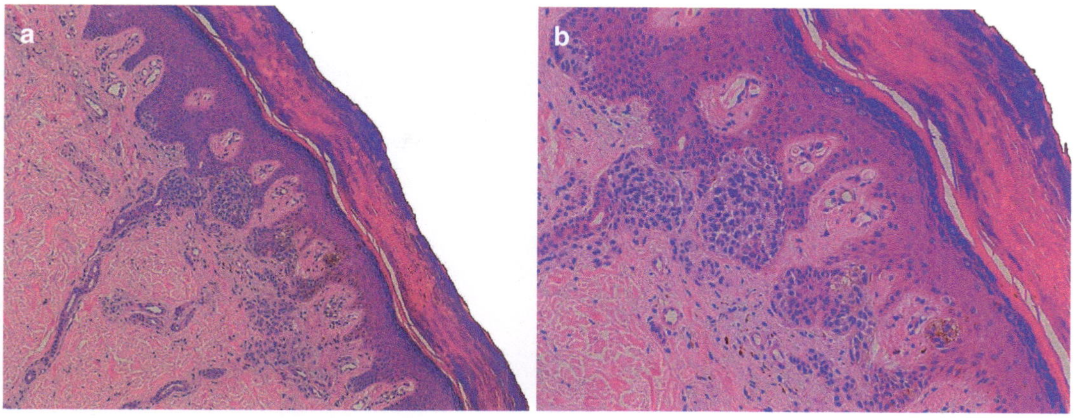

Fig. 7.3 (**a**, **b**) Cryobiopsy. Compound melanocytic nevi. Absence of the artifactual changes. Hematoxylin-eosin stained. Original magnification: 1: 100×; 2: 200×

cannot be obtained after the fixation process because it is a dynamic feature. On the other hand, an equivalent image is acquired after histopathologic manipulation. This manipulation consists of fixation, inclusion, cutting, and staining. Fixation is the most important step in this complex procedure. As one can see, the main purpose of the histopathologic technique is to strive to have the equivalent image be as similar as possible to the real image.

Fixatives are classified in two distinct groups: (a) fixatives by physical methods and (b) fixatives by chemical methods. In the first case, freezing is employed on a tissue as a method of stopping the autolysis and putrefaction.

In general, when temperature decreases too much, intracellular and extracellular water is crystallized. The key of a successful fixation by tissue freezing lies in freezing and taking the sample as quick as possible. All physiological processes are immobilized in the ice crystals by the quick-freezing methods, and every component of the cells and tissues are maintained in situ at the time of freezing. Thus, ischemic or anoxic effects are minimized [3].

When the tissue specimens are frozen for an extended period of time, the ice microcrystals enlarge, puncturing the membranes of the cells and cellular organelles and causing histopathologic changes. Unlike slow freezing of fixed tissue which affects specimens frozen, for instance, on a cold winter day [4], the rapid freezing of tissue to a temperature below −15 °C in cryoanesthesia is associated with the uniform production of ice microcrystals within the tissues of the cells and within the extracellular space. When the frozen tissue is thawed slowly, the formation of large vacuoles and circular structures represents artifact vacuolization from nuclear retraction and presence of ice microcrystals secondary to inadequate fixation in formalin [5].

However, the quick freezing of tissue followed by correct fixation in formalin prevents the accumulation of large ice crystals and membrane micropuncture, reducing morphological artifacts and thus avoiding visible tissue defects through the light microscope [6] (Fig. 7.3a, b).

Current studies have also demonstrated that the stability of human epidermal cells to low temperature relates to their stage of differentiation. The epidermal stem cells and transitory cells are more stable than differentiated cells [7].

Our experience is based on the study of 20 cases corresponding to actinic keratosis, melanocytic nevi, basal cell carcinomas, squamous carcinomas, seborrheic keratosis, and pyogenic granulomas. In all of them, the cryobiopsy technique was correctly performed by the same operator with immediate formalin fixation. In order to achieve a more objective evaluation, no information was given to the pathologist about the procedure carried out. In all cases, the material was suitable for histology study, the diagnosis was correct, and no artifacts were described. A second

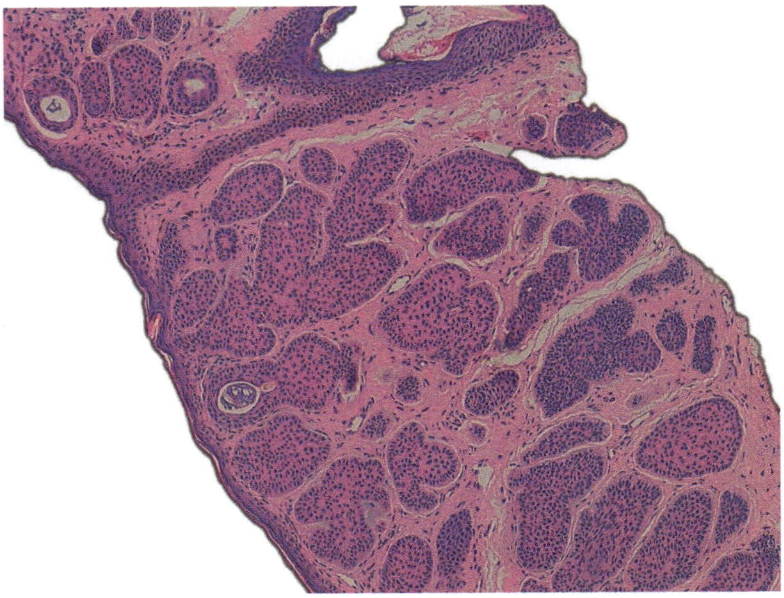

Fig. 7.4 Cryobiopsy. Basal cell carcinoma. Absence of the artifactual changes. Hematoxylin-eosin stained. Original magnification, 100×

pathologist confirmed the absence of artifacts in all the cases (Fig. 7.4).

The use of cryobiopsy in medicine is not limited to the dermatology field. For example, cryo-needle is used to obtain large histological specimens of high quality from intrathoracic lymph nodes [8].

7.2.1 Technique

7.2.1.1 Spraying or Open Technique

This technique is probably the most commonly used technique. A superficial spraying of 4–5 s over the lesion intended to be biopsied should leave a whitened area of certain consistency. Shaving is performed right away – since freezing is superficial, thawing is quite fast (Fig. 7.5a–d). If the tissue is too hard, the scalpel will not cut through; as thawing begins, shaving is performed on a tissue that still offers some resistance. Ideally, the base of the shaved area will still be slightly frozen (white) by the time the shaving is done. Before thawing is complete, apply a topical hemostatic solution to stop any bleeding from small, cut capillaries. Any hemostatic solution will work [9]: it will reduce bleeding caused by post-freezing vasodilation.

Care should be taken when applying certain hemostatic substances. Some sting, such as silver nitrate sticks. If there is a need to use them, apply them alternating with wet gauze soaked in fresh saline solution. This helps reduce the stinging sensation.

Cryotweezers work very well on protruding lesions. Grasp the lesion with the frozen cryotweezer (Fig. 7.6) and allow the freezing front to reach the skin surface. Then cut the lesion out with a scalpel or fine scissors (Fig. 7.7a, b).

7.3 Cryoanalgesia

Cryosurgery has been used to reduce neuralgic pain. One common condition is postherpetic neuralgia.

7.3.1 Trigeminal Neuralgia

This is a common consequence of a postherpetic infection. Up to 16 % of patients less than 60 years of age and up to 47 % of patients over 60 can have persistent pain. Many medical and surgical treatments have been proposed [10].

Cryoablation has been used for neuralgic pain with the probe placed over the area and either sonographically guided [11] or CT-guided [12]. Cryosurgery is an excellent treatment option for genuine trigeminal neuralgia. The first treatments required exposing the nerve and placing a probe over it for direct freezing of the nervous fibers. Newly developed cryoprobes for peripheral

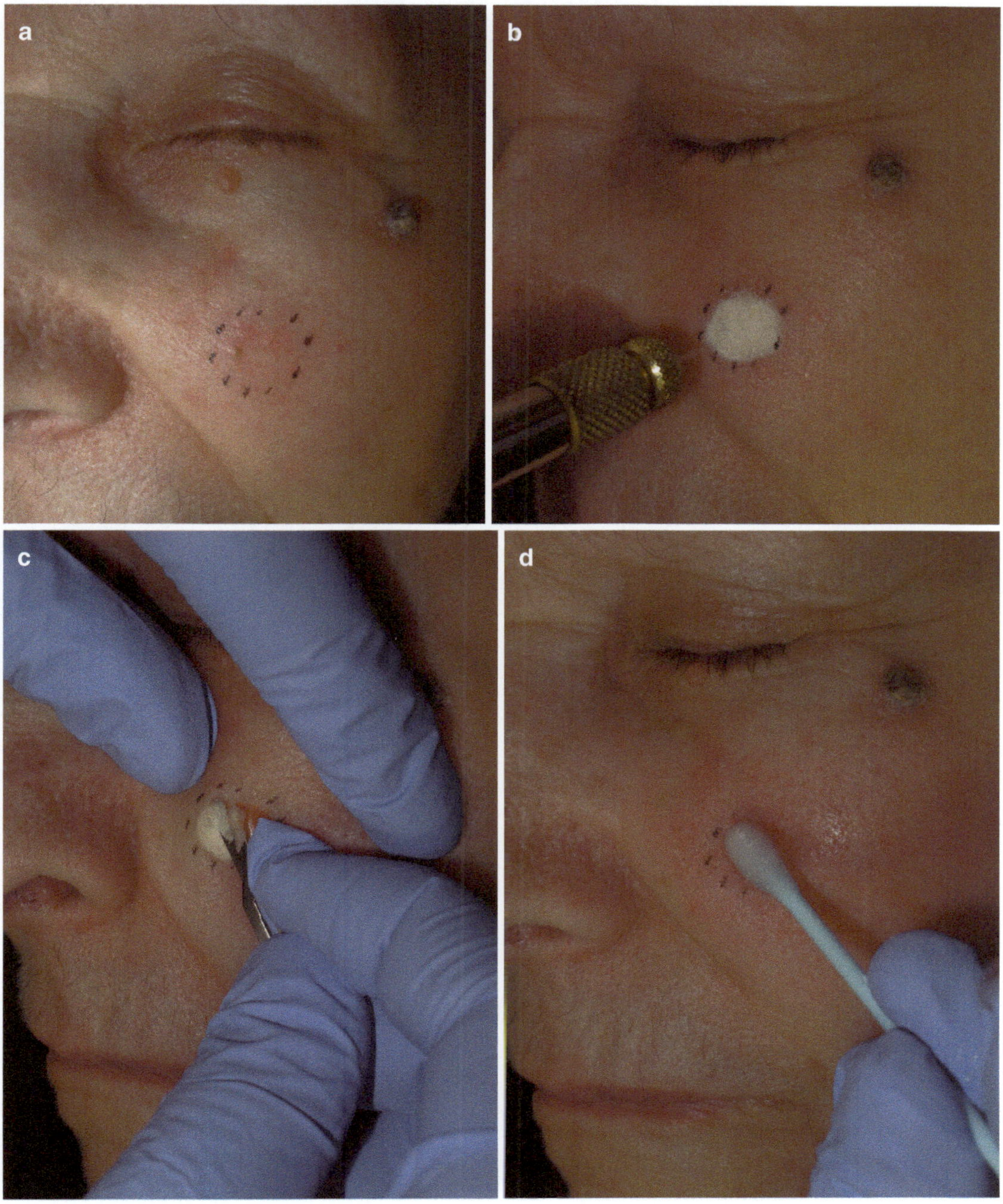

Fig. 7.5 (**a–e**) Cryobiopsy using the spraying technique. (**a**) Chosen lesion; (**b**) superficial spraying; (**c**) shaving with tissue slightly frozen showing the bottom still white; (**d**) hemostatic solution applied immediately after shaving and with tissue still frozen to avoid bleeding; (**e**) immediately after hemostatic solution

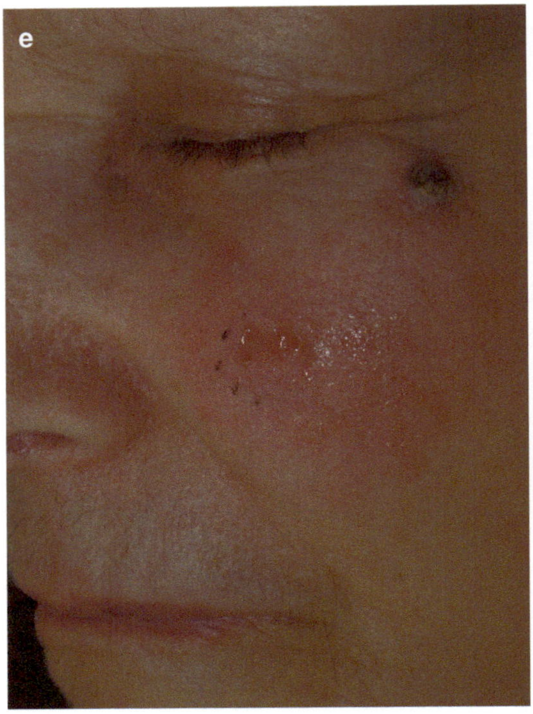

Fig. 7.5 (continued)

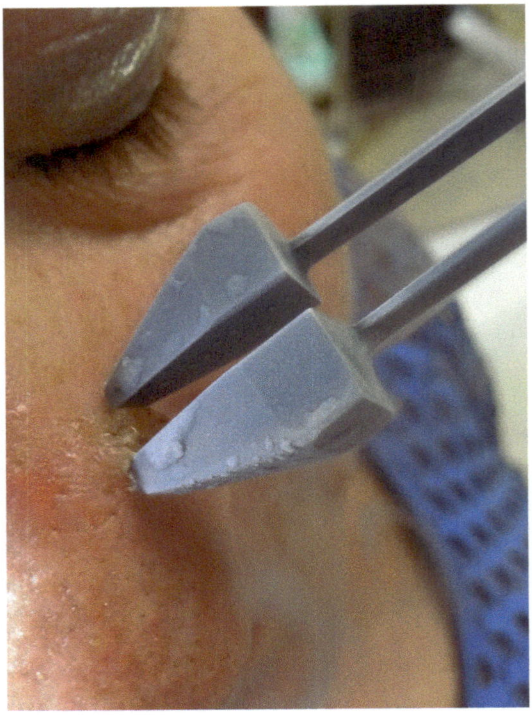

Fig. 7.6 Grabbing a verrucous lesion on the dorsum of the nose with cryotweezers for shaving biopsy

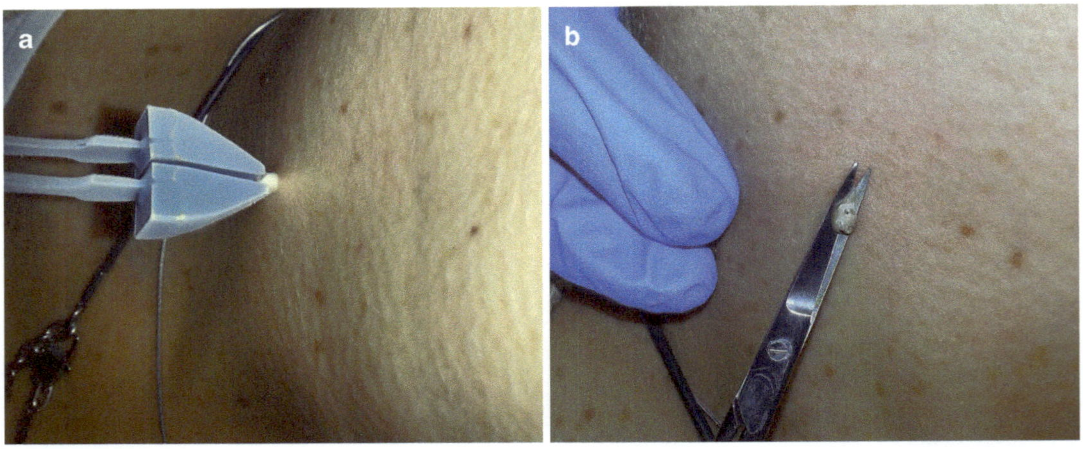

Fig. 7.7 (**a**) Freezing with cryotweezers of a protruding lesion. (**b**) Cutting it out for speedy recovery and biopsy material (if needed)

nerves allow the freezing of branches of the trigeminal nerve without exposing the nerve or damaging the surrounding tissue. They are designed to be inserted transmucosally. It is a non-stressful procedure that can be repeated as needed [13].

A "non-freezing technique" (NFT) has been proposed by Calandria [14] for neuralgic pain. This technique consists of spraying topically over the affected dermatome without freezing, perpendicularly to the skin at a distance of 15 cm for 30 s. The mean number of sessions is 5.

Essential Tidbits

- Cryobiopsy is a modified shaving technique that has the advantage of requiring no local anesthesia.
- Spraying or cryotweezers can be used for cryobiopsy.
- Frozen tissue needs to be partially thawed for scalpel shaving or scissor cutting.
- Apply hemostatic solution before complete thawing.
- Make sure complete thawing has occurred and no superficial bleeding is present before covering the lesion.

References

1. Mutalik S. How to make local anesthesia less painful. J Cutan Aesthet Surg. 2008;1(1):37–8.
2. Stańczyk M, Telega JJ. Thermal problems in biomechanics – a review. Part III. Cryosurgery, cryopreservation and cryotherapy. Acta Bioeng Biomech. 2003;5:3–22.
3. Ohno S, Ohno N, Terada N, et al. In vivo cryotechniques for preparation of animal tissues for immunoelectron microscopy. Methods Mol Biol. 2010;657: 167–79.
4. Elenitsas R, Halpern AC. Biopsy techniques. In: Elder D, Elenitsas R, Jawoksy C, Johnson Jr B, editors. Lever's histopathology of the skin. 8th ed. Philadelphia: Lippincott Williams & Wilkins; 1997. p. 2–3.
5. Walling HW, Swick BL. Simulation of cutaneous Bowen's disease by freeze artifact in tissue briefly fixed in formalin. Int J Dermatol. 2011;50:757–8.
6. Luck L, Longley BJ. Cutaneous cryoanesthesia does not affect histopathology of biopsy specimens. Cutis. 1999;64:225–6.
7. Raidan M, Shubin NA, Blinova MI, et al. The effect of low temperatures on the viability of human epidermal keratinocytes found at different stages of differentiation. Tsitologiia. 2011;53:22–30.
8. Franke KJ, Nilius G, Rueble KH, et al. The cryoneedle: a new tool for histological biopsies. A feasibility study. Lung. 2013;191:611–7.
9. Glick JB, Kaur RR, Siegel D. Achieving hemostasis in dermatology – part II: topical hemostatic agents. Indian Dermatol Online J. 2013;4(3):172–6.
10. Jainkittivong A, Aneksuk V, Langlais RP. Trigeminal neuralgia: a retrospective study of 188 Thai cases. Gerodontology. 2012;29(2):e611–7.
11. Friedman T, Richman D, Adler R. Sonographically guided cryoneurolysis: preliminary experience and clinical outcomes. J Ultrasound Med. 2012;31(12):2025–34.
12. Dar SA, Love Z, Prologo JD, Hsu DP. CT-guided cryoablation for palliation of secondary trigeminal neuralgia from head and neck malignancy. J Neurointerv Surg. 2013;5(3):258–63.
13. Pradel W, Hlawitschka M, Eckelt U, Herzog R, Koch K. Cryosurgical treatment of genuine trigeminal neuralgia. Br J Oral Maxillofac Surg. 2002;40(3):244–7.
14. Calandria L. Cryoanalgesia for post-herpetic neuralgia: a new treatment. Int J Dermatol. 2011;50(6):746–50.

Cryosurgery for Common Benign Lesions

8

Miguel Alejandro Lopez Blanco,
Anthony Panagiotopoulos, and Paola Pasquali

Contents

M.A. Lopez Blanco, MD
Department of Dermatology, Hospital Militar Carlos Arvelo, Caracas, Venezuela
e-mail: miguelalejandrolb@yahoo.com

A. Panagiotopoulos, MD
Department of Cryosurgery, Hospital Andreas Syggros, Athens, Greece
e-mail: antonispan2004@yahoo.com

P. Pasquali, MD (✉)
Department of Dermatology, Pius Hospital de Valls, 43800 Tarragona, Spain
e-mail: pasqualipaola@gmail.com

Key Points

- Benign lesions are the most commonly treated lesions with cryosurgery.
- Many medical and surgical specialties share their interest in treating benign lesions with cryosurgery.
- As a general rule, in benign lesions, it is better to undertreat a lesion than to overtreat it, in order to achieve a better cosmetic result.

8.1 Introduction

By far, benign lesions are the most common crysurgically treated lesions [1]. Operators include family physicians, nurses, physician assistants, and gynecologists, in addition to dermatologists. Seborrheic keratosis, warts, skin tags, and molluscum contagiosum are among the

P. Pasquali (ed.), *Cryosurgery: A Practical Manual*,
DOI 10.1007/978-3-662-43939-5_8, © Springer-Verlag Berlin Heidelberg 2015

Table 8.1 Most common benign conditions amenable to cryosurgical treatment

	Suggested technique
Noninfectious conditions	
Acne (cysts)	S
Alopecia areata	S
Benign pigmentary lesions: lentigines, lentigos simplex, solar lentigos, ephelides	S
Dermatofibroma	P, SO
Ingrowing toenail	P, S
Granuloma annulare	P, S
Keloids	S, P, IL
Lichen planus	S
Myxoid cysts	P, S, SO
Prurigo nodularis	S
Seborrheic keratosis	S
Sebaceous hyperplasia	P
Skin tags	T, S
Trigeminal neuralgia	P, S
Pearly penile papule	S, P
Vascular lesions (see Chap. 12)	P, S
Infectious conditions	
Chromomycosis	S
Molluscum contagiosum	P, SO
Leishmaniasis	S
Larva migrans	P, S
Warts (see Chap. 9)	S, SO

Techniques: *S* spray (open), *P* probe (closed), *T* cryotweezer, *SO* cone (semi-open)

most popular conditions, and these conditions are where most experience exists. The best results will be obtained when the proper lesion, skin type, anatomical area, and cryosurgical technique are selected. Some benign lesions are destroyed for curative reasons (as in molluscum, warts, or leishmaniasis), while others are treated for cosmetic (lentigines) or functional (lesions in areas of friction) reasons. As a general rule, undertreatment is preferred to overtreatment since there will always be the chance to repeat the treatment if needed and because overtreatment can leave non-cosmetic scars.

As far as the technique goes, open technique (spraying) is by far the most utilized, followed by semi-open (cone-limited LN). Close contact, tweezers, and intralesional are also used. Cryochambers (semi-closed technique) should be avoided because the resulting freezing front is too deep.

Some of the conditions amenable to cryosurgical treatment are shown in Table 8.1.

8.2 Acne

Although cryosurgery is not a first treatment modality in acne cysts, it can be the sole alternative when dealing with patients with severe cystic forms of acne that cannot be treated either with oral or with topical medication. Such is the case in pregnancy [2].

Cold has an initial inflammatory effect, but 24–48 h after freezing the lesion an anti-inflammatory effect becomes evident and a faster reabsorption of the lesion occurs. A superficial spraying for 5–7 s is usually enough: freezing beyond the margin of the lesion is not necessary. In order to avoid LN insufflations, spraying before draining the lesion is advisable.

8.3 Rhinophyma

Cryosurgery has been an excellent option [3–5] for rhinophyma where good cosmetic results have been reported. Two or three freeze-thaw cycles of 15–30 s separated by 1 min are recommended. Sessions can be repeated every 2 weeks for up to seven sessions [6]. Another alternative is to shave the excess tissue (previous local anesthesia) using electrosurgery and later deep spray, freezing the base of the lesion.

8.4 Alopecia Areata

Some authors report the use of cryosurgery in alopecia areata. LN can be applied either by cotton swab technique [7] or by superficially spraying the lesion until the skin turns slightly pinkish red. No blister should be induced. Besides the slight discomfort from cold, pain is not a major complaint. Apparently it works by inducing local vasodilation or even by cold immunomodulation.

8.5 Benign Pigmentary Lesions: Lentigines, Lentigos Simplex, Solar Lentigos, and Ephelides

Freezing for 5–7 s, using a superficial spray technique (open method), until the whole pigmented area and an additional 1–2 mm margin are included in the treatment zone is recommended [8].

The aim is to cause a sloughing of the superficial pigmented epidermis. No destruction of melanocytes occurs because freezing is very light. Likewise, recurrence can occur if no proper sun protection follows treatment, just as it occurs with any other surgical treatment of pigmented lesions. Lentigos in the dorsum of the hand leave very satisfactory results although the patient must be warned that the complete healing process can take over a month. Lentigos in the dorsum of the hands have to be spray-freezed for a few seconds each. The crusts can take up to a month to fall off and the pink residual spots can take up to 2 months.

Special consideration should be taken in darker skin types as even a light freezing can result in hyperpigmentation. Do not ever use it in melasma.

8.6 Dermatofibroma

Although it is possible to treat dermatofibroma with cryosurgery, this lesion has a deep dermal fibrous component that requires a deep freezing (contact/probe). In certain skin types, hyper- or hypopigmentation can make the result unsatisfactory. Lesions located on the legs require healing times that may exceed 2 months, making a simple excision with conventional surgery a better technique. Dermatofibromas that respond well to a cryosurgical treatment include lesions that are small, not too elevated, and nonpigmented lesions located above the waistline [9].

8.7 Ingrown Toenail

Ingrown toe nail or onychocryptosis is related to congenital or to acquired defect of the toenail (inadequate shoes or improper nail cut). This condition might be present at birth but frequently makes itself evident in early adulthood. In patients with congenital conditions in whom the presence of granulomas is persistent or recurrent, a partial or total surgical nail removal or a surgical ablation of laterals and/or distal nail folds is the best therapeutic approach. A conservative approach is an option for those granulomas that are present in acquired cases. Cryosurgery is an excellent option that avoids the need for conventional nail surgery. If skin infection is present, a previous topical antibiotic is recommended. One cycle of cryosurgery with a previously frozen probe (closed method) or one cycle of LN spraying (open method) with a 1 mm margin is usually enough to destroy the granuloma. Combination treatments (cryosurgery plus matrixectomy) have been reported with good results [10].

8.8 Granuloma Annulare

Single lesions of granuloma annulare sometimes disappear after biopsy. Sometimes this phenomenon is also observed when freezing a portion of the border of the lesion, using a probe or spraying LN directly into the lesion. It is an option in children with lesions that do not respond to topical treatment [11].

8.9 Keloids and Hypertrophic Scars

These scars are considered benign proliferations of fibrous tissue composed mainly of collagen. For keloids, the stimulus that triggers could be any type of trauma to the skin and may not even be present or evident. Keloids have an accelerated growth pattern and by definition occupy a much larger area than that of the corresponding area of trauma or initial stimulus. Keloids tend to grow, creating finger-like projections or pseudopods. In the case of hypertrophic scars, a history of trauma to the skin is present and the fibrous tissue becomes bulky, but generally it does not exceed the corresponding area of the initial trauma [12].

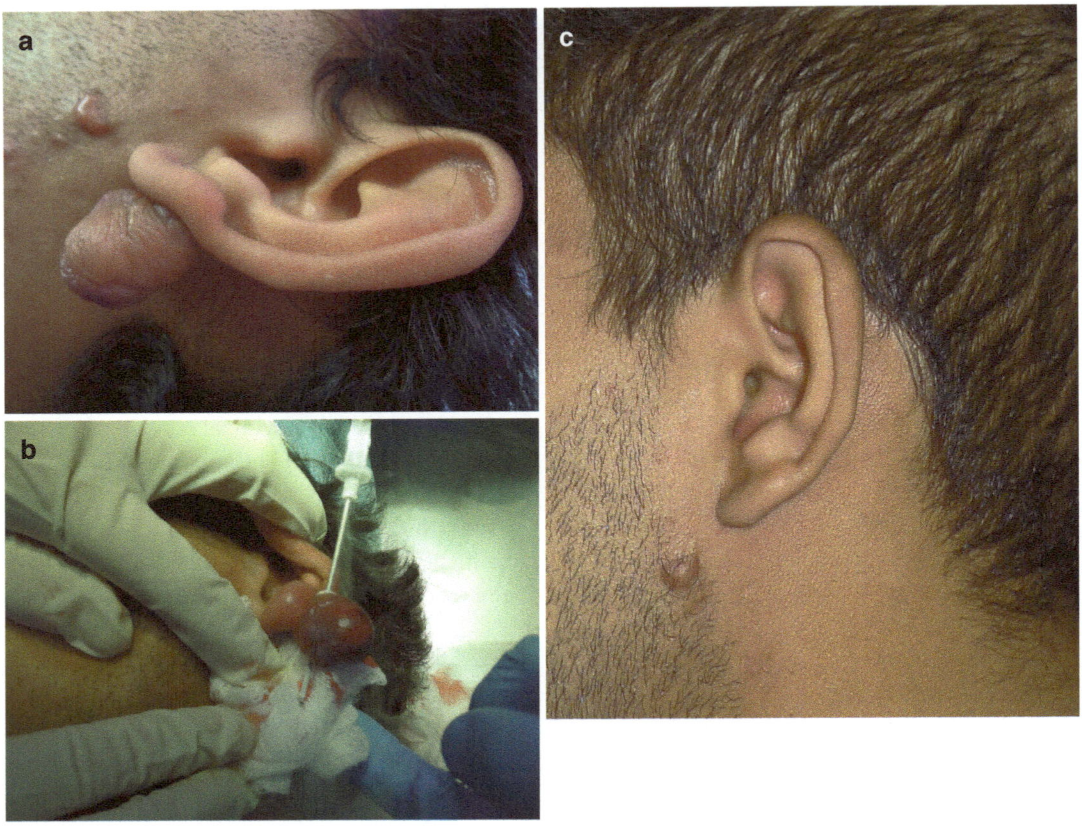

Fig. 8.1 (**a**) Large keloid on the earlobe. (**b**) Intralesional cryosurgery followed by corticosteroid infiltration. (**c**) End results

It is known that keloids are more common in people with darker skin phototypes, but they have been reported in all races. Keloids have a predilection to appear in certain anatomical regions such as ears, chest, shoulders, neck, and abdomen, among others [12].

Whichever method is used, the treatment of keloids is difficult and sometimes unrewarding due to the high recurrence rate. When treated with simple surgical excision, recurrence rates of approximately 55 % have been reported [12].

Cryosurgery has proved to be useful in the management of both keloids and hypertrophic scars. It has been observed in vitro that freezing human living skin modifies collagen synthesis by promoting the differentiation of keloid fibroblast into normal phenotype fibroblasts. Recurrence varies with reports, but better results are obtained when used in combination with intralesional steroids, which decreases collagen synthesis and increases its degradation [13, 14].

The form of application varies according to the size of the lesion and its anatomical location. In small lesions, an open method or spray can be used. Choosing an adequate tip that allows a sufficient cryogen flow is important to achieve a rapid and solid freezing. Repeat the procedure 2–3 times for better results. In large and bulky lesions and in certain anatomical regions such as ear lobes, a thick needle or cryoneedle can be inserted in and through the lesion. The needle is attached to a cryosurgery device directly or using a Luer-Lock adapter; as the cryogen passes through the needle, the freezing of the lesion occurs from the center to the periphery allowing a solid freezing, including the center of the lesion. A mild bleeding at the puncture sites might occur which can be controlled by applying pressure for a few minutes (Fig. 8.1a–c) [12, 13].

Using intralesional corticosteroids after the cryosurgery seems to warrant better results and diminishes the risk of recurrence. Some authors suggest that the benefit of using this combined treatment is due to the sum of the mechanisms of action of both therapeutic methods. However, it seems easier to infiltrate the corticosteroid into the fibrous tissue a few minutes (10–15 min) after the last freeze-thaw cycle, apparently due to keloid tissue edema. A higher volume of the drug can be injected into the tissue after the freezing compared with the amount that can be injected without a previous cryosurgery. Triamcinolone is the preferred corticosteroid; infiltration of the maximum amount of undiluted triamcinolone (10 mg/ml) that the tissue can sustain is advisable. Figueroa et al. reported 80–100 % reduction in 75 % of the lesions, 50–80 % reduction in 16 % of the lesions, and one patient with a recurrent lesion after 1 year of follow-up, using a technique that included shaving, cryosurgery with an open method, and intralesional steroid injections [15]. Zouboulis et al. reported an excellent response in 32.3 %, a good response in 29 %, and a poor response in 9.7 % of patients treated with a contact method with freeze-thaw cycles of 30 s and repeating the procedure every 20–30 days if needed; there were no recurrences [16].

An important tissue necrosis is an unavoidable event since a solid and complete freezing is of paramount importance in treating this kind of lesions. However, achromic and hypopigmented scarring of the skin may be present in the final cosmetic result. Notifying patients in advance of this postoperative possibility is very important.

8.10 Myxoid Cysts

Myxoid cysts (in hand or toes) can be treated with cryosurgery using LN spray [17] (open technique) or probe (closed technique) [18]. A double freeze-thaw cycle is recommended by some authors [19]. Local infiltrative or troncular block anesthesia is recommended. A small incision is made in the center of the lesion in order to drain its content-a viscous mucous-like material. It also confirms the diagnosis. A previously frozen probe or a warm probe (to help fix into place) is applied with pressure. Freezing should extend 1 mm beyond the borders of the lesion. Generally, one cycle is sufficient (Fig. 8.2a–d). Recurrences are possible.

8.11 Prurigo Nodularis

One cycle of LN superficial spraying is usually enough. It is an option used in other inflammatory conditions such as psoriasis and lichen planus among others [20].

8.12 Seborrheic Keratosis (SK)

SK is probably the most gratifying lesion to treat with cryosurgery (Fig. 8.3a, b). In fact, cryosurgery stands as the first treatment option, and one can hardly think of any other surgical alternative that gives such results. Many lesions can be treated at once, with low cost and in a time-saving procedure to the patient. SK can have many presentations as far as morphology: thin, thick, large, small, and hyperpigmented. Sometimes, they can mimic malignancies (Fig. 8.4a) (as basal cell carcinomas or melanomas) and vice versa (Fig. 8.4b). This enhances the importance of having a correct diagnosis before freezing. Dermoscopy plays an important role in making the right choice with these patients, since dermoscopic characteristics of SK are distinctive and allow for a correct diagnosis in most of the cases. A biopsy is mandatory in cases when the clinician is unsure about the diagnosis.

The most commonly used technique is open or spraying [21, 22]. Depending on the size of the lesion, a thin aperture will work best for precise freezing while a large aperture works best for fast freezing of very large lesions. For small lesions, always spray in the center of the lesion and allow the freezing front to advance toward the periphery until a 1 mm margin is included. For large lesions, segmental cryosurgery is the correct

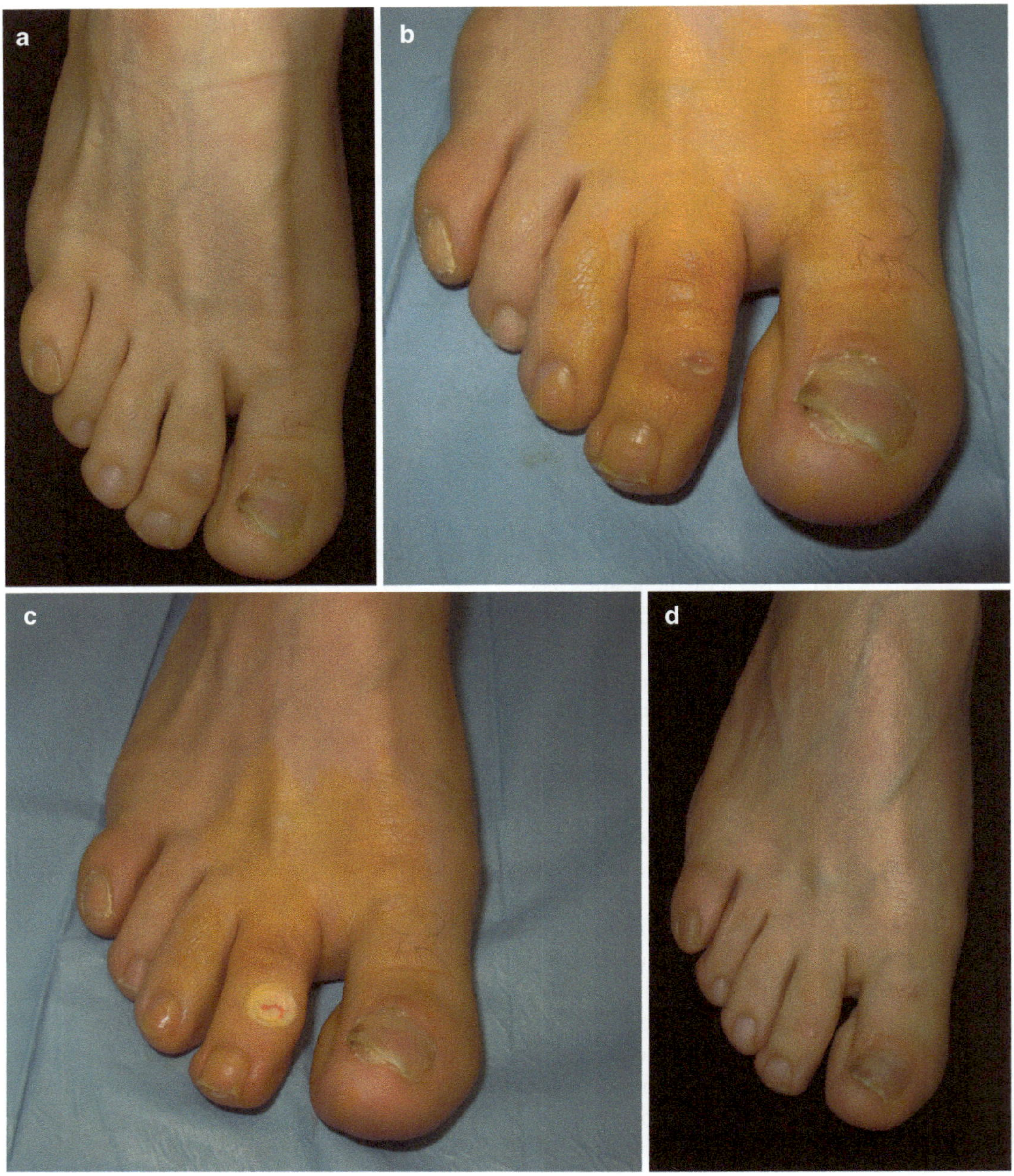

Fig. 8.2 (**a**) Myxoid cyst on second toe of right foot. (**b**) Drainage of viscous content to confirm diagnosis. (**c**) One cycle deep probe freezing with 4 mm probe. (**d**) Four months later

technique to use. Segmental cryosurgery consists of freezing a large lesion by sectors: a large area is divided by imaginary lines, and freezing is done on each sector. Overlapping of the margins will avoid the chances of leaving untreated areas.

Once the SK is frozen (one single freeze cycle), there are two options: (a) Let the lesion thaw and let it follow its normal cycle of natural sloughing off in a period of time that will depend on the anatomical area of location or (b) let thawing begin and curette the lesion off with a scalpel or curette. This will reduce the healing time. If this second option is chosen, care should be taken with post-cryosurgical vasodilation

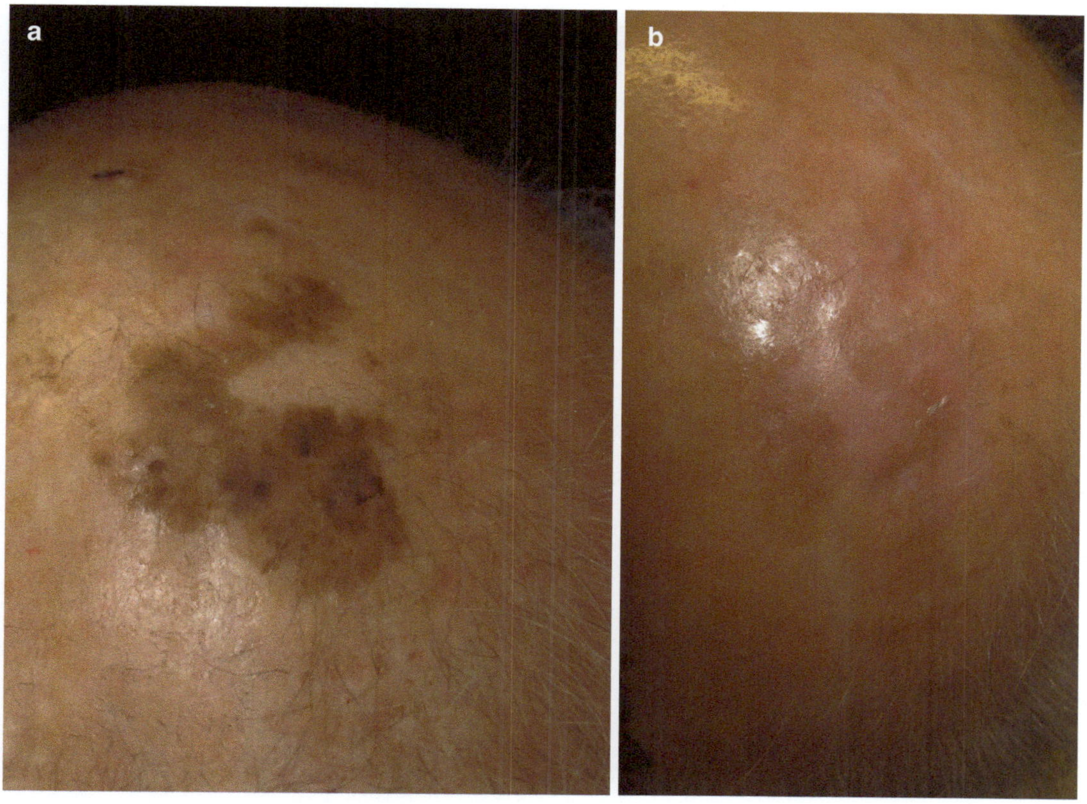

Fig. 8.3 (**a**) Seborrheic keratosis of the scalp. (**b**) Three months after treatment, one freeze-thaw cycle, open technique

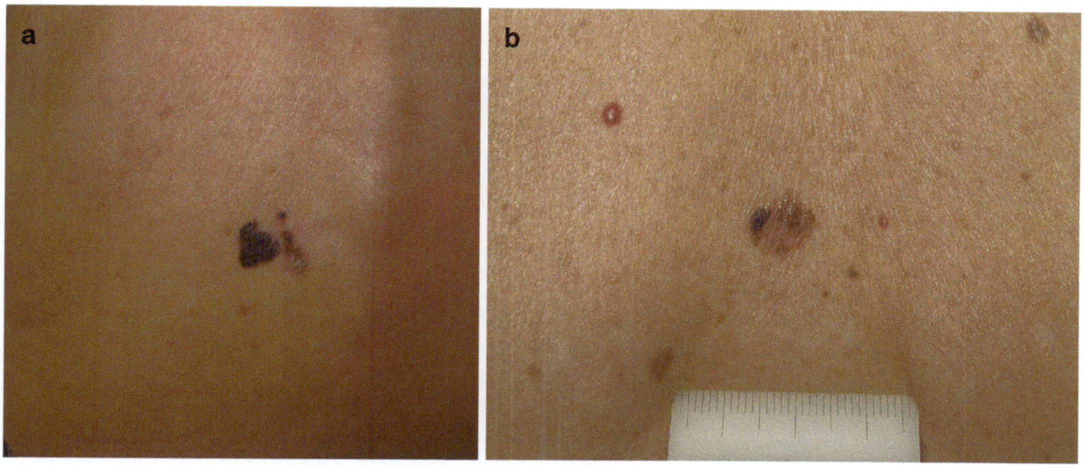

Fig. 8.4 (**a**) Seborrheic keratosis mimicking a malignant melanoma. (**b**) Malignant melanoma mimicking a seborrheic keratosis (**b**, Courtesy of Dr. Giuseppe Argenziano)

which will cause some bleeding at the base (Fig. 8.5a–d). The latter can be resolved by simple application of hemostatic solutions or by applying pressure for a few minutes.

Once complete healing has occurred, the base of the lesion will look pink for some weeks (Fig. 8.6a, b). Sun protection is extremely important during this period of time.

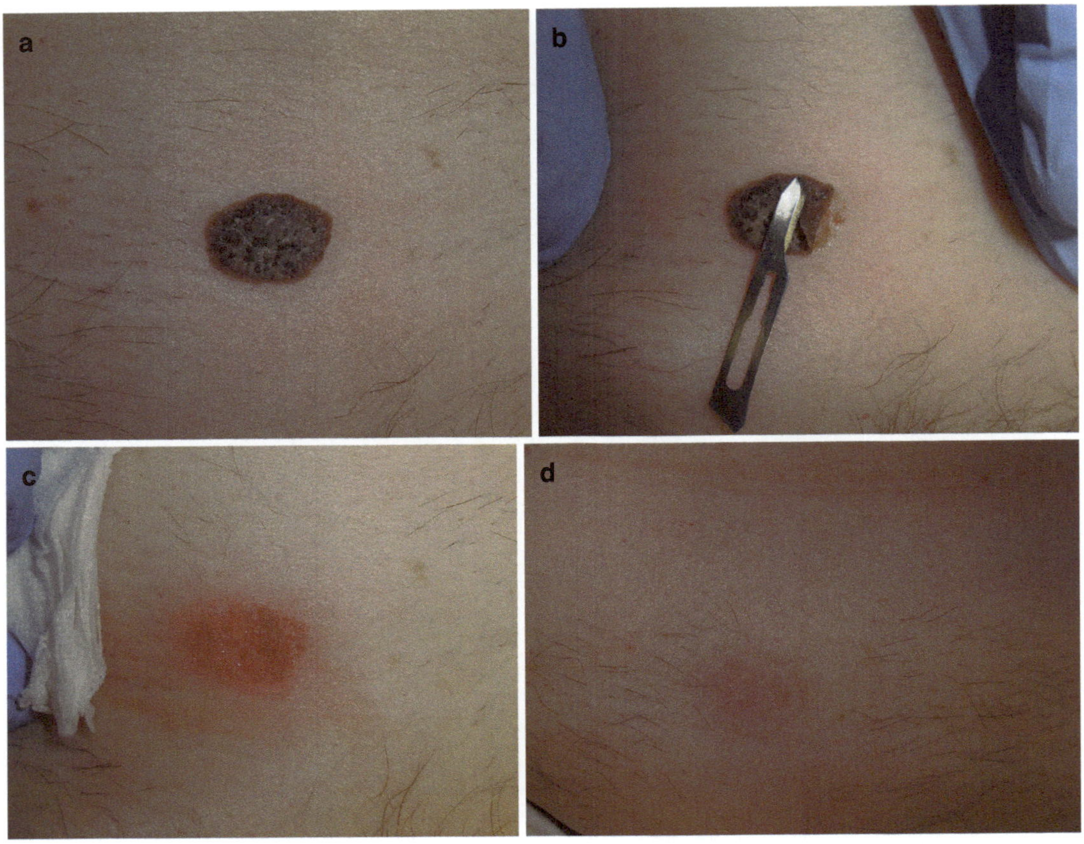

Fig. 8.5 (**a**) Seborrheic keratosis during thawing time. Center is still frozen. (**b**) Curettage with scalpel during thawing (still partially frozen lesion). (**c**) Vasodilation of the base with complete thawing and once the lesion has been completely curetted. (**d**) Three months post cryosurgery

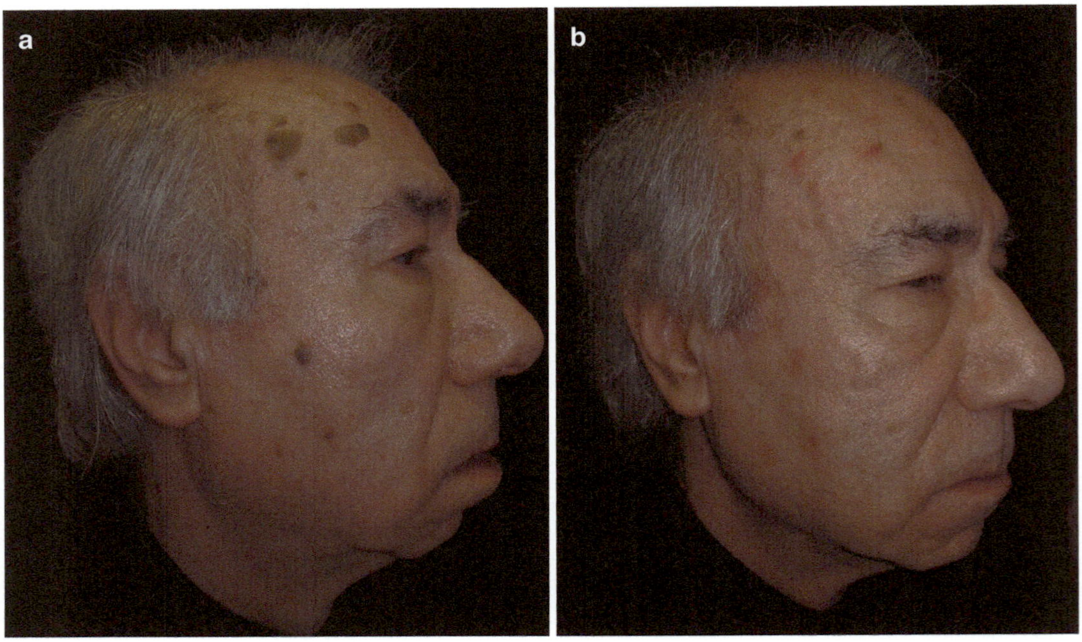

Fig. 8.6 (**a**) Multiple seborrheic keratosis on the face. One single cycle, spraying technique. (**b**) One month after treatment. Pink coloration still visible in treated areas

8.13 Sebaceous Hyperplasia

Sebaceous hyperplasia responds well to one cycle of closed technique (probe) cryosurgery. A 2 mm probe is ideal for treating these lesions. No local anesthesia is required. Since these are facial lesions, complete healing usually takes 1 week. Sun protection is extremely important during this period of time.

8.14 Skin Tags

Skin tags are ideally treated with tweezers (Fig. 8.7). Once the lesion is grabbed with a previously frozen tweezer, the freezing front is allowed to advance up to the skin surface (Fig. 8.8) and at maximum one extra millimeter. Spraying is only recommended in sessile lesions, and the use of cones is recommended to avoid freezing healthy perilesional skin. In order to avoid residual hyperpigmentation, protecting the perilesional skin is particularly important in type III or darker skin.

8.15 Pearly Penile Papules

Pearly penile papules, when protruding, are easily treated by cryotweezers, and one single treatment is usually enough. Other options include cryospraying the lesions with a C tip (treatment has to be repeated after a month) [23, 24]. No local anesthesia is required. No secondary effects have been reported.

8.16 Chromomycosis

This is a very difficult disease to treat [25]; it is often refractory to various therapeutic approaches and relapses are frequent. One option is cryosurgery [26]; a positive experience with a monthly cryospray session of the entire lesion combined with oral itraconazole (300–400 mg/day) for 6–8 months has been reported [27].

8.17 Molluscum Contagiosum

For most dermatologists, cryosurgery is the treatment of choice in molluscum contagiosum [28]. Many treatment regimens have been proposed [29, 30]. Depending on the lesion size, molluscum can be treated with open (spray) for large lesions, semi-open (cone) for intermediate size, and closed (probe) technique for small lesions. Spraying with tip D and intermittent spraying helps the operator gain precision. In children, previous topical anesthesia will reduce discomfort. Care should be taken to limit freezing to the lesion in order to avoid secondary

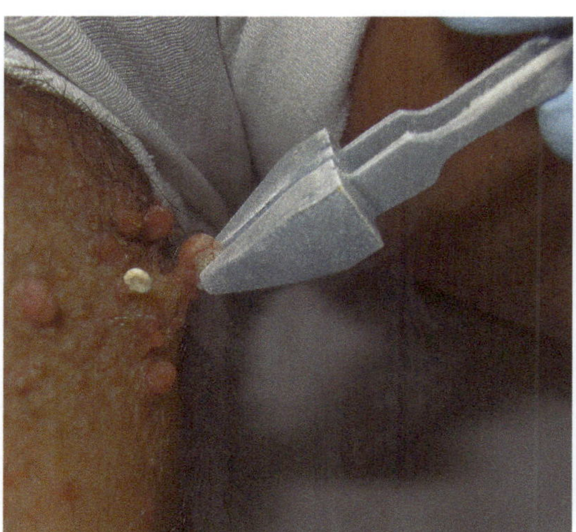

Fig. 8.7 Frozen cryotweezers grasping skin tag on inner thigh

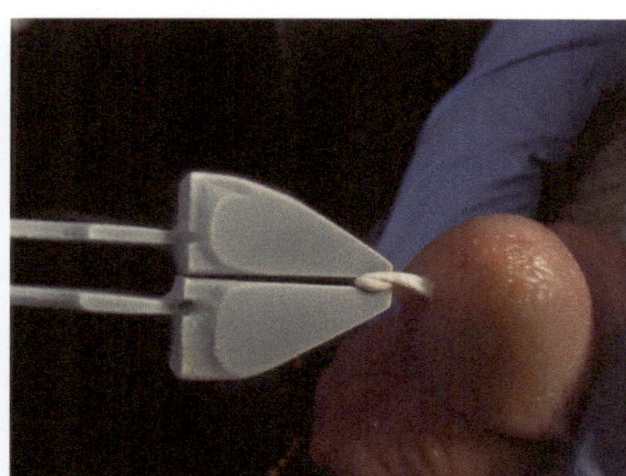

Fig. 8.8 Freezing with cryotweezers just to the base of the lesion. The lesion can be left to thaw and fall off in a few days or shaved at the base for biopsy

hyperpigmentation of the healthy skin. For protruding lesions, cryotweezers can be an excellent alternative technique.

8.18 Leishmaniasis

Cryosurgery is effective for eradication of acute cutaneous leishmaniasis. All leishmania species are very thermosensitive. Cryosurgery provides the lethal subzero temperature. Freezing can reach deep into the skin and mucous membranes [31]. Cryosurgery for cutaneous leishmaniasis displays many advantages. It is a simple method, has no need for anesthesia, produces rapid destruction of the leishmania organisms, is comparatively inexpensive, and is not associated with serious complications [32]. Various techniques with liquid nitrogen and carbon dioxide probe and slush have been used [33–35]. Liquid nitrogen is the cryogen of choice for the treatment of cutaneous leishmaniasis, and it is applied either in the open spray technique or in CryoProbe. Single or double freeze-thaw cycles are used with a freezing time of 10–30 s. Dipstick technique has been also used with freezing times of 15–20 s and a thaw time of 1 min in 2–3 sessions [36] (Fig. 8.9a–c).

A solid freezing is necessary to cause a bullous reaction. Healing and cosmetic results are excellent with negligible scar formation. Cryosurgery of cutaneous leishmaniasis has been combined with intralesional stibogluconate injection, providing superior results to either modality used separately [37].

8.19 Larva Migrans Cutanea (LMC)

Several treatment options have been proposed for LMC [38]. Although cryosurgery is not the first treatment option in LMC, it has been used in combination with oral medication [39], and it is an excellent alternative [40] for those patients who cannot receive the indicated topical or oral medication (thiabendazole, albendazole, ivermectin). A frequent reason for requiring use of cryosurgery is the lack of availability of the medication of choice. Oral treatment is occasionally not available or economically not feasible; this is usually the case in countries where LMC is endemic. Closed (contact) is the ideal technique [41] in order to avoid spraying and damaging healthy perilesional skin. Freezing should be performed at both ends of the larva trail. One freeze-thaw cycle is sufficient.

8.20 Cryosurgery and Other Benign Conditions

Results have been reported for conditions such as fibrous papules in tuberous sclerosis [42], lymphocytoma cutis [43], and granuloma faciale [44, 45], among others.

8.21 Postoperative Considerations

See Chap. 22. No major care is required after cryosurgery for benign lesions. Since it tends to be a superficial procedure, daily washing with water and soap and eventual application of an antibiotic ointment is sufficient.

Essential Tidbits

- The best treatment is the one you only need to do once. Still, in benign lesions it is best to undertreat and repeat treatment in a residual lesion than overtreat.
- Seborrheic keratosis (SK) can be frozen (one freeze-thaw cycle) and allowed to fall off, or the freeze-curette-local hemostasis approach (faster healing) can be used.
- Earlobe keloids respond better to cryosurgery when compared to other locations.
- In keloid treatment, do not remove the crust. Let it fall off spontaneously when dry.

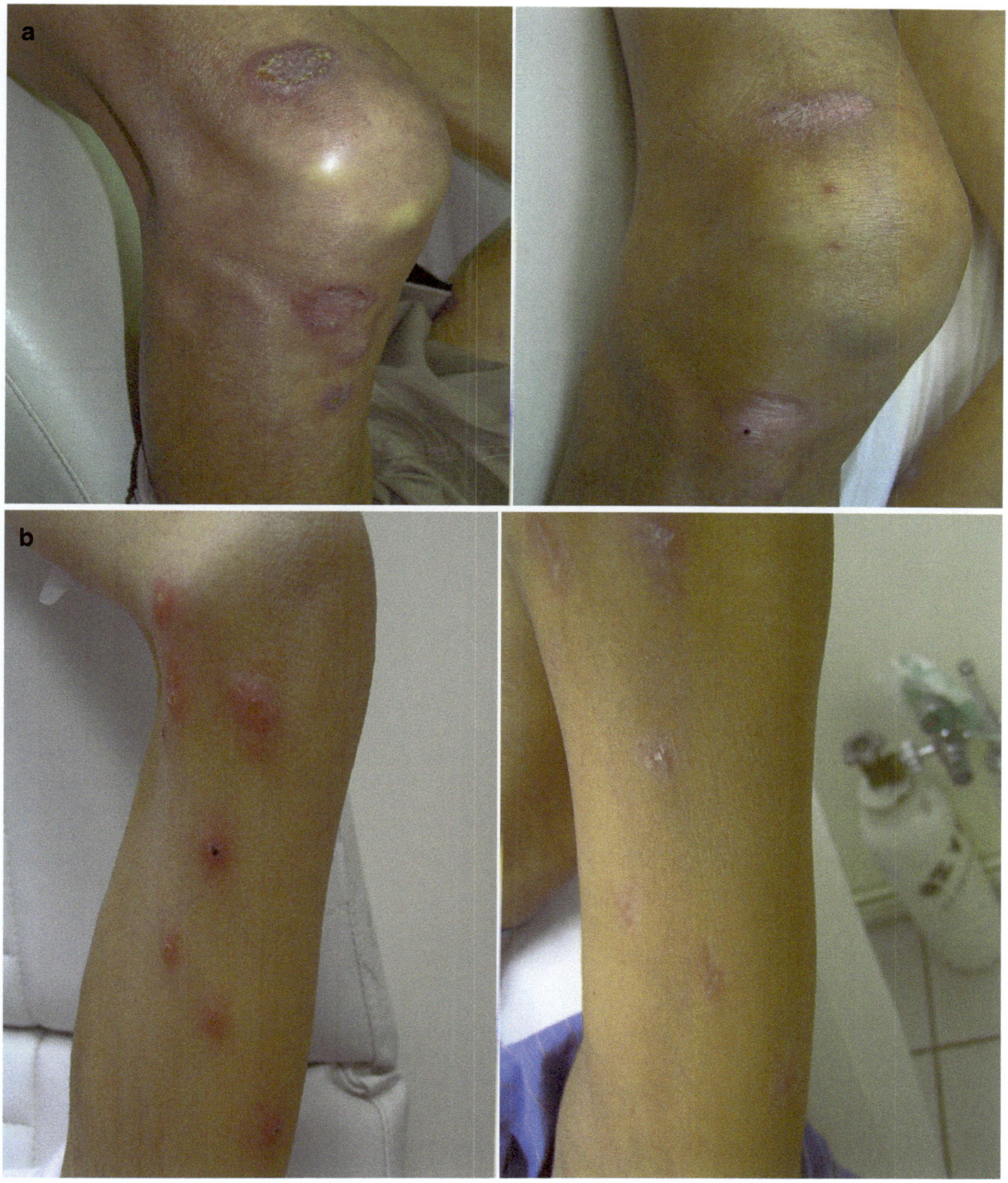

Fig. 8.9 (a–c) Leishmaniasis treated with cryosurgery. The freezing time for the three cases shown was of 15–20 s. Double freeze-thaw cycle, in two sessions

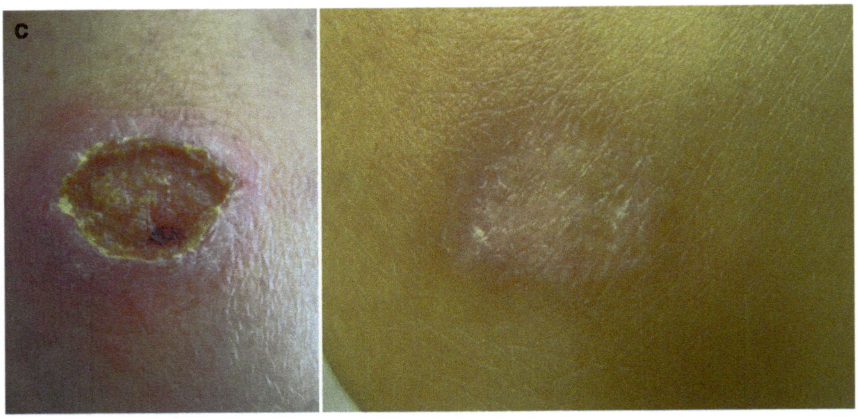

Fig. 8.9 (continued)

Conclusions

Most cryosurgery is performed on benign lesions. It is a technique relatively simple to learn, fast to perform, and with excellent cosmetic and curative results. In dark skin types, it is preferable to first test the procedure on small and hidden lesions in order to see the response and make sure no undesired hyperpigmentation occurs [46]. As a general rule, in benign lesions, it is best to undertreat than to leave a non-cosmetic pigmentation change or even a scar.

With proper training, dermatologist, family physicians [47], physician assistants, and nurses can perform most of the procedures as long as there is complete certainty of the diagnosis [48].

Glossary

LMC Larva migrans cutanea
LN Liquid nitrogen
P Probe or closed technique
S Spray or open technique
SK Seborrheic keratosis
SO Semi-open technique or cone technique
T Cryotweezer

References

1. Graham GF. Advances in cryosurgery during the past decade. Cutis. 1993;52(6):365–72.
2. Pasquali P. Cryosurgery. In: Robinson JK, Hanke CW, Siegel DM, Fratila A, editors. Surgery of the skin procedural dermatology. 2nd ed. Edinburgh/New York: Elsevier; 2010. p. 153–66.
3. Nolan JO. Cryosurgical treatment of rhinophyma. Case report. Plast Reconstr Surg. 1973;52(4):437–8.
4. Wiecko J, Sonnenberg Z. Nasal rhinophyma. Combined surgical treatment and cryotherapy. Otolaryngol Pol. 1985;39(3):204–10. [Article in Polish].
5. Sonnex TS, Dawber RP. Rhinophyma-treatment by liquid nitrogen spray cryosurgery. Clin Exp Dermatol. 1986;11(3):284–8.
6. Kempiak SJ, Lee PW, Pelle MT. Rhinophyma treated with cryosurgery. Dermatol Surg. 2009;35(3):543–5.
7. Machońko T, Grabowski T. Liquid nitrogen treatment of alopecia areata. Przegl Dermatol. 1981; 68(5–6):607–9. [Article in Polish].
8. Almond-Roesler B, Zouboulis CC. Successful treatment of solar lentigines by brief gentle cryosurgery using a Kryomed device. Br J Dermatol. 2000;143(1):216–8.
9. Wetmore SJ. Cryosurgery for common skin lesions. Treatment in family physicians' offices. Can Fam Physician. 1999;45:964–74.
10. Küçüktaş M, Kutlubay Z, Yardimci G, Khatib R, Tüzün Y. Comparison of effectiveness of electrocautery and cryotherapy in partial matrixectomy after partial nail extraction in the treatment of ingrown nails. Dermatol Surg. 2013;39(2):274–80.
11. Blume-Peytavi U, Zouboulis CC, Jacobi H, Scholz A, Bisson S, Orfanos CE. Successful outcome of cryosurgery in patients with granuloma annulare. Br J Dermatol. 1994;130(4):494–7.
12. Johnson BL. Keloids. In: Johnson BL, Moy R, White G, editors. Ethnic skin, medical and surgical. 1st ed. St. Louis: Mosby; 1998. p. 167–70.
13. Weshahi AH, Abdel HR. Intralesional cryosurgery and intralesional steroid injection: a good combination therapy for treatment of keloids and hypertrophic scars. Derm Ther. 2012;23:273–6.
14. Har-Shai Y, Amar M, Sabo E. Intralesional cryotherapy for enhancing the involution of hypertrophic scars and keloids. Plast Reconstr Surg. 2003;111(6):1841–52.
15. Careta MF, Fortes AC, Messina MC, Maruta CW. Combined treatment of earlobe keloids with

shaving, cryosurgery and intralesional steroid injection: a 1-year follow up. Dermatol Surg. 2013;39:734–8.
16. Zouboulis CC, Blume U, Büttner P, Orfanos CE. Outcomes of cryosurgery in keloids and hypertrophic scars: a prospective consecutive trial of case series. Arch Dermatol. 1993;129(9):1146–51.
17. Dawber RP, Sonnex T, Leonard J, Ralfs I. Myxoid cysts of the finger: treatment by liquid nitrogen spray cryosurgery. Clin Exp Dermatol. 1983;8(2):153–7.
18. Kuflik EG. Specific indications for cryosurgery of the nail unit. Myxoid cysts and periungual verrucae. J Dermatol Surg Oncol. 1992;18(8):702–6.
19. Böhler-Sommeregger K, Kutschera-Hienert G. Cryosurgical management of myxoid cysts. J Dermatol Surg Oncol. 1988;14(12):1405–8.
20. Waldinger TP, Wong RC, Taylor WB, Voorhees JJ. Cryotherapy improves prurigo nodularis. Arch Dermatol. 1984;120(12):1598–600.
21. Herron MD, Bowen AR, Krueger GG. Seborrheic keratoses: a study comparing the standard cryosurgery with topical calcipotriene, topical tazarotene, and topical imiquimod. Int J Dermatol. 2004;43(4):300–2.
22. Wood LD, Stucki JK, Hollenbeak CS, Miller JJ. Effectiveness of cryosurgery vs curettage in the treatment of seborrheic keratoses. JAMA Dermatol. 2013;149(1):108–9.
23. Ocampo-Candiani J, Cueva-Rodriguez JA. Cryosurgical treatment of pearly penile papules. J Am Acad Dermatol. 1996;35(3 Pt 1):486–7.
24. Porter WM, Bunker CB. Treatment of pearly penile papules with cryotherapy. Br J Dermatol. 2000;142(4): 847–8.
25. Queiroz-Telles F, Santos DW. Challenges in the therapy of chromoblastomycosis. Mycopathologia. 2013;175(5–6): 477–88.
26. Ameen M. Chromoblastomycosis: clinical presentation and management. Clin Exp Dermatol. 2009;34(8): 849–54.
27. Torres-Guerrero E, Isa-Isa R, Isa M, Arenas R. Chromoblastomycosis. Clin Dermatol. 2012;30(4): 403–8.
28. Hughes CM, Damon IK, Reynolds MG. Understanding U.S. healthcare providers' practices and experiences with molluscum contagiosum. PLoS One. 2013;8(10): e76948.
29. Handjani F, Behazin E, Sadati MS. Comparison of 10% potassium hydroxide solution versus cryotherapy in the treatment of molluscum contagiosum: an open randomized clinical trial. J Dermatolog Treat. 2014;25(3):249–50.
30. Gamble RG, Echols KF, Dellavalle RP. Imiquimod vs cryotherapy for molluscum contagiosum: a randomized controlled trial. Arch Dermatol. 2012;148(1):109–12.
31. Leibovici V, Homayoun A. Cryotherapy in acute cutaneous leismaniasis. Int J Dermatol. 1986;25:473–5.
32. Panagiotopoulos A, Stavropoulos P, Hasapi V, Papakostantinou AM, Petridis A, Katsambas A. Treatment of cutaneous leishmaniasis with cryosurgery. Int J Dermatol. 2005;44:749–52.
33. Bassiouny A, El Meshad M, Talaat M, et al. Cryosurgery in cutaneous leismaniasis. Br J Dermatol. 1982;107:467–74.
34. Faber WR. Cryosurgery for cutaneous leismaniasis. J Dermatol Surg Oncol. 1983;9:354–6.
35. Al-Qubati Y, Janiger EJ, Swartz RA. Cutaneous leismaniasis: cryosurgery using carbon dioxide slush in a resourse-poor country. Intern J Dermatol. 2012;51: 1217–20.
36. Al Majali O, Mehari Routh H, et al. A 2-year study of liquid nitrogen therapy in cutaneous leismaniasis. Int J Dermatol. 1997;36:460–2.
37. El Darouti MA, Rubaie SM. Cutaneous leismaniasis treatment with combined cryotherapy and intralesional stibogluconate injection. Int J Dermatol. 1990;29:56–9.
38. Albanese G, Venturi C, Galbiati G. Treatment of larva migrans cutanea (creeping eruption): a comparison between albendazole and traditional therapy. Int J Dermatol. 2001;40(1):67–71.
39. Kapadia N, Borhany T, Farooqui M. Use of liquid nitrogen and albendazole in successfully treating cutaneous larva migrans. J Coll Physicians Surg Pak. 2013;23(5):319–21.
40. Kamińska-Budzińska G, Krauze E, Pierzchała E, Lis A, Brzezińska-Wcisło L. Cutaneous larva migrans–an unusual case. Pol Merkur Lekarski. 2002;12(69):232–4. [Article in Polish].
41. Pasquali P, Trujillo B. Perlas Quirúrgicas: Opción crioquirúrgica ante infestación por larva migrans cutánea (Surgical Pearl: cryosurgical option in larva migrans cutánea) (Spanish). Dermat Venezolana. 2005;43. Available http://svdcd.org.ve/revista/2005/43/2/DV-2-05-Com2-LarMig.pdf
42. Dvir E, Hirshowitz B. The use of cryosurgery in treating the fibrous papules of tuberous sclerosis. Ann Plast Surg. 1980;4(2):158–60.
43. Kuflik AS, Schwartz RA. Lymphocytoma cutis: a series of five patients successfully treated with ryosurgery. J Am Acad Dermatol. 1992;26(3 Pt 2):449–52.
44. Dowlati B, Firooz A, Dowlati Y. Granuloma faciale: successful treatment of nine cases with a combination of cryotherapy and intralesional corticosteroid injection. Int J Dermatol. 1997;36(7):548–51.
45. Maillard H, Grognard C, Toledano C, Jan V, Machet L, Vaillant L. Granuloma faciale: efficacy of cryosurgery in 2 cases. Ann Dermatol Venereol. 2000;127(1):77–9. [Article in French].
46. Seirafi H, Fateh S, Farnaghi F, Ehsani AH, Noormohammadpour P. Efficacy and safety of long-pulse pulsed dye laser delivered with compression versus cryotherapy for treatment of solar lentigines. Indian J Dermatol. 2011;56(1):48–51.
47. Andrews MD. Cryosurgery for common skin conditions. Am Fam Physician. 2004;69(10):2365–72.
48. Graells J, Espinola A, Barrio C, Muñoz MD, Román A, Parellada N. Minor cutaneous ambulatory surgery and cryotherapy. Comparative study between a dermatologist and family physicians. Actas Dermosifiliogr. 2007;98(3):171–7. Spanish.

Cryosurgery for Warts

9

David Buckley

Contents

D. Buckley, MB, BCh, NUI, MRCGP
Solas Dermatology and Laser Clinic,
The Ashe Street Clinic, Tralee, County Kerry, Ireland
e-mail: info@asctralee.com

Key Points

- Never treat a lesion with cryosurgery unless certain of the diagnosis upon clinical assessment. If unsure of the diagnosis, refer the patient to a more experienced colleague or take a biopsy.
- The easiest and most successful way to treat most warts is by using liquid nitrogen via a closed handheld cryogun and the open spray technique.
- De-bulking warts with a surgical blade under local anaesthetic will lead to a far higher cure rate and a quicker postoperative recovery and is more comfortable for the patient.

9.1 Introduction

Warts (verruca vulgaris) are benign epidermal skin tumours that affect almost everyone at some stage in their life. There are many types of warts (Table 9.1) and over 100 subtypes of the human papillomavirus (HPV) that can affect various parts of the body (Table 9.2). HPV is not highly contagious and most warts will not penetrate intact skin. They usually need a portal of entry such as a crack or a cut in the skin to gain access. Diagnosis is usually obvious especially in children but warts can be more difficult to diagnose in certain areas such as the feet (Table 9.3) and genital areas. Warts are less common in the

P. Pasquali (ed.), *Cryosurgery: A Practical Manual*,
DOI 10.1007/978-3-662-43939-5_9,

Table 9.1 Names given to different types of warts

Types of warts	
Common term	Specific term
Common warts	Verruca vulgaris
Flat (plane) warts	Verruca plana
Filiform warts	
Periungual warts	
Plantar warts	Verruca plantaris
Butcher's warts	
Kissing warts	
Mosaic plantar warts	
Anogenital warts	Condyloma acuminata

Table 9.2 The most common subtypes of HPV causing warts

HPV subtypes causing warts	
Wart type	HPV subtype
Common	1,2,4,57
Plantar	1,2,4,57
Mosaic	2
Plane	3,10
Oral	6,11,32
Anogenital	6,11,16,18,31,33,35,55,56,58

Table 9.3 How to differentiate a plantar wart from a corn

Plantar wart	Corn
On any part of the sole of the foot	Over pressure points
Thrombosed capillaries	No vascular structures
More tender when squeezed	More tender when pressed
Well demarcated (white ring)	Poorly demarcated
More common in young people	More common in those >50 years old

elderly and can be confused with a basal cell (BCC) or squamous cell (SCC) carcinoma (Fig. 9.1). If in doubt, a biopsy should be taken or the patient referred for a second opinion.

Apart from anogenital warts, which are a risk factor for cervical cancer, most warts are harmless and 60 % clear spontaneously within 2 years without any treatment, especially in children and immunocompetent adults [1]. However, sometimes warts can continue to grow and spread to other parts of the body. The most common indication to treat warts is for cosmetic or comfort reasons. Warts in children are probably best left untreated unless they are particularly unsightly (i.e. warts on the face) or pain (i.e. large plantar warts). Doctors often underestimate the amount of embarrassment patients suffer with their warts, especially if they are on exposed areas (hands or face) (Fig. 9.2) and/or the patient is working with the public or is a food handler. There are many unanswered questions about the simple common wart. Why do some people appear to be immune, while other apparently healthy individuals can be plagued by persistent and recurrent warts?

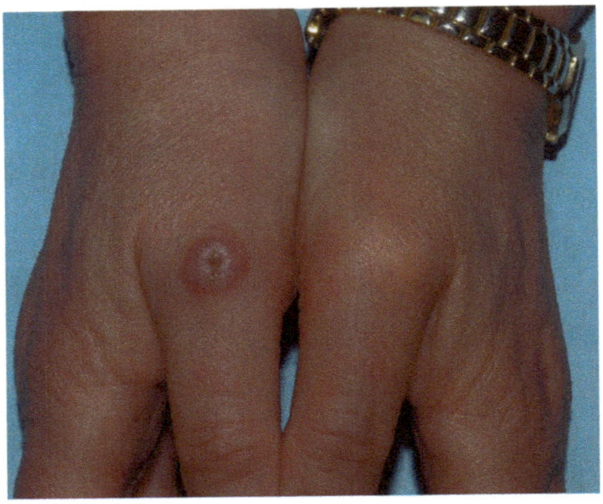

Fig. 9.1 A "warty"-looking growth on a 56-year-old woman's hand that was a squamous cell carcinoma in situ

Patients with a depressed immune system (poorly controlled diabetes, HIV, chemotherapy, lymphoma, transplant patients) are more vulnerable to warts, find it more difficult to clear them and often relapse after treatment (Fig. 9.3). In older patients, particularly if they are immunosuppressed, such as transplant patients, the wart virus may have oncogenic potential and can predispose to skin cancer such as squamous cell carcinomas.

Research into warts and their treatment are scanty and most of what is published is of poor quality and design. A recent Cochrane systemic review of 60 trials on warts showed that 46 (77 %) were classified as low quality, heterogeneity between trials was high and analysis was often inappropriate or misleading [2]. Comparison of different treatments is often difficult to assess, as the exact techniques used for treatment of the warts is not always described.

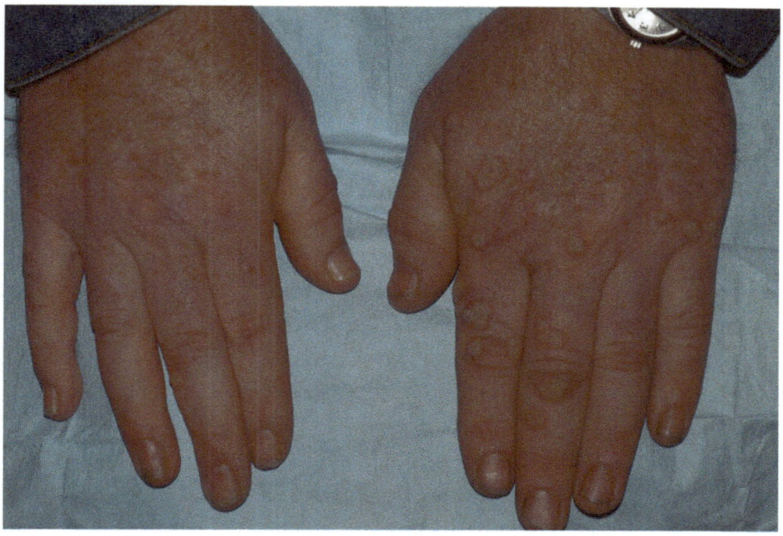

Fig. 9.2 Multiple hand warts

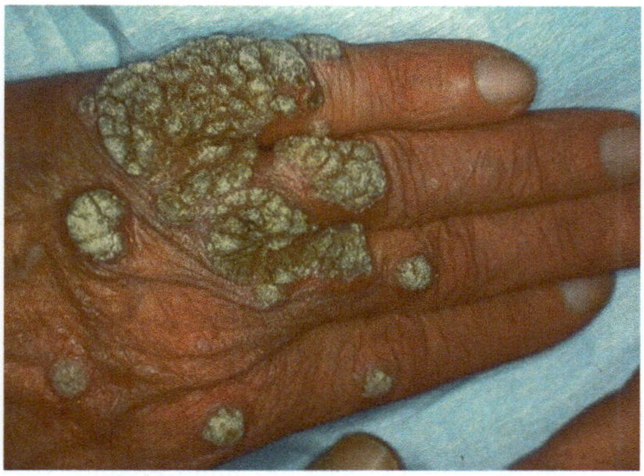

Fig. 9.3 Warts in an immunosuppressed patient

9.2 Nonsurgical Treatment

The decision to treat warts has to be made on a case-by-case basis according to the experience of the doctor, patient's preference and the application of evidence-based medicine (Table 9.4). If warts have to be treated (for pain or cosmetic concerns), the first line of treatment is usually with topical treatments with salicylic acid or a traditional cure. Traditional cures probably get their reputation by the fact that most warts will regress and clear spontaneously within time. A placebo has a 27 % success rate [2]. However, one should never underestimate the power of persuasion, wishful thinking and the ability of mind to cure the body.

Table 9.4 Most common treatment modalities used for the treatment of warts

No treatment
Traditional cure/placebo
Topical salicylic acid
Topical glutaraldehyde
Cryosurgery
5 % imiquimod
Topical podophyllotoxin
3 % formalin soaks
Monochloroacetic acid crystals embedded in 50 % salicylic acid
Pulse dye laser
Photo dynamic therapy
Curettage and cautery
Systemic retinoids
Intralesional bleomycin
Intralesional interferon
Intralesional immunotherapy

There are many over-the-counter topical agents used to treat warts in children and adults. Some of these are keratolytic such as salicylic acid which has a cure rate of up to 75 % if used daily for 12 weeks [3]. Others are verucidal such as glutaraldehyde. There is very little evidence to recommend one over the other. Success in treatment is often more dependent on the enthusiasm and persistence of the patient or parent. Most will work better if applied after paring down the keratin with an emery board or blade every night before applying the gel and continuing the treatment for at least 6–12 weeks. Most patients and parents give up long before this, unless is it clearly outlined to them how to apply the treatment and how long the treatment will take.

The 3 % formalin soaks daily for 6–12 weeks can sometimes help clear mosaic plantar warts. The plantar wart should be pared down nightly with an emery board or file, and then the wart is soaked in a bowl of formalin or cotton wool soaked in formalin for 10–20 min. The surrounding healthy skin can be protected with Vaseline® if necessary.

Monochloroacetic acid crystals embedded in 50 % salicylic acid cream can be helpful in isolated plantar warts, less than 10 mm, in patients who are not suitable for cryosurgery or other topical agents. The cream and crystals are held in place over the wart using a corn plaster and tape for 3 days. It causes a sterile abscess which lifts the wart from the surrounding skin. The abscess needs to be incised and drained (which can be difficult in children), and the plantar wart can be shelled out leaving a clean ulcer which will usually heal in 2–3 weeks.

Photodynamic therapy (PDT) has been used for treating warts, but it is time consuming and expensive, and results are variable.

Pulse dye lasers can be effective when treating warts that are not too bulky. Removing the thick keratin is important before laser treatment, as the light will not penetrate thick dark keratin. Like cryosurgery, this can be painful and may require local anaesthetic. One of the advantages is that there is little or no swelling or blistering; post laser treatment, bruising can last 1 week. It is thought to work by blocking the small feeding capillaries, thus causing an ischemic necrosis.

Intralesional bleomycin or interferon can be an effective treatment for resistant warts but is again expensive, very painful and only available in some hospital dermatology departments.

Intralesional immunotherapy using various antigens such as the MMR (measles, mumps, rubella) vaccine or candida skin test antigen causes a delayed-type hypersensitivity reaction increasing the ability of the immune system to recognise and clear the HPV. This has an 85 % cure rate [4].

9.3 Cryosurgical Treatment

Some patients (or their parents) with unsightly or painful warts do not want to use a cumbersome, uncomfortable, time-consuming treatment with topical agents such as salicylic acid that may only have a 75 % per cent cure rate after 12 weeks [3]. They will often prefer a 10 s treatment with cryosurgery (with local anaesthetic if necessary) with an over 90 % success rate, and the wound usually heals up in 2–3 weeks without scarring (Fig. 9.4a, b).

9.3.1 Warts

Cryosurgery is a method of selectively destroying unwanted tissue using cold liquids or gasses. The aim is to cause maximum tissue destruction in the target lesion with minimal collateral damage to the surrounding healthy structures. Cryosurgery does not kill the wart virus; in fact viruses can survive and be preserved in liquid nitrogen. Cryosurgery destroys the cells that are infected with the wart virus by creating intracellular ice crystal formation that ruptures the cell, thus allowing clean, healthy, uninfected cells to take their place. Post cryosurgery, there is a lot of swelling which blocks the small feeding vessels, causing ischaemic necrosis to the frozen area, enhancing cell death. In addition, cryosurgery has the unique action of "cryoimmunostimulation", whereby some of the wart virus is released from the frozen wart after cryosurgery, presenting the wart to the immune system. This acts like a vaccine, helping the body to fight off the HPV in the treated and sometimes even distant untreated warts. As a personal observation, occasionally patients clear their hand warts spontaneously while being treated for their plantar warts. Patients who have a suppressed immune system are less likely to benefit from "cryoimmunostimulation". Combining imiquimod (Aldara®) with cryosurgery may enhance this response.

There is only one important rule in cryosurgery: never freeze any lesion unless one is 100 % sure of the diagnosis. If a confident named

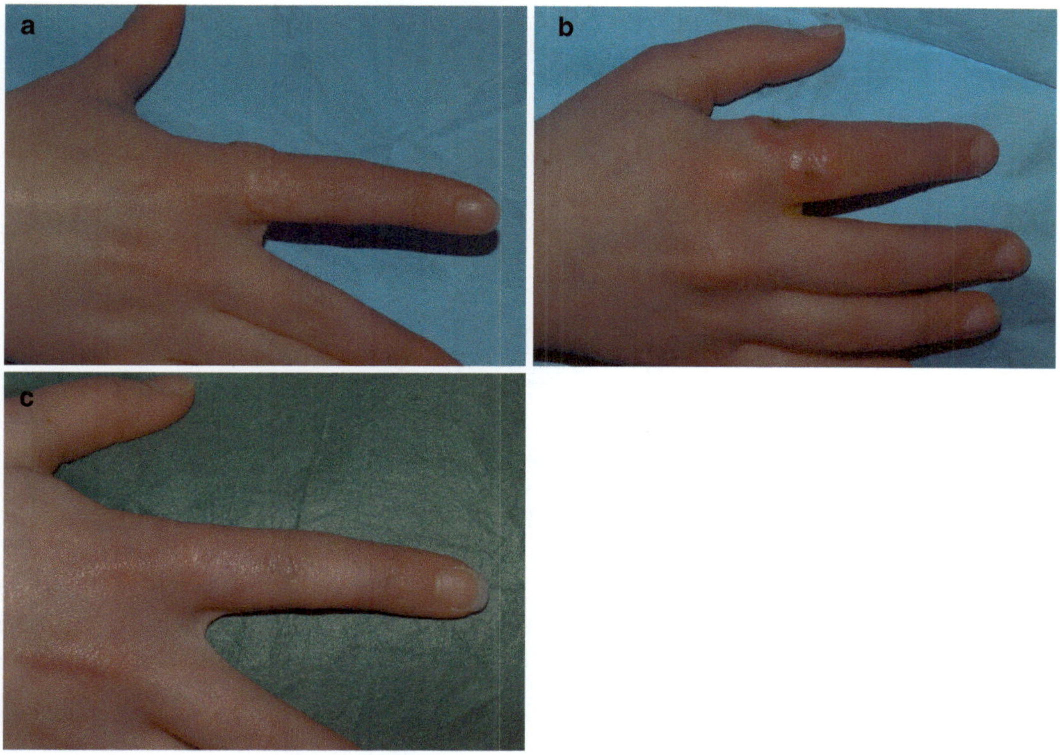

Fig. 9.4 Hand warts (**a**) before, (**b**) 1 week and (**c**) 2 months post cryosurgery

clinical diagnosis cannot be made do not freeze – take a biopsy or refer the patient for another opinion.

Success in cryosurgery is dependent on four main factors:

- Cryogen
- Delivery system
- Patient selection
- Technique

9.3.1.1 Cryogen

Maximum cell destruction is achieved by a rapid freeze, achieving temperatures of less than −40 C at the base of the lesion; a slow thaw; and carrying out at least two freeze-thaw cycles (Fig. 9.5). This can generally only be achieved by using liquid nitrogen which is the coldest (−196 °C), most versatile, cheapest cryogen available (Table 9.5). Over-the-counter cryogens such as home freezers like Wartner®, which contain a mixture of dimethyl ether and propane (DMEP), are much less effective as most only get down to −30 °C at the surface of the wart with a very slow freeze. Handheld medical devices such as the Histofreezer® or the DermaFreeze® also contain DMEP and are equally ineffective and far too expensive per unit cost to make them practical in clinical practice. Most of these devices are limited as they can only apply the cryogen via a bud applicator which is of a predefined shape and size, whereas warts come in all different shapes and sizes. Nitrous oxide gas, while not as cold as liquid nitrogen, can reach −89 °C and can give reasonably good results provided there is meticulous attention to technique.

Liquid nitrogen is cheap, safe and easily available and is the cryogen of choice for treating warts. A 21 liter extended holding time Dewar's flask will usually hold enough liquid nitrogen to last 10 weeks of frequent use.

9.3.1.2 Equipment

While the handheld cryogun is the best way to apply liquid nitrogen, cotton buds soaked in liquid nitrogen and applied to a pared-down wart are still far superior to home freezers such as the

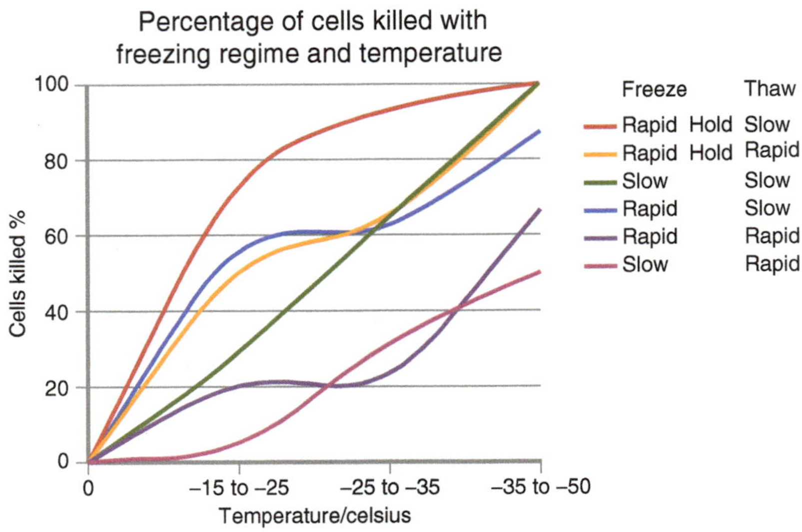

Fig. 9.5 Maximum cell destruction achieved by a rapid freeze-thaw cycle

Table 9.5 Different cryogens and their temperatures

Cryogens	Temp °C
Ice (water)	0
Ice (saturate salt and water mix)	–25
Dimethyl ether and propane in a cotton bud	–30
Nitrous oxide	–89
Liquid nitrogen	–196

Histofreezer® or nitrous oxide gas, particularly if the wart is well pared down or debunked before treatment. When using the cotton bud technique, do not use commercially available cotton buds. Make up your own by winding a large bud of cotton wool around the end of an orange stick and tapering it near the end. This will allow you to have a reservoir of liquid nitrogen which will slowly drip down to the tip when applying it to the wart for a long enough time (usually 10–20 s) before the liquid nitrogen eventually evaporates from the cotton bud. The cotton bud can be re-dipped into the liquid nitrogen to replenish it before each freeze of the warts. Liquid nitrogen should be stored in a polystyrene cup for this technique, and everything should be safely disposed of (the cup, the liquid nitrogen and the cotton buds) to prevent cross infection between patients (Fig. 9.6).

Liquid nitrogen cryosurgery via a closed, handheld cryogun is the safest, most effective, most versatile method to deliver a freeze. A cryogun is a surgical instrument just like a scalpel. Like a scalpel, a cryogun in one doctor's hands can work wonders, while in another doctor's hands it can cause a lot of harm.

9.3.1.3 Patient Selection

Patient selection is crucial in delivering effective cryosurgery. Children under the age of six do not make good candidates for cryosurgery for warts, and doctors should resist parental pressure to freeze warts in this age group. The only exception is freezing molluscum contagiosum, which usually clear up with a tiny, almost painless, three second freeze. Children between the ages of 6 and 12 years are generally poor candidates for cryosurgery unless the child (and not the parent) is highly motivated, can understand what is involved and is determined to have the treatment. As a personal opinion, I avoid treating children with cryosurgery for warts greater than 4 or 5 mm in diameter or a cluster of warts together, unless the child can tolerate a local anaesthetic injection. Other poor candidates for cryosurgery are needle phobics and patients with immunosuppression such as poorly controlled diabetics.

9.3.1.4 Technique

There is a limit to the depth of freeze one can achieve with cryosurgery. Hypertrophic warts are often covered with thick keratin, which acts as a

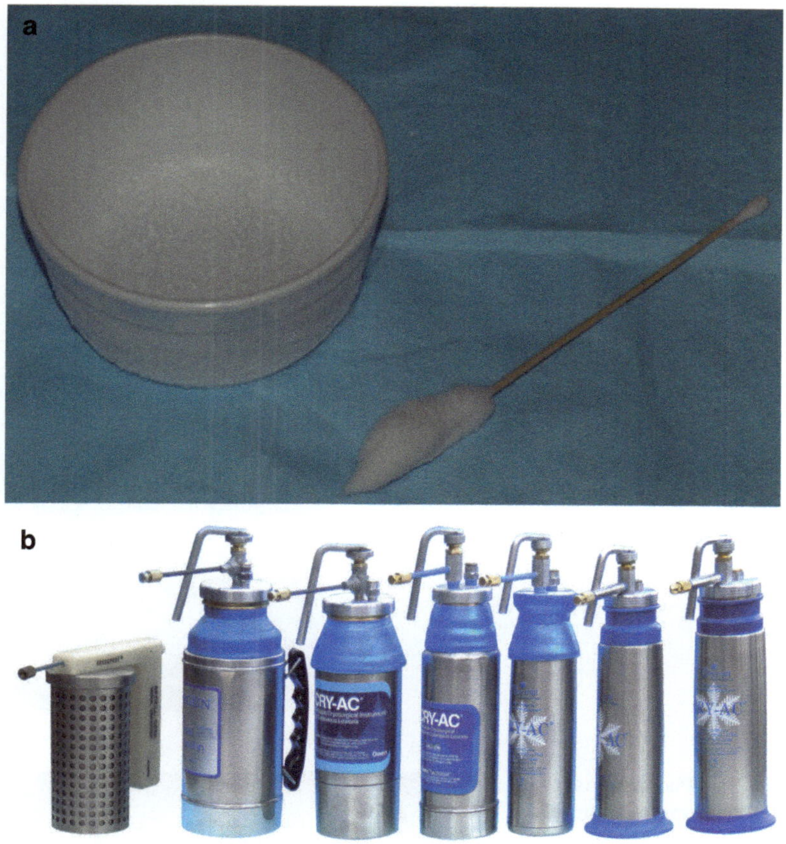

Fig. 9.6 (**a**) Equipment for the cotton bud technique for treating warts with liquid nitrogen (**b**) Development of cryoguns over the past 50 years (Used courtesy of Brymill Corporation)

thermal insulator. This has to be removed with a blade to allow the freeze to penetrate to the base of the wart. Even after removing keratin, many large warts can be 4 or 5 mm deep (Fig. 9.7). Success with cryosurgery is increased dramatically when a wart is de-bulked. Generally this can only be achieved by applying local anaesthetic and surgical paring down the wart. For hand warts, pare them down with a scalpel blade until they are flush with the surrounding skin before beginning cryosurgery. For plantar warts, pare them out leaving a crater to freeze into. In this way, probably 75–90 % of the wart is removed even before starting the freeze. Another bonus is that the local anaesthetic makes the whole procedure far more tolerable for the patients and more enjoyable for the doctor.

For most warts greater than 4 or 5 mm in diameter, or for a cluster of warts together, the discomfort of a prick with a 30 gauge needle with local anaesthetic is generally a lot less painful than trying to treat the wart using cryosurgery without local anaesthetic.

Emla® or Ametop® topical anaesthetic is not sufficient on its own to give good analgesia for treating ordinary warts. However, topical anaesthetics are useful in children and needle phobics, as it will allow injecting the local anaesthetic needle with little or no pain or discomfort. The biggest drawback with topical anaesthetics is that they take 30–60 min to work on the skin. Topical anaesthetics on their own work extremely well on mucous membranes (perianal, genital, lip and nostril) and usually work within 10–15 min on mucous membranes.

Local anaesthetic infiltrated with a 30 gauge needle around and under a wart is relatively painless, and it takes 2–3 min to work. Ring block anaesthesia can take 10 min to work. Use local anaesthetic with adrenaline everywhere except on the fingers, toes and the tip of the penis, as local anaesthetic with adrenaline lasts longer and reduces bleeding during and after treatment.

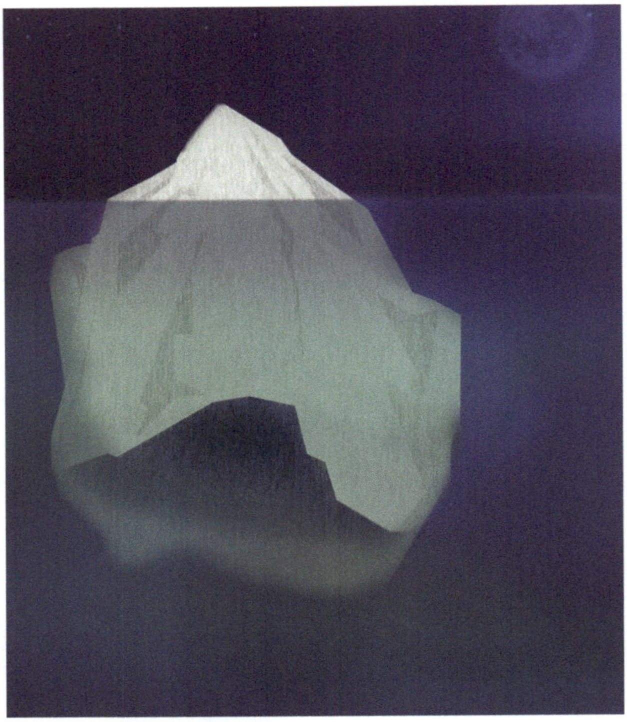

Fig. 9.7 Plantar warts are like icebergs. What you see on the surface is only a small part of the wart (Used with permission of the artist PaulGuzzo/Shutterstock.com.)

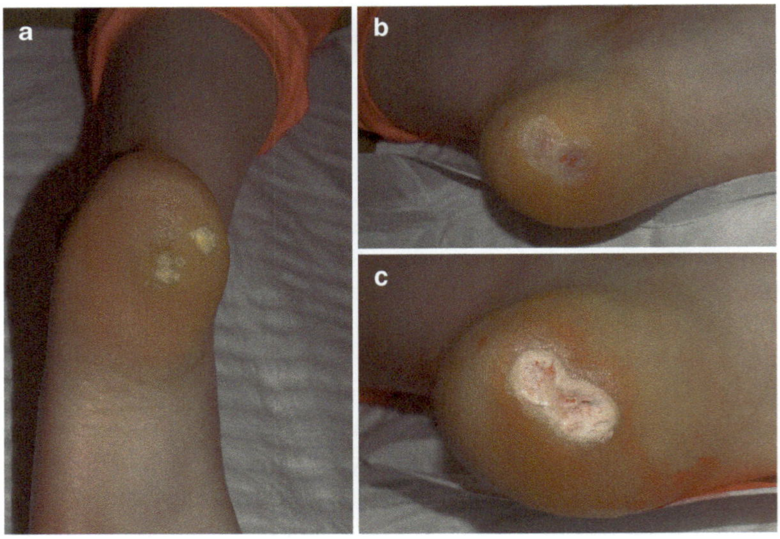

Fig. 9.8 Plantar warts (**a**) before paring, (**b**) immediately post paring and (**c**) immediately after one session of cryosurgery

With local anaesthetic, de-bulking the wart is easy and the cryosurgeon can deliver an adequate length of freeze and two freeze-thaw cycles without fear of the patient becoming distressed. Using this technique, clearing of 92.5 % of plantar warts can be achieved and 90 % of these clear with one single treatment [5] (Fig. 9.8a, b). Another advantage to de-bulking is that there is less necrotic tissue to die off post cryosurgery.

A possible disadvantage is that there can be bleeding while shaving the wart. Stop any bleeding before starting to freeze to maintain local low freezing temperatures. Use alginate dressings, aluminium chloride or cautery to control bleeding. Be careful not to contaminate the cryogun with blood. Put on a fresh glove just before picking it up for freezing.

Postoperative bleeding can usually be controlled with a pressure dressing and elevation. The

Table 9.6 Suggested freeze time and thaw cycles for some common viral skin conditions

Freeze-thaw cycles		
Type of wart	Freeze times (s)	Freeze-thaw cycles
Molluscum contagiosum	3	1
Periungual warts	7	1
Filiform warts	10	1
Anogenital warts	10	1–2
Common warts	10	2
Plantar warts	10–15	2
Mosaic plantar warts	15	2

warts swell up after cryosurgery, compressing the small capillaries, and the risk of bleeding is generally reduced after 24 h. Postoperative pain can usually be controlled by giving paracetamol immediately after the session of cryosurgery, before the local aesthetic has had time to wear off.

Most bulky warts require two freeze-thaw cycles (Table 9.6).

Freeze-Thaw Cycle

- Start freezing as quickly as possible until the whole wart is frozen.
- Continue freezing until a halo of normal uninfected skin, 1 or 2 mm, around the wart is also frozen.
- Continue to freeze (at a slower rate to avoid excessive lateral spread) for 10 s.
- Let the wart thaw out completely without heating, before starting a second freeze-thaw cycle exactly the same way, if required.

Most warts are best treated with the open spray technique which is quick and does not require any equipment or probes to be autoclaved between patients. For smaller warts, less than 10 mm, use the C or E spray tip, freezing with two consecutive 10 s freeze-thaw cycles. For larger warts, one could use the B spray tip. The contact probe technique is useful when needing to protect the underlying structure such as around the eye or nose. It is also slightly less painful. Applying a small amount of ultrasound gel to the tip of the probe allows the probe to stick to the wart during the freeze so that you can elevate the wart from the surrounding structures during the freeze. Any probes that touch the skin need to be autoclaved between patients.

Freezing down the auroscope (otoscope) cone is a useful technique for plantar warts, which allows getting a deeper penetration of the freeze, without too much lateral spread. This leads to a higher success rate with lower morbidity. Use local anaesthetic for plantar warts greater that 4 or 5 mm and de-bulk the area with a blade.

The auroscope cone needs to be 1 or 2 mm larger than the plantar wart and has to be pressed firmly on the target. Spray down the auroscope cone with a C or E spray tip for 10 s only as this is a much more concentrated form of cryosurgery than using the open spray technique. Most plantar warts require two freeze-thaw cycles with the auroscope cone technique. Start the second freeze as soon as the wart is completely thawed out after the first freeze.

Flat warts (plain warts) are usually quite superficial and so are much easier to treat. They do not usually require paring or de-bulking because they are usually small and can often be treated without local anaesthetic. Genital and mucous membrane warts are usually soft with no keratin, and again they do not usually require paring or de-bulking before cryosurgery.

The maximum number of times to freeze any one wart is two to three times. If they are not cleared after this, there is little point in persisting with cryosurgery. It is not infrequent to find patients that have undergone a series of suboptimal painful freezes on the same wart without local anaesthetic, with no de-bulking of the lesions, over the course of many weeks or months, resulting in a very low cure rate. This should not be done.

9.3.2 Anogenital Warts

Anogenital warts present unique problems as they are usually sexually transmitted and may predispose to cervical cancer, especially in smokers. All patients with genital warts should have a full STI screen and contact tracing. It is usually best carried out within an STI clinic. However, the warts can be treated by a GP/dermatologist/ob-gyn who has experience in wart therapies.

Podophyllotoxin (Warticon® or Condyline®), which has antimitotic activity, was the most common way to treat genital warts. However, nowadays most genital warts are treated with 5 % imiquimod cream (Aldara®) as it will help clear the clinical and subclinical warts. Aldara® is a topical immune response modifier that stimulates the patient's own immune response to help clear HPV. It should be applied overnight three times a week, for 6–12 weeks. Patients should be warned that the warts can become quite painful during this treatment. Recent surveys have shown that combining imiquimod with cryosurgery seems to be more effective that either treatment alone in the treatment of skin cancer ("cryoimmunostimulation") [6]. Combination of imiquimod followed by cryosurgery is recommended when there are large and numerous genital warts. Use imiquimod for the first 2 weeks; then treat the warts with gentle cryosurgery under topical anaesthetic (10 s freeze, one freeze-thaw cycles); then continue imiquimod post cryosurgery for another 4 weeks.

Special care should be taken with anal warts in immunosuppressed patients. Numerous, large or suspicious lesions have to be biopsied before any further treatment [7] to rule out malignancies (Fig. 9.9).

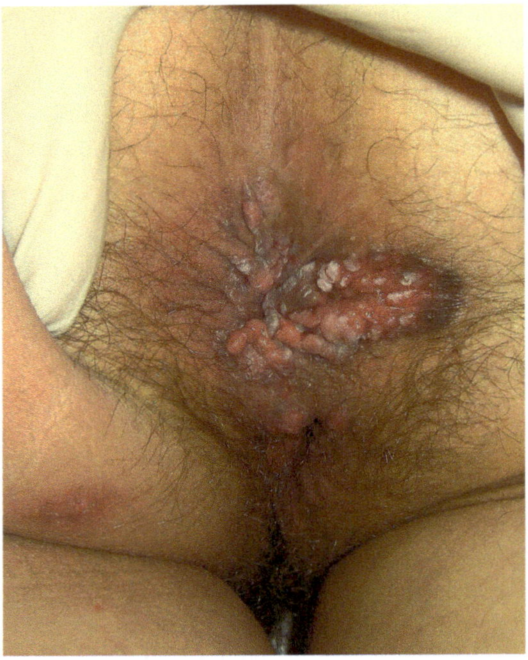

Fig. 9.9 Squamous cell carcinoma on an HIV + female patient with multiple anal condilomas (Courtesy of Paola Pasquali, MD)

When treating multiple penile condilomas, care should be taken not to freeze on the same day lesions all around the foreskin as oedema can cause a paraphimosis. Treat one side first. On the second session, treat the other side.

9.3.3 Periungual Warts

Periungual warts usually occur as a result of damage to the cuticle, which is normally self-inflicted from biting, picking or constantly wetting the hands. Harsh soaps, shampoos and washing-up liquids can also damage the cuticles. Periungual warts can be very difficult to manage, as periungual skin is very delicate.

The first treatment should be topical agents such as salicylic acid to be applied nightly for 6–12 weeks after paring down the wart. Treat with cryosurgery the remaining lesion.

Be careful in the periungual area as too aggressive a freeze may damage the nail plate, which could cause permanent damage to the nail. Use local anaesthetic (either a ring block or local infiltration using a 30-gauge needle and local anaesthetic without adrenalin) as it is a very painful area to freeze. De-bulk as much as possible with a blade, attempting to remove 75–90 % of wart. Sometimes part of the nail will have to be cut to allow proper de-bulking and adequate cryosurgery. Treat the base with a 5–7 s freeze and only one freeze-thaw cycle. If the wart has damaged the cuticle, there may be secondary nail dystrophy in the nail distal to the site of the wart. It is important to document this before starting cryosurgery; otherwise, the patient may blame cryosurgery for the damage to the nail plate. The nail dystrophy usually resolves once the wart clears and the cuticle regenerates, but this can take months (Fig. 9.10a–c).

9.3.4 Complications

Patients should be warned in advance that frozen warts will swell up, may blister and will take 2–4

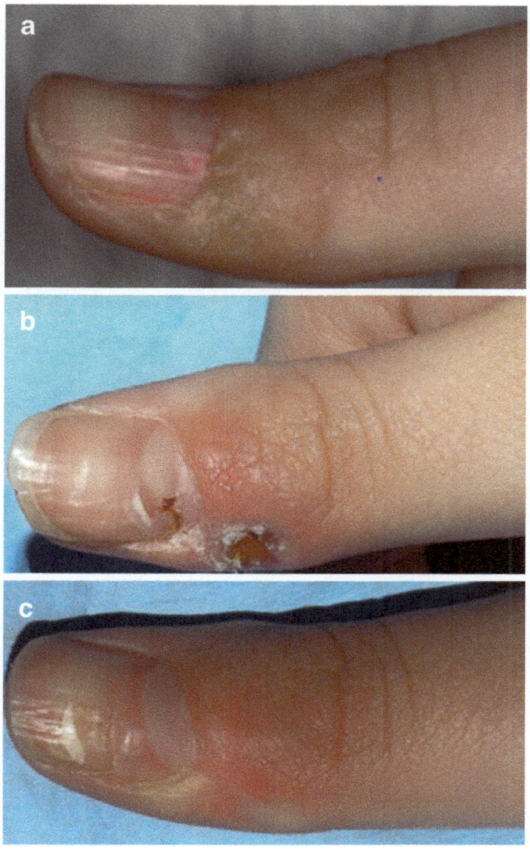

Fig. 9.10 Periungual warts (**a**) before, (**b**) 1 month after and (**c**) 2 months after cryosurgery

weeks to heal. Large mosaic plantar warts sometimes take 2 months to heal and can be very painful to walk on for at least the first few weeks. Patients should be instructed to wash the wound with an antiseptic every day and to burst any blisters with a sterile pin, leaving the roof of the blister to act as a natural dressing on the healing wart. Some cryosurgeons prefer to remove the blister completely.

For patients with multiple lesions in both feet and/or hands, a sound advice could be to treat one hand or one foot at a time and only do five to ten small warts per session. If patients have multiple warts, it may take three or four sessions to treat them all. Treat the large, unsightly or uncomfortable warts, and you may leave the other smaller warts for topical treatment, especially in children.

With more aggressive cryosurgery, swelling, blistering and pain is more likely. Provide verbal and written instructions on how to manage the wound post cryosurgery. Melanocytes are very sensitive to cold, and pigmented changes (hypopigmentation or hyperpigmentation) can sometimes occur particularly in dark-skinned patients. Pigment usually comes back after a few months, particularly when the freeze time is not more than 10 s with no more than two freeze-thaw cycles. Alopecia is a risk but this does not usually occur with the type of freeze-thaw cycles used for warts (10 s, two freeze-thaw style cycles). The myelin sheet of the nerve is relatively insensitive to cold. However when freezing over a nerve, for example, the digital nerve on the side of the finger, temporary numbness may occur but usually resolves after a few months. This has the added advantage of reducing postoperative pain after cryosurgery. Collagen and fibroblasts are the least sensitive to the cold, and this is why the skin usually heals without scarring when treating warts with cryosurgery.

The wart virus can display the Köbner phenomenon. The wart seeds in to a scratch or scar. This is sometimes helpful in diagnosing warts, such as a line of plain warts in a scar. The Köbner phenomenon can also cause warts to recur in the scar of previous surgery such as cautery, excision or cryosurgery, if the initial treatment is suboptimal and does not clear all the warts (Fig. 9.11a–c). This is another good reason to treat warts aggressively from the onset and attempt to kill all the wart-infected cells in one single session by combining surgical de-bulking followed by cryosurgery under local aesthetic.

Essential Titbits

- Keratin is a bad conducting material. De-bulking lesions prior to freezing will allow better penetration of the freezing front, reducing freezing time.
- Previously wet keratin (using a wet gauze applied for 1 min) will increase permeability and allow a better freezing procedure.
- Combination treatment with imiquimod enhances the response.

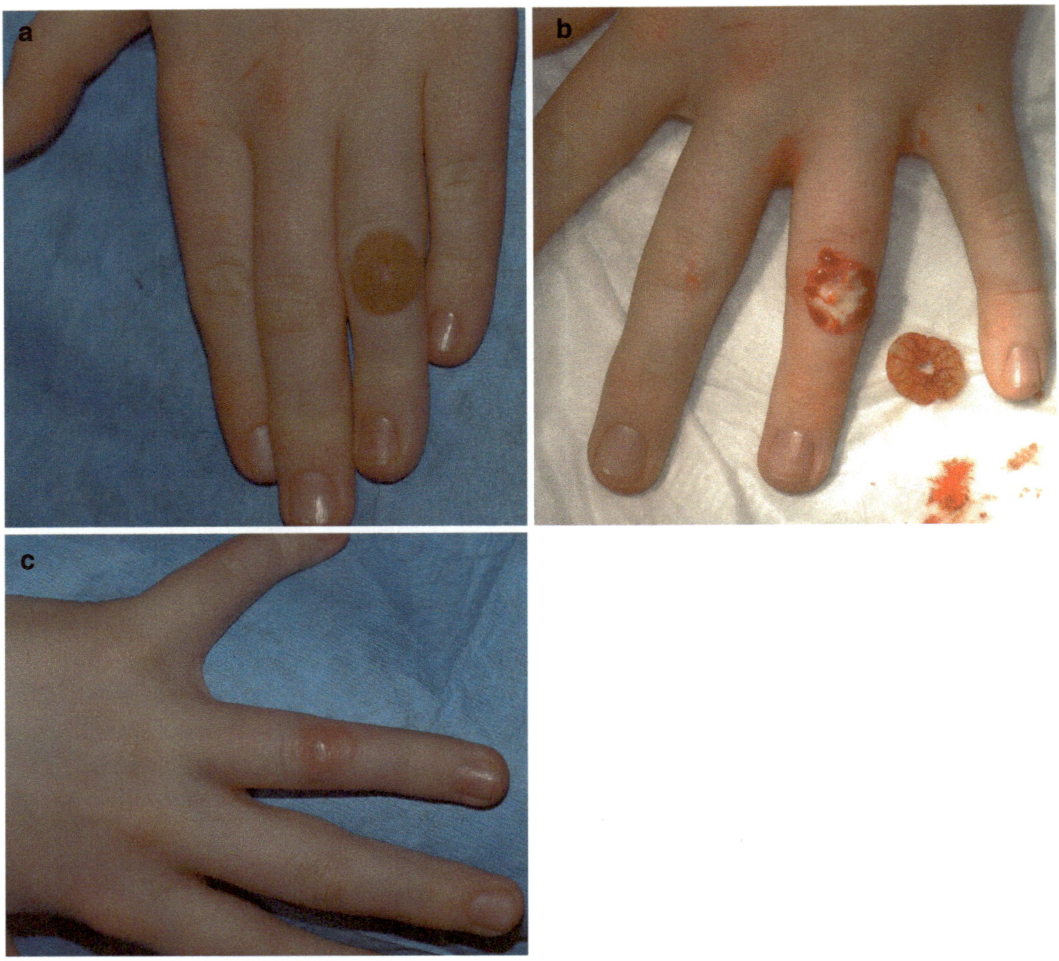

Fig. 9.11 (**a**) Wart recurring in the scar of a previous suboptimal freeze. (**b**) De-bulking of wart under local anaesthetic. (**c**) Shown 6 weeks post cryosurgery

9.4 What's Next in the Approach to Cryosurgery for Warts?

Combining imiquimod (Aldara®) with gentle cryosurgery has been shown to enhance the results of treatment for some skin cancers (immunocryosurgery, Chap. 20). This combination may also help in the treatment of recalcitrant viral warts (Fig. 9.12a, b).

Additional clinical studies aimed to establish differences between treatment wart modalities and recurrence rates are warranted.

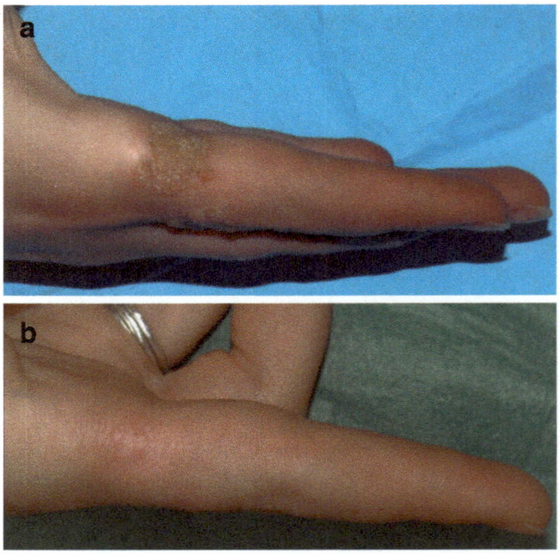

Fig. 9.12 Recalcitrant warts (**a**) before and (**b**) after two sessions of cryosurgery combined with imiquimod 5 % (Aldara®)

Glossary

Alopecia Hair loss

Cryogen Liquids or gasses used to lower temperature in tissues

Cryosurgery The controlled application of ultralow temperatures to tissues in order to achieve selective tissue necrosis

Cryoimmunostimulation Stimulation of the immune system by the release of tumour-specific antigens resulting in the production of anti-tumour antibodies after cryosurgery

De-bulked Surgical removal of part of a tumour so as to enhance the effectiveness of other treatments such as cryosurgery

DMEP Dimethyl ether and propane

HPV Human papillomavirus

Hypertrophic warts Warts with a lot of overlying thick hard keratin

Immunocryosurgery The combination of immuno-modulators and cryosurgery to enhance the cryoimmunostimulation response

Isotherms Lines linking areas of similar temperature

Keratin The hard outer layer of the skin

Molluscum contagiosum A viral infection for the skin caused by the poxvirus

Mosaic plantar warts A cluster of warts that coalesce to form one single large lesion

Mucus membranes Membranes lining body cavities and canals that lead to the outside of the body such as the respiratory, digestive and urogenital tracts

Nail dystrophy Misshaped, damaged, infected or discoloured nails

Necrotic Death of cells of tissues through injury or disease

Numbness When you cannot feel anything in part of your body or skin

Periungual warts Warts around the proximal end of the nail

Recalcitrant warts Warts resistant to standard therapies

Suboptimal Being below an optimal level or standard

Warts Benign epithelial tumours caused by infection by the human papillomavirus

References

1. Glover MG. Plantar warts. Foot-Ankle. 1990;11(3):172–8.
2. Gibbs S, Harvey I. Topical treatments for cutaneous warts. Cochrane Database Syst Rev. 2006;(3):CD001781.
3. Gibbs S, Harvey I, Sterling J, Stark R. Local treatments for cutaneous warts: systematic review. BMJ. 2002;325(7362):461.
4. Nofal A, Nofal E. Intralesional immunotherapy of common warts: successful treatment with mumps, measles, and rubella vaccine. J Eur Acad Dermatol Venerol. 2010;24:1166–70.
5. Buckley D. Cryosurgery treatment of planter warts. Ir Med J. 2000;93(5):140–3.
6. Gaitanis G, et al. Immunocryosurgery for basal cell carcinoma; results of a pilot, prospective, open-label study of cryosurgery during continued imiquimod application. J Eur Acad Dermatol Venerol. 2009;23:1427–31.
7. Kutlubay Z, Engin B, Zara T, Tüzün Y. Anogenital malignancies and premalignancies: facts and controversies. Clin Dermatol. 2013;31(4):362–73.

Cryosurgery for Benign Oral Lesions

10

Panagiota Loumou and Eleni A. Georgakopoulou

Contents

P. Loumou, MD, DDS, PhD (✉)
Second Department of Dermatology, University Hospital Attikon, 44 Nefelis Street, Athens 11853, Greece
e-mail: ploumou@yahoo.com

E.A. Georgakopoulou, MD, DDS, MSc
Department of Histology and Embryology, Medical School of Athens, 4 Fokaias str, 14232 Nea Ionia, Athens 14232, Greece
e-mail: eageorgakopoulou@gmail.com

Key Points

- Cryosurgery is a simple method for oral medicine with very short healing time.
- It is very effective in selected benign oral lesions especially in warts, mucocele, fibromas, and vascular lesions (venous lakes, hemangiomas, lymphangiomas).
- Both liquid nitrogen (LN) and nitrous oxide (NO) can be used as cryogens.

10.1 Introduction

In oral medicine, cryosurgery has been used for over 40 years. It is a simple, easy-to-use, and effective method which can contribute to the treatment of some diseases of the oral mucosa. Cryosurgery reduces the tissue temperatures to such a level that local cellular damage is evoked [1].

The therapeutic approach of many diseases of the oral mucosa has been influenced by the treatment of similar skin diseases, so cryosurgery has been applied as an alternative therapy in various lesions of the oral cavity.

The purpose of this chapter is to describe the indications and the cryosurgical techniques of benign oral lesions.

P. Pasquali (ed.), *Cryosurgery: A Practical Manual*,
DOI 10.1007/978-3-662-43939-5_10,

10.2 Oral Cryosurgery

The basis of safe and adequate application of cryosurgery on the oral mucosa is making the right diagnosis, carefully choosing prospective patients, specifying its indications, and applying the right technique [2]. Histologic examination is required to confirm the clinical diagnosis if it is needed.

Cryosurgery in the treatment of benign lesions of the oral cavity competes favorably with other therapeutic methods. Benign lesions usually require superficial freezing. As a general rule, it is better to undertreat than to overtreat and, if it is necessary, then to reapply. Local anesthesia usually is not required.

Both liquid nitrogen (LN) and nitrous oxide (NO) can be applied on oral lesions [2, 3].

Freezing time will depend on the type, size, and location of the lesion, and it usually varies between 5 and 20 s. One single or double freeze-thaw cycle can be used.

10.3 Advantages of Cryosurgery on the Oral Mucosa

The advantage of applying cryosurgery on the oral mucosa is due to the ability of the cryogen to agglutinate on the tissues and lead to controlled necrosis, aseptic inflammation, hemostasis, and topical anesthesia.

Some of the advantages of cryosurgery specifically in the oral cavity are summarized in Table 10.1 [3, 4]. The indications of cryosurgery in benign oral diseases are summarized in Table 10.2 [5–8].

Table 10.1 Advantages of cryosurgery in the oral cavity

Oral cavity is easily accessible
The moisture of the mouth and the soft tissue favor the rapid spread of ice ball
Possibility of using a local cream for anesthesia
Ease of postoperative follow-up and possibility of reapplication in case of residual disease
Minimum risk of postoperative bleeding
Postoperative infections are rare
Complications are rare
Healing is good
Cure rates are high

Table 10.2 Cryosurgery in benign oral diseases

Disease	Indications	Freezing time
HPV disease (Warts, condylomata acuminata, papillomas, focal epithelial hyperplasia)	+ + +	10–20 s
Fibroma	+ +	15–20 s
Mucocele	+ +	10–20 s
Pyogenic granuloma (as long as it is a confirmed diagnosis)	+	20–30 s
Venous lake	+++	15–30 s
Palatal papillary hyperplasia	+	30 s
Melanocytic macules of the lower lips	++	3–5 s
Lymphangioma	++	15–20 s
Hemangiomas (mostly small)	+++	15–20 s
Familial acanthosis nigricans	+++	15–20 s
Median lip fissure	+	10 s

10.4 Cryosurgical Techniques for Oral Cavity

Generally, for a *lege artis* cryosurgical procedure, a proper diagnosis, a good understanding of the basic principles of cryosurgery, a written consent from the patient, adequate illumination, use of sterilized equipment (probes, tips), and a chronometer are required.

For cryosurgery with LN as cryogen, we use the dipstick technique, the open (spray) or semi-open (cone) technique, and mainly the close (probe) technique [2].

Selection of the candidate lesion, its location in the oral cavity, its size, and the number of lesions are critical for a favorable result.

Selection of cryogen (liquid nitrogen vs. nitrous oxide) depends on several reasons. In general, nitrous oxide (NO) is preferred for benign oral lesions. Selection of a cryogen will depend on the experience of the cryosurgeon, availability of cryosurgical equipment, and location, size, and infiltration of the lesion. For instance, in lesions on the lips and posterior oral cavity, both cryogens can be used. For lesions located in the posterior oral cavity NO is used (better control of the technique, avoidance of the liquefaction of LN).

For small and superficial lesions, nitrous oxide is preferred. For example, NO is used for superficial mucoceles in children, while LN–CryoProbe technique is preferred for venous lake in the lips [9, 10].

10.5 Cryosurgery as First-Choice Treatment in the Oral Cavity [4, 5, 7, 11, 12]

There are a number of lesions where cryosurgery stands as the first choice of treatment. It gives extremely satisfactory results in less than a week with almost no scar. The postoperative procedure is very simple, and no local anesthesia is required. It is an office procedure that takes very little time. The treatment protocol is suggested in Table 10.3.

The lesions are:

1. Venous lake
2. Small hemangiomas (Fig. 10.1a–c)
3. Lymphangioma
4. Mucocele (Figs. 10.2a–d and 10.3a, b)
5. HPV (Fig. 10.4a, b)
6. Fibroma
7. Familial acanthosis nigricans
8. Focal epithelial hyperplasia

10.5.1 Venous Lake

Venous lake of the lips responds favorably to cryosurgery with the close (probe) technique yielding excellent cosmetic results. The freezing time can range between 15 and 30 s. Usually a single freeze-thaw cycle is sufficient [5, 13]. No local anesthesia is needed, and the patient has to be warned of the local edema which will last a few days.

Table 10.3 Treatment protocol

Name
Address
Date
Clinical photograph (before treatment)
Diagnosis
Location and size of the lesion
Histologic examination (if needed)
Technique
Freezing and thaw time
Cryogen used
Complications
Follow-up
Clinical photograph (after treatment)

10.5.2 Small Hemangiomas

Small hemangiomas can respond well to cryosurgical technique. A probe is used with a single or double freeze-thaw time of 10–20 s. Both liquid nitrogen (LN) or nitrous oxide (NO) can be used [14].

10.5.3 Lymphangiomas

Lesions especially on the tongue have been controlled by repeated applications of close (probe) technique. The probe has to be firmly applied until a halo of 1–2 mm appears [13]. The treatment can be repeated, in due time, as many times as necessary.

10.5.4 Mucocele

Mucocele responds favorably to cryosurgery. Mucocele of the lip can be frozen solidly with slight pressure until a normal frozen rim appears outside the border of the lesion. The lesion is first de-roofed for evacuation of the gelatinous material. Repeat treatments may be required in 8 week intervals [13].

10.5.5 HPV Lesions

Warts respond favorably to cryosurgery. The spray technique is used. The entire lesion is frozen with a slight amount of base and surrounding rim [4, 10]. Condylomata acuminata also respond well to cryosurgery with both liquid nitrogen and nitrous oxide [5, 13]. Focal epithelial hyperplasia is especially suited for cryosurgery. Freezing time varies from 10 to 20 s [15].

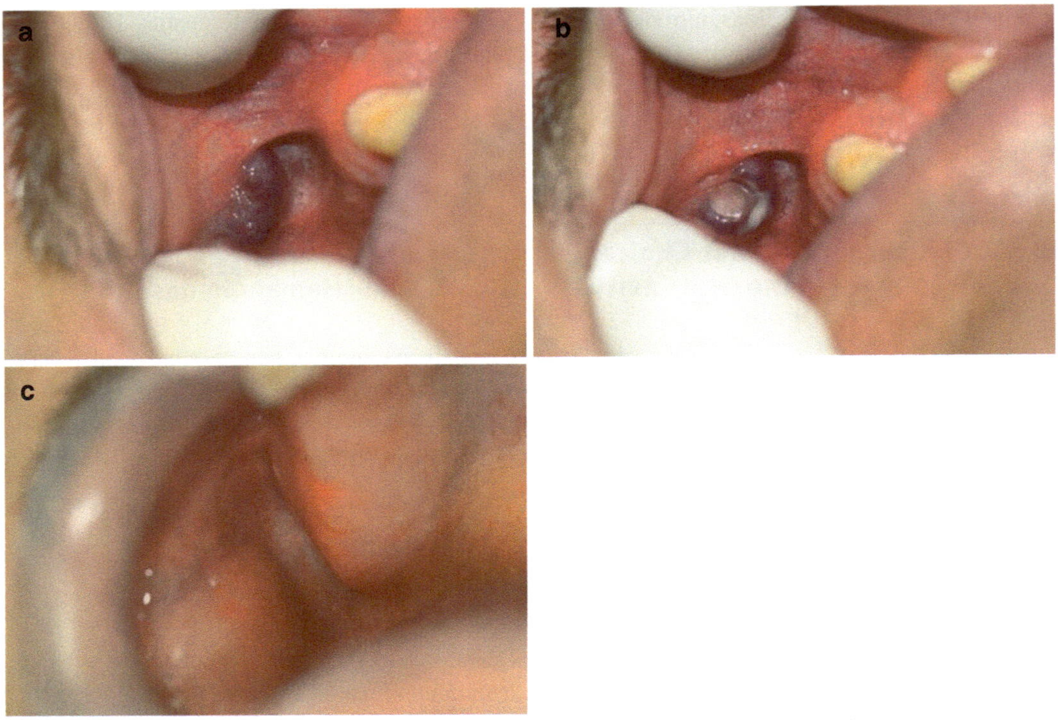

Fig. 10.1 (**a**) Hemangioma on the right buccal mucosa. (**b**) Treatment with close (probe) technique, freezing time: 15 s; double freeze-thaw cycles. (**c**) 1 year later

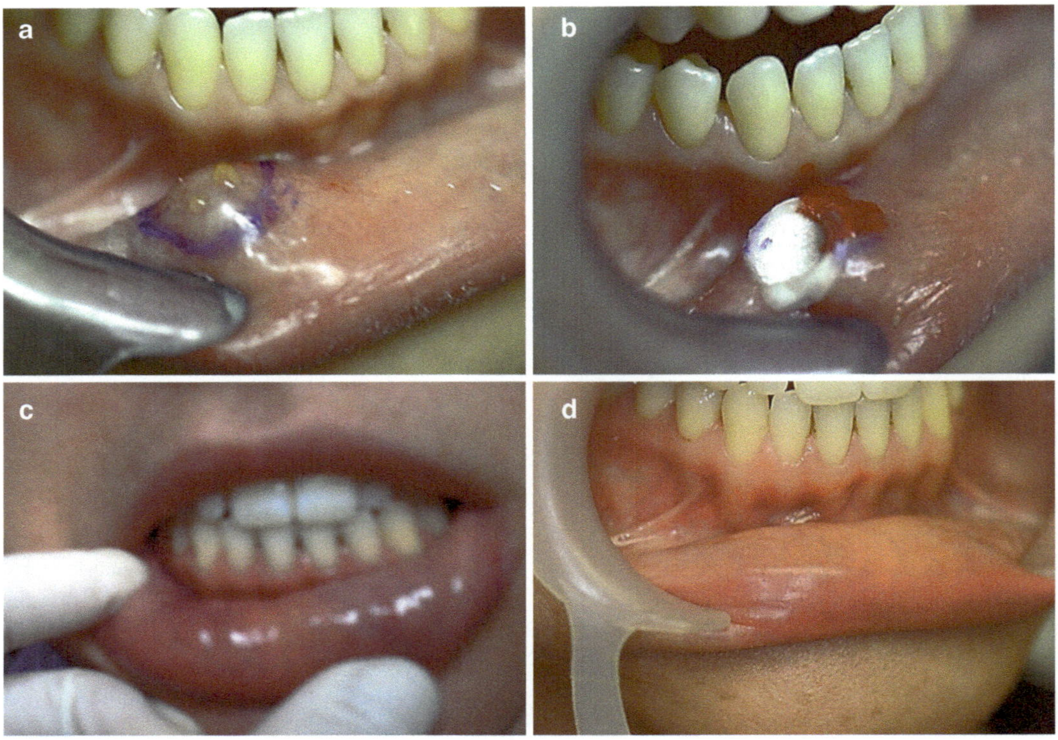

Fig. 10.2 (**a**) Mucocele on the lower lip. (**b**) Close technique (probe), freezing time: 15 s; double freeze-thaw cycles. (**c**) 1 year later. (**d**) 4 years later

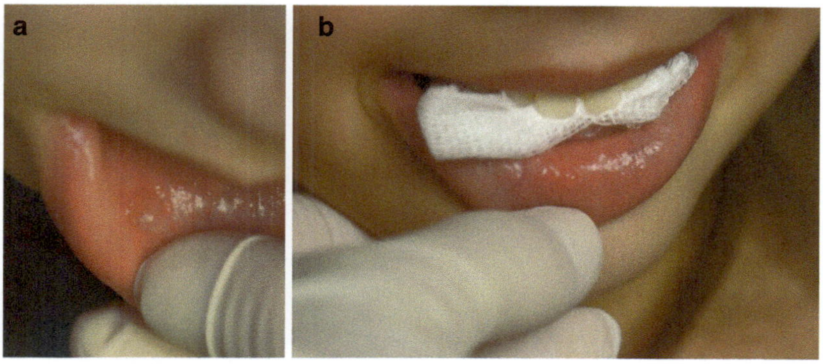

Fig. 10.3 (**a**) Mucocele on the lower lip. (**b**) Open spray technique, nitrous oxide FT: 5 s; double freeze-thaw time

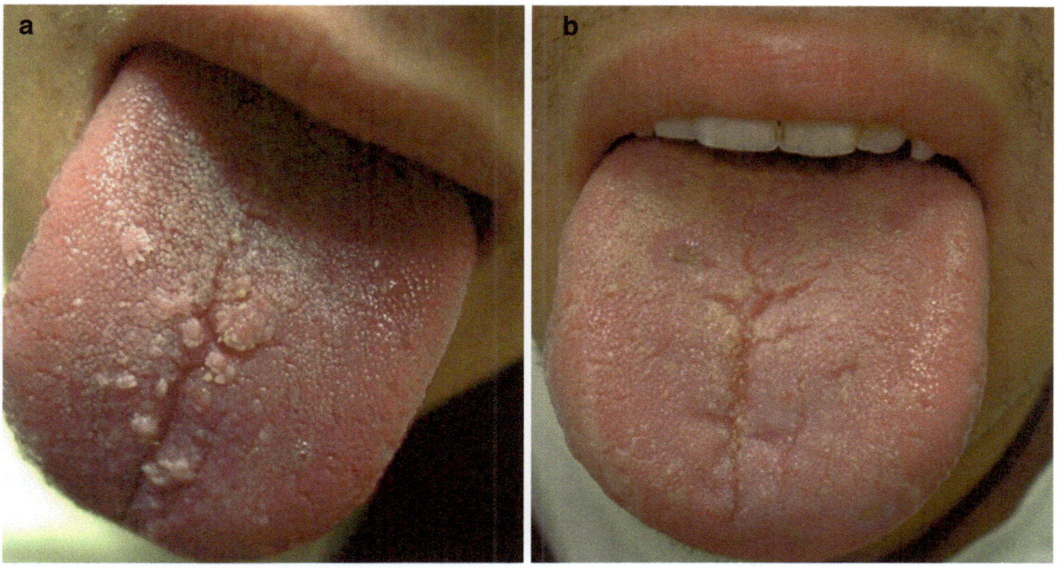

Fig. 10.4 (**a**) Condylomata acuminata. (**b**) Open spray technique, liquid nitrogen FT: 10 s; double freeze-thaw time in 5 sessions

10.5.6 Fibroma

Fibroma is the most common benign tumor of the oral cavity. Clinically, it looks like a well-defined, firm, sessile, or pedunculated tumor with a smooth surface of normal epithelium. The open spray technique is used. Freezing time varies between 10 and 15 s [4, 5].

10.5.7 Familial Acanthosis Nigricans

Cryosurgery is effective in the treatment of familial acanthosis nigricans. The open (spray) technique is used with a freezing time of 15–20 s. For a proper follow-up of patients, it is necessary to register the whole cryosurgical procedure.

10.6 Special Tips for Oral Cryosurgery

For minimizing complications (Table 10.4) of oral cryosurgery, the basic principles of cryosurgery and these special tips should be applied carefully:

- Cryosurgery is better used in anterior oral cavity and lips.
- Contact with the cryogen or liquefaction of the nitrogen in the posterior oral cavity could induce trauma, ulceration, or edema [4].

Table 10.4 Complications of oral cryosurgery

Swallowing liquid nitrogen drops
Damage of healthy tissue from unexpected freezing
Tooth pain
Tearing of the mucosa due to violent detachment of the cryogen
Pain
Edema
Sialadenitis
Discoloration of the skin in the borders of the lips
Notching of the vermillion border of the lip [3]

- In the oral cavity, application of probe technique is safer compared to other techniques [16, 17]
- Always protect the healthy mucosa from unexpected damage [11] (Fig. 10.5).
- In contact technique (liquid nitrogen), the probe is previously frozen and retracted gently at the end of the freezing time [3, 18]. Never force the probe out. Let it thaw and then remove it.
- In the event that the probe gets stuck and the operator desires to remove the probe to avoid excessive freezing, running some warm water helps remove it.
- Only small hemangiomas should be treated with cryosurgery in order to avoid development of excessive edema [4, 6].
- When cryosurgery is applied in the corners of the mouth, the required freezing time should be shorter because of the risk of constriction [5].
- The ducts of the major salivary glands should be protected to avoid sialadenitis [4, 17].
- A local antibiotic ointment is used on the treated lesion of the lips for 10 days [13].
- In treating mucocele, it is better to evacuate the content of the cyst before treatment [13] (Fig. 10.6).

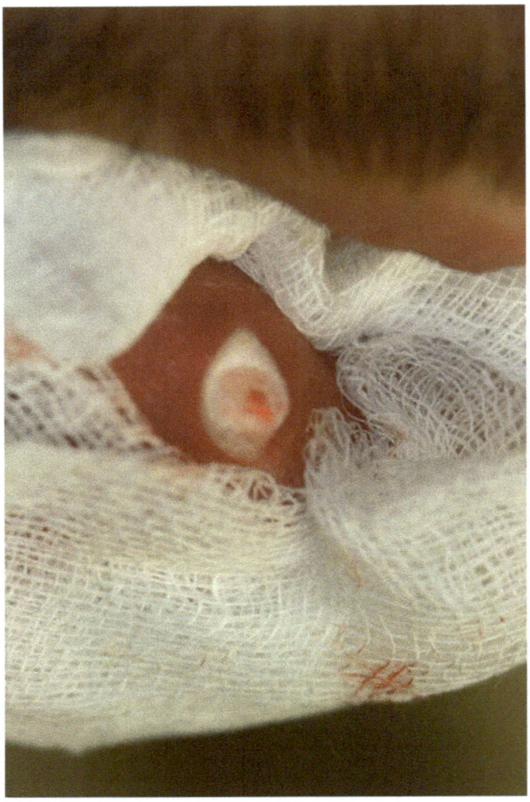

Fig. 10.5 Protection of the healthy mucosa

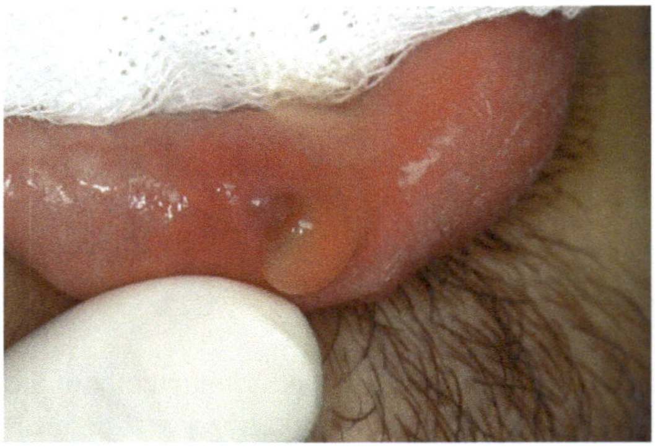

Fig. 10.6 Mucocele: evacuation of the gelatinous material

10.7 Posttreatment Care

It is better to provide written instructions after application of a cryosurgical procedure (Table 10.5) [13, 16, 19]. Patients must be informed about the edema, especially when treatment has been done to the lips. Although it will last just a few days, it can be a cause of concern.

Table 10.5 Instructions after cryosurgical treatment in oral diseases

Dear Sir or Madam:
You have been treated with cryosurgery
If you have any pain, you should take analgesics
You have to eat cold and soft foods for 2 days
No brushing if the wound is on the gums
A local antibiotic cream must be applied for 7–10 days if the wound is on the lips
Use antiseptic mouthwashes for 1 or 2 weeks period
In case of bleeding, you have to press solidly with wet oxygenated gauze for several minutes
In case of serious edema, you should seek medical advice
Your follow-up is in … days.

Essential Tidbits

- In probe (close) technique on mucosa, keep warm water at hand. If unable to detach the probe, let some warm water run until the frozen probe detaches.
- Most procedures do not require local anesthesia.
- Pre-freezing the probe will reduce the possibility of having it stuck to the mucosal surface. When using probes, make sure the patient stays still. Sudden movements can accidentally break a frozen tissue stoke to a probe.

Conclusions

Cryosurgery is a simple, easy, effective, and well-tested method. It is the first treatment option for many common lesions and can constitute a useful treatment alternative for a variety of diseases of the oral mucosa. The basic principles for safe and proper cryosurgery generally (and particularly in the mouth) are proper selection of patients, correct diagnosis, and good knowledge of cryosurgical techniques adapted to the oral cavity.

Glossary

Lege artis Doing something exactly according to fixed and approved rules of the artist and not by any improvised method

Nitrous oxide A cryogen with a boiling point of −88.48 °C. The temperature achieved at site is sufficient for benign lesions of the oral mucosa

References

1. Farah CS, Savage NW. Cryotherapy for treatment of oral lesions. Aust Dent J. 2006;51(1):2–5.
2. Sunitha J. Cryotherapy – a review. J Clin Diagn Res. 2010;4:2325–9 [serial online].
3. Dawnber RPR, Grover G, Jackson A. Cutaneous cryosurgery. London: Martin Dunitz; 1994.
4. Ishida C, Ramos-Silva M. Cryosurgery in oral lesions. Int J Dermatol. 1988;37:283–5.
5. Kufflik E. Cryosurgery updated. J Am Acad Dermatol. 1994;31:925–44.
6. Turjansky E,Stolar F. Lesiones de piel y Mucosas. Tecnicas Terapeuticas. Buones Aires: EDAMA ediciones; 1990.
7. Scully C, Bagan J, Eisen D, Porter S, Rogers R. Dermatology of the lips. Oxford: Isis Medical Media; 2000.
8. Cage A, Carnava J, Graham G. A comparison of instruments. Methods of monitoring freezing in cryosurgery. J Dermatol Surg Oncol. 1983;9:209–14.
9. Abbasi F, et al. Cryosurgical treatment of exophytic lesions of oral mucosa. Res J Biol Sci. 2008;3:899–900.

10. Ravi N, Bhavna M. Role of cryosurgery in the management of benign and premalignant lesions of the maxillofacial region. Ind J Dent Sci. 2012;4:63–6.
11. Graham F. Cryosurgery. Clin Plast Surg. 1993;20:131–47.
12. Regezi JA, Sciubba JJ, Jordan RC. Oral pathology. Philadelphia: Saunders; 2008.
13. Torre D, Lubritz R, Kufflik E. Practical cutaneous cryosurgery. Norwalk: Appleton and Lange; 1998.
14. Gongloff R. Treatment of intraoral hemangiomas with nitrous oxide cryosurgery. Oral Surg Oral Med Oral Pathol. 1983;56:20–4.
15. Vera-Iglesias E, García-Arpa M, Sánchez-Caminero P, Romero-Aguilera G, de la Cortina Calle P. Focal Epithelial Hyperplasia. Actas Dermosifiliogr. 2007;98:621–3.
16. Sailer H, Pajarolo G. Oral surgery for general dentist. Thieme. 1999;29:276–7.
17. Scala M, Margarino G, Meteu P, Giponi M. Cryosurgery in otorhynolaryngology. In: Korpan N, editor. Basics of cryosurgery. Wien/New York: Springer; 2001.
18. Cryotherapie RI. Le point sur les indications en stomatologie. Actuelle Odonto-Stomatologiques. 1984;164:251–63.
19. Cage A. Cryosurgery: mechanisms and applications. Paris: International Institute of Refrigeration; 1995.

Cryosurgery for Benign Eyelid Lesions

11

Raimo Suhonen and Paola Pasquali

Contents

R. Suhonen, MD, PhD
Department of Dermatology, Ikioma Medical Center, Kalevankatu 22, Mikkeli FI 50100, Finland
e-mail: raimos@iki.fi

P. Pasquali, MD (✉)
Department of Dermatology, Pius Hospital de Valls, 43800 Tarragona, Spain
e-mail: pasqualipaola@gmail.com

Key Points

- Cryosurgery is the treatment of choice for many common benign lesions on eyelids and conjunctiva.
- It is a safe, low-cost, and office-based procedure that provides excellent cosmetic results.
- Proper training and a high degree of knowledge about the anatomical structures of the eye are mandatory.

11.1 Introduction

For the treatment of lesions around the eye, an operator has to feel confident working around this area. Such confidence only comes with experience and deep knowledge of the anatomy. Many benign tumors or conditions can be present in the eye area. Some are common to other anatomical areas (like seborrheic keratosis), while others are specific to the eye (like trichiasis). Working in the eye area requires a high degree of knowledge about the anatomic structures. In the eyelid, many of these tumors can be removed with cryosurgery thanks to the excellent curative and cosmetic results. It is a safe and low-cost, office-based procedure; its versatility allows treatment of protruding, flat, or cystic lesions.

Several cryosurgical techniques can be used to treat these lesions [1, 2]. Open spray and tweezer

P. Pasquali (ed.), *Cryosurgery: A Practical Manual*,
DOI 10.1007/978-3-662-43939-5_11,

Table 11.1 Most common eyelid and conjunctival tumors amenable to cryosurgical treatment

	Anatomical location	Types of tumors	Suggested cryosurgical treatment
Eyelid	Benign tumors of the eyelid (Epidermis)	Eyelid squamous papilloma	T
		Eyelid seborrheic keratosis	S, P, SO
		Eyelid keratoacanthoma	S, P, SO, SC, T
		Eyelid cutaneous horns	T
	Premalignant tumors of the eyelid epidermis	Eyelid actinic keratosis	S, SO
	Eyelid sebaceous gland tumors	Eyelid sebaceous hyperplasia	P
	Eyelid sweat gland tumors	Eyelid syringoma	P
	Vascular tumors of the eyelid	Eyelid congenital capillary hemangioma	P
		Eyelid acquired hemangioma (cherry hemangioma)	P, S
		Eyelid varix	P
		Eyelid lymphangioma	P
		Eyelid pyogenic granuloma	P, S, T
	Eyelid histiocytic, myxoid, and fibrous lesions	Xanthelasma	S
	Eyelid cystic lesions simulating neoplasms	Eyelid eccrine and apocrine hidrocystoma	P
	Eyelid inflammatory lesions simulating neoplasms	Eyelid molluscum contagiosum infection	P, T
	Others: lid margin (hair structure)	Trichiasis	P, S
Conjunctiva	Vascular tumors and related lesions of the conjunctiva	Conjunctival capillary hemangioma	P
		Conjunctival pyogenic granuloma	P

Open or spray (*S*), close or probe (*P*), semiopen or cone (*SO*), semiclosed or cryocamera (*SC*), cryotweezer (*T*)

technique are the most commonly used. Probes are preferred when there is a need for compression, such as for hemangiomas or cysts. Based on the classification by Shield [3], some of these are presented in Table 11.1 and in the text that follows, and each condition will be discussed individually.

In benign lesions, deep freezing treatments should be avoided for patients with dark skin due to the risk of hypopigmentation.

11.2 Preparation

Proper protection of the eye is mandatory. Eye protectors should be plastic or wooden, never metal. If a spoon or spatula is going to be used, any sharp, casting, or protruding element must previously be eliminated (Fig. 11.1).

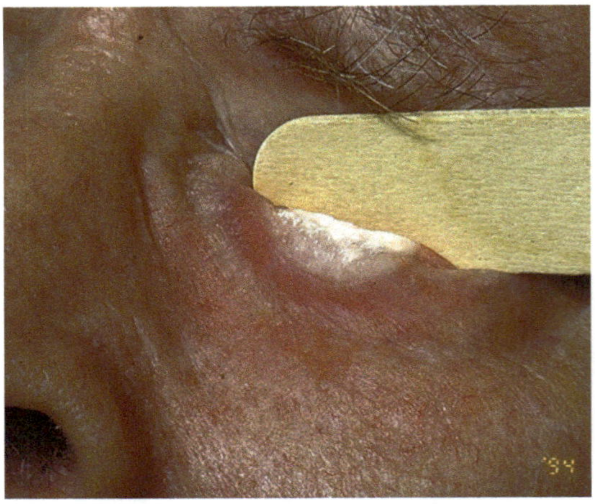

Fig. 11.1 Protection of the eyelid must be made of wood or plastic (never metal)

Touching the eye surface should be avoided at all times in order to prevent epithelial damage. For lower eyelid surgery, the upper eyelid can be pushed down to the lower conjunctival fornix and kept there for extra protection of the eye. Previous eye drops of

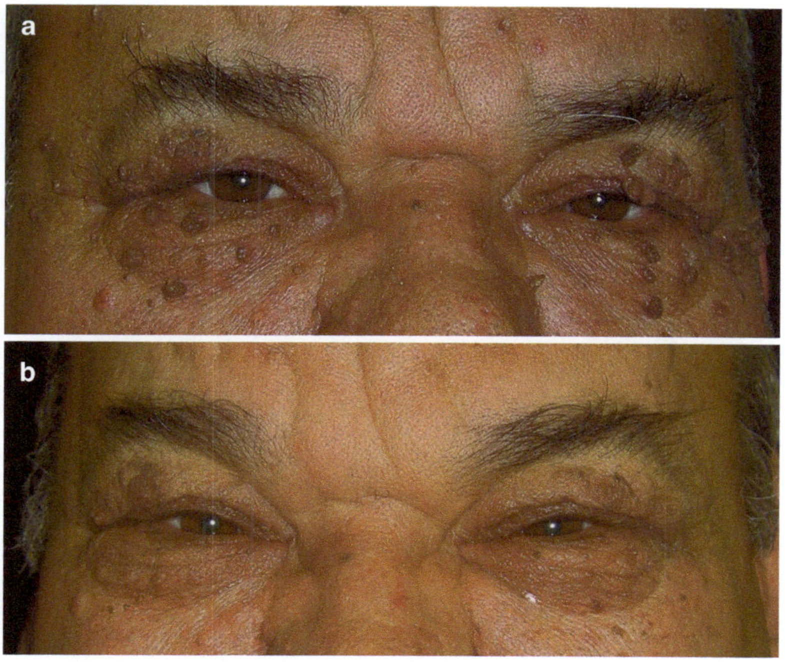

Fig. 11.2 (**a**, **b**) Multiple skin tags of the eyelids treated with one cycle cryotweezers (before and after treatment)

oxybuprocaine or tetracaine will be sufficient to anesthetize the conjunctival surface.

It is necessary to have a good binocular loupe or a 3D microscope [4] as well as a whole set of probes, cones, spraying tips, eye protectors, and high-quality forceps (the latter, for trichiasis/distichiasis treatment).

11.3 Tumors of the Eyelids

11.3.1 Benign Tumors of the Eyelid (Epidermis)

11.3.1.1 Eyelid Squamous Papilloma

These are also called fibroepithelial polyps, acrochordons, or skin tags. They are very common, can have different sizes, can be protruding, occur as single units or as multiples, and present in the upper and lower lids as well as on the lateral sides of the eye. Sometimes they impair the field of vision; for some patients, they are of cosmetic concern. Cryotweezers are probably the best treatment option because they are painless, multiple lesions can be treated in one session, and there is no risk of hyperpigmentation because freezing is done only to the base of the lesion and no further. This is an important consideration because skin tags are very common in 3/5 skin types (Fig. 11.2a, b). Eyelid warts are also a form of squamous papilloma. They are very common and present as solitary with a filiform/digitated shape. These are best treated by grasping them with a cryotweezer until the freezing front reaches the bottom of the lesion. One cycle is sufficient. Larger lesions can be sprayed with LN.

11.3.1.2 Eyelid Seborrheic Keratosis

These can be thin or thick, gray or brownish, or highly hyperpigmented, and there is usually a family tendency to present with them. They can be located anywhere in the lids (Fig. 11.3a, b) and sometimes occupy the lid margin (Fig. 11.4a, b), impairing the field of vision. Spraying with a small aperture should include a 1 mm margin of healthy skin to avoid ring-shaped recurrences or residual tumor. For lesions in the lid margin, it is best to use an appropriate size probe. The moisture in the area will help to fix the probe and control the advancing freezing zone. For those situations in which one desires to stop freezing and wants to detach the probe, a warm saline solution will do the job. One should not ever perform any forceful movements in the

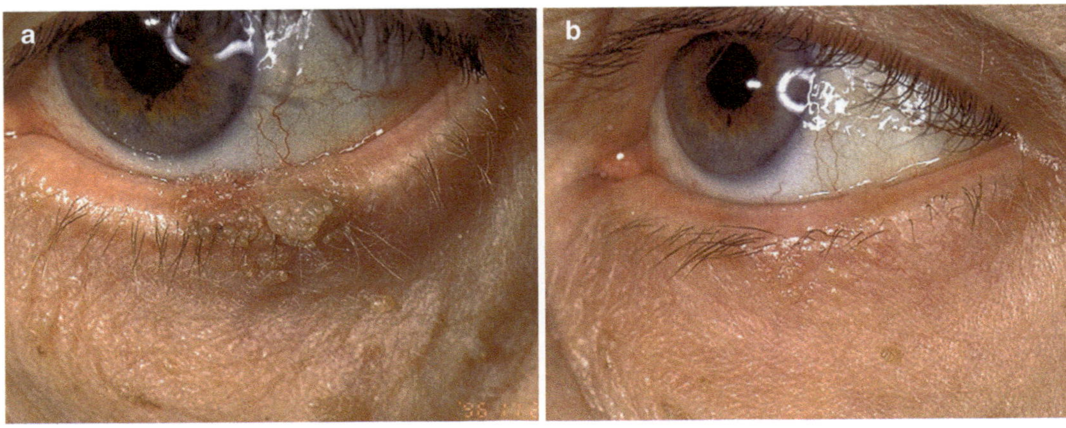

Fig. 11.3 (**a**, **b**) Seborrheic keratosis on the lower lid margin (before and after treatment). One cycle open (spraying) technique with protection of the eye

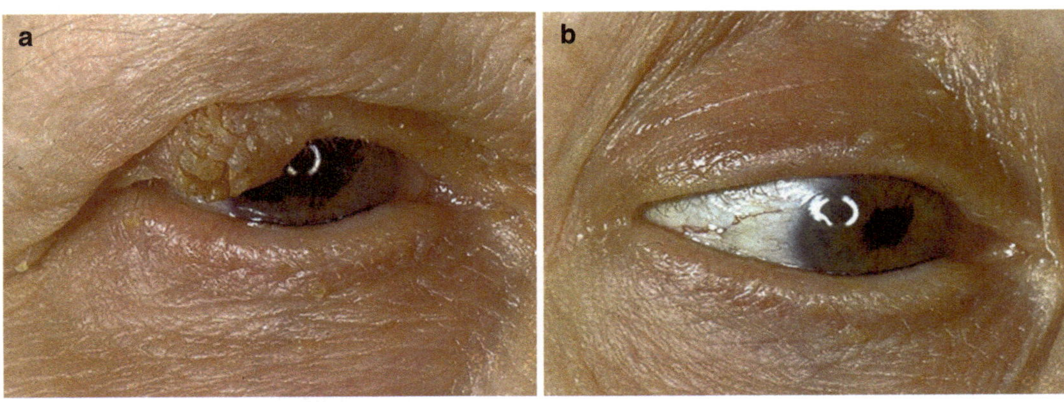

Fig. 11.4 (**a**, **b**) Seborrheic keratosis on the upper lid margin that impaired the field of vision (before and after treatment). One cycle close (contact probe) technique

eyelid. The freezing with a fixed probe is best done when the patient is in a lying position.

11.3.1.3 Eyelid Keratoacanthoma and Cutaneous Horns

In most dermatology reference books, keratoacanthomas are classified as well-differentiated squamous cell carcinomas. Eyelid keratoacanthomas are relatively frequent and have a typical dome-shaped appearance with a central crater or horn (Fig. 11.5). Cutaneous horns are classified by some as nonspecific keratosis. As a general recommendation, a biopsy of all cutaneous horns should be taken since some can have squamous cell carcinoma cells at the bottom. One technique that works very well for both lesions is to grab the lesion with

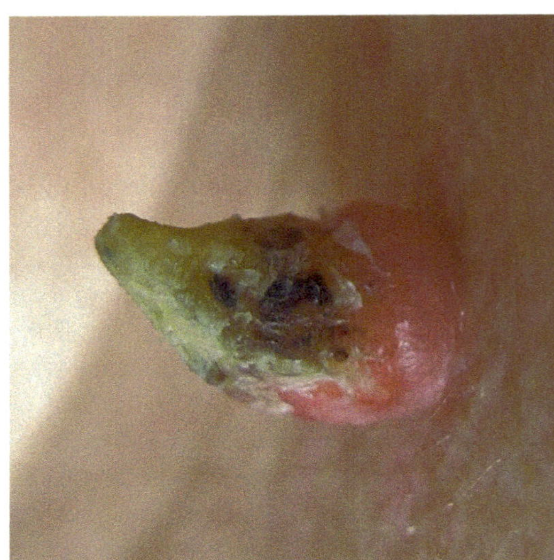

Fig. 11.5 Close-up look of keratoacanthoma of the eyelid

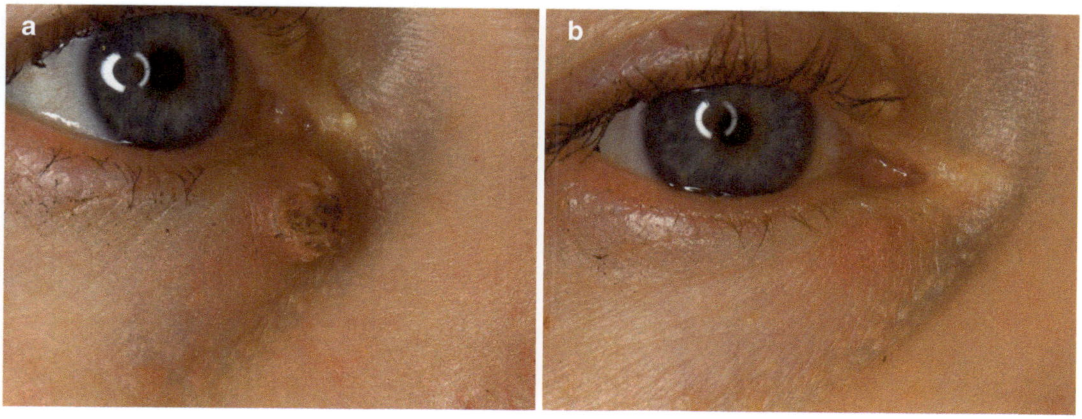

Fig. 11.6 (**a**, **b**) Keratoacanthoma on the inner angle of the lower eyelid, one freeze-thaw cycle with close (probe) technique. Before and after treatment

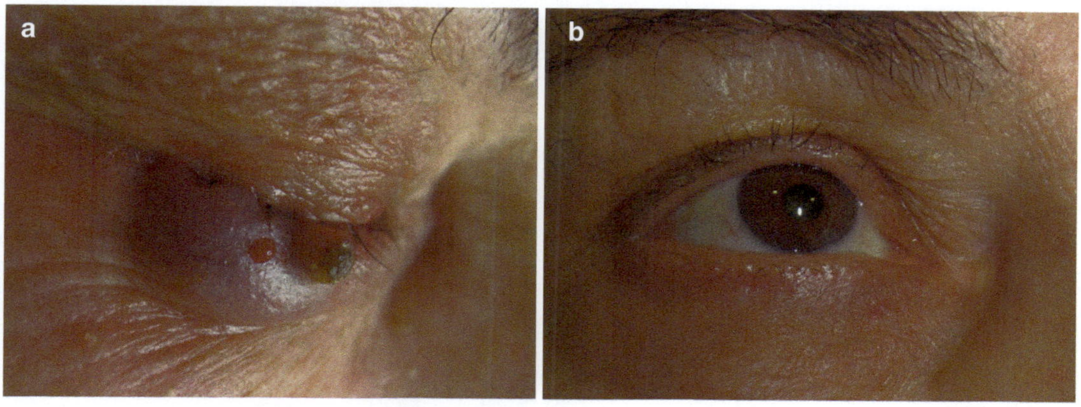

Fig. 11.7 (**a**, **b**) Keratoacanthoma of the lower eyelid. Local anesthesia was applied (hematoma formation from the puncture). Cryotweezer of the lesion, shaving of the frozen block and one freeze-thaw cycle with close (contact probe) technique. Before and after treatment

a previously frozen cryotweezer and allow the freezing front to advance just to the bottom. Then shave the frozen block (for the histopathology study) and probe freeze the bottom of the lesion. By freezing the bottom part with a probe, any residual cells are destroyed and there will be no need for further treatment (Figs. 11.6a, b and 11.7a, b).

11.3.2 Premalignant Tumors of the Eyelid Epidermis

11.3.2.1 Eyelid Actinic Keratosis

Actinic keratosis (AK) is not very common in the eyelid. Since most topical treatment options used for KA can be irritating to the conjunctiva, spray cryosurgery remains as the best option.

11.3.3 Eyelid Sebaceous Gland Tumors

11.3.3.1 Eyelid Sebaceous Hyperplasias

These are yellowish papules that can be single or multiple. They occasionally mimic basal cell carcinomas, and dermoscopy can then be extremely helpful in differentiating between them. They are best treated with contact probes.

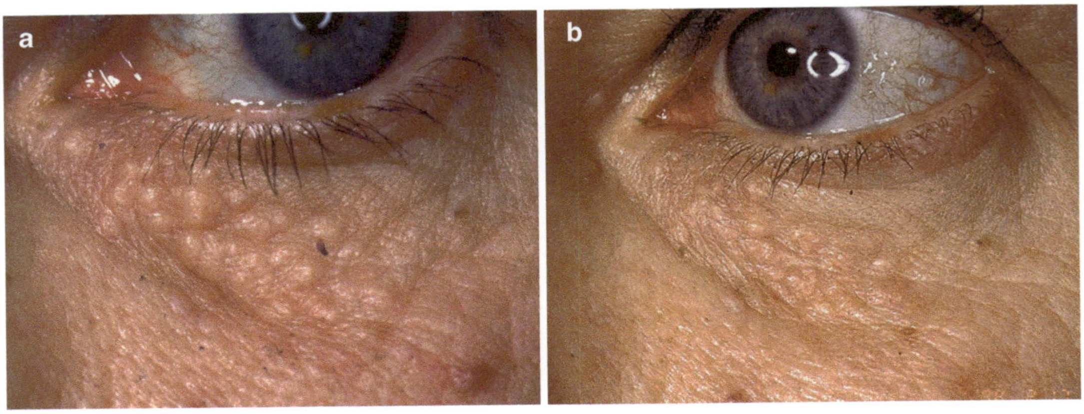

Fig. 11.8 (a, b) Eyelid syringomas treated with close (probe) technique, one freeze-thaw cycle, 2 mm margin (before and after treatment)

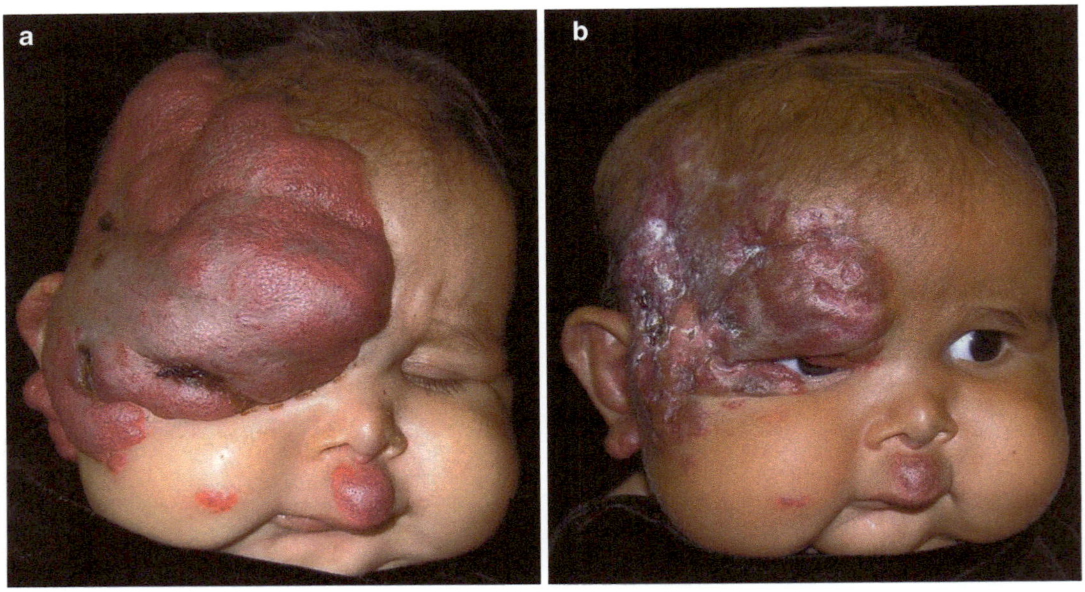

Fig. 11.9 (a, b) Huge capillary hemangioma that covered the right eye entirely. The child was treated with oral medication, laser therapy, and local corticoid infiltration. The aperture of the eyelid was obtained after several sessions of close technique, with precooled probes applied with pressure (before and after treatment)

11.3.3.2 Eyelid Syringomas

These are sweat gland tumors typically found clustered in the eyelids. They are best treated with very small probes, leaving a 2 mm margin (Fig. 11.8a, b).

11.3.4 Vascular Tumors of the Eyelid

11.3.4.1 Eyelid Congenital Capillary Hemangioma

These usually appear 1 week after birth. They have a fast growing period that usually lasts up to 6 months and a slow involution that can last as long as 6–7 years. Because their final size is not predictable, they are best treated if present in orifices or breathing areas. In babies, obstruction of an otherwise normal eye can cause amblyopia by deprivation. This form of amblyopia is considered the most severe and can cause blindness. They are real emergencies (Fig. 11.9a, b) and are ideally treated when still small and actively growing (Fig. 11.10a, b). Combination treatments are sometimes required [5]. They are best treated with a precooled probe applied with pressure, one freeze-thaw cycle for a few seconds.

11.3.4.2 Eyelid-Acquired Hemangioma (Cherry Hemangioma)

These common vascular tumors usually appear in middle age. They are usually solitary and vary in size, from a few millimeters up to 1 cm. They are best treated with previously frozen probes of the appropriate size, with pressure, just like hemangiomas. Very protruding lesions can also be treated with spray (Fig. 11.11).

11.3.4.3 Spider Telangiectasias

Freezing of the central vessel is sufficient to eliminate this lesion. Very thin probes need to be used and pressed against the center to empty the content. A few seconds is sufficient. A non-precooled probe helps for more exact positioning of the probe (Fig. 11.12).

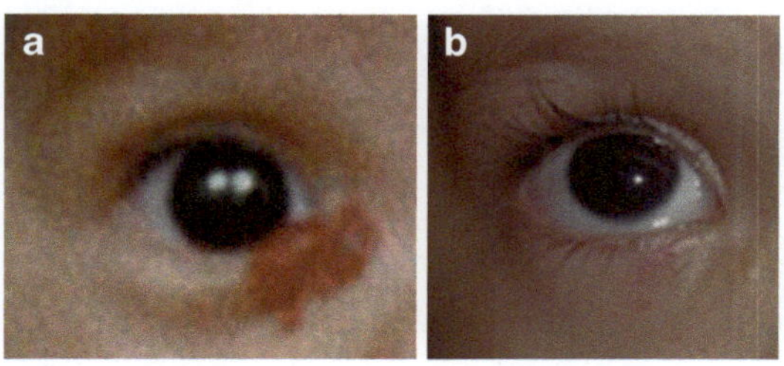

Fig. 11.10 (**a, b**) Actively growing capillary hemangioma on the lower eyelid treated with one freeze-thaw cycle close (probe). No anesthesia was required. The probe was precooled and applied with pressure for a few seconds. One single treatment. Before and after treatment

11.3.4.4 Eyelid Varix

It is possible to treat a small varix just as a hemangioma, with a precooled probe applied with pressure.

11.3.4.5 Eyelid Lymphangioma

These lesions usually are small and occur in multiples. Treatment is noncurative as new lesions keep appearing. They can have blood on the inside and then are called hemolymphangiomas. They are best treated with previously frozen (precooled) probes applied with pressure. Probes have to fit as best as possible or be slightly smaller for ideal cosmetic results.

11.3.4.6 Eyelid Pyogenic Granuloma

This is a common acquired vascular tumor that can occur in children, during pregnancy, and in areas of previous trauma. They are best treated with the probe technique, with a previously frozen probe (precooled) applied with pressure (as in hemangiomas), but open spray technique can work as well. For small lesions, the cryotweezer technique is an option (Fig. 11.13a, b).

11.3.5 Eyelid Histiocytic, Myxoid, and Fibrous Lesions

11.3.5.1 Xanthelasma

These are demarcated areas of fat beneath the skin. They can be present in lower or upper eyelids.

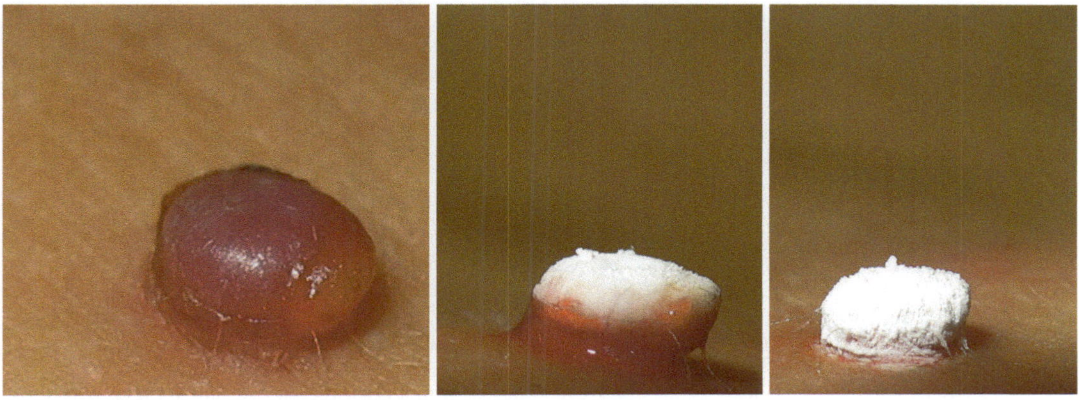

Fig. 11.11 A small cherry angioma treated with one cycle spraying technique. A 1 in. × 20 g straight spray was used for better control of freezing spray. The freezing front was allowed to reach just to the surface of the skin avoiding excess freezing. Before and after treatment

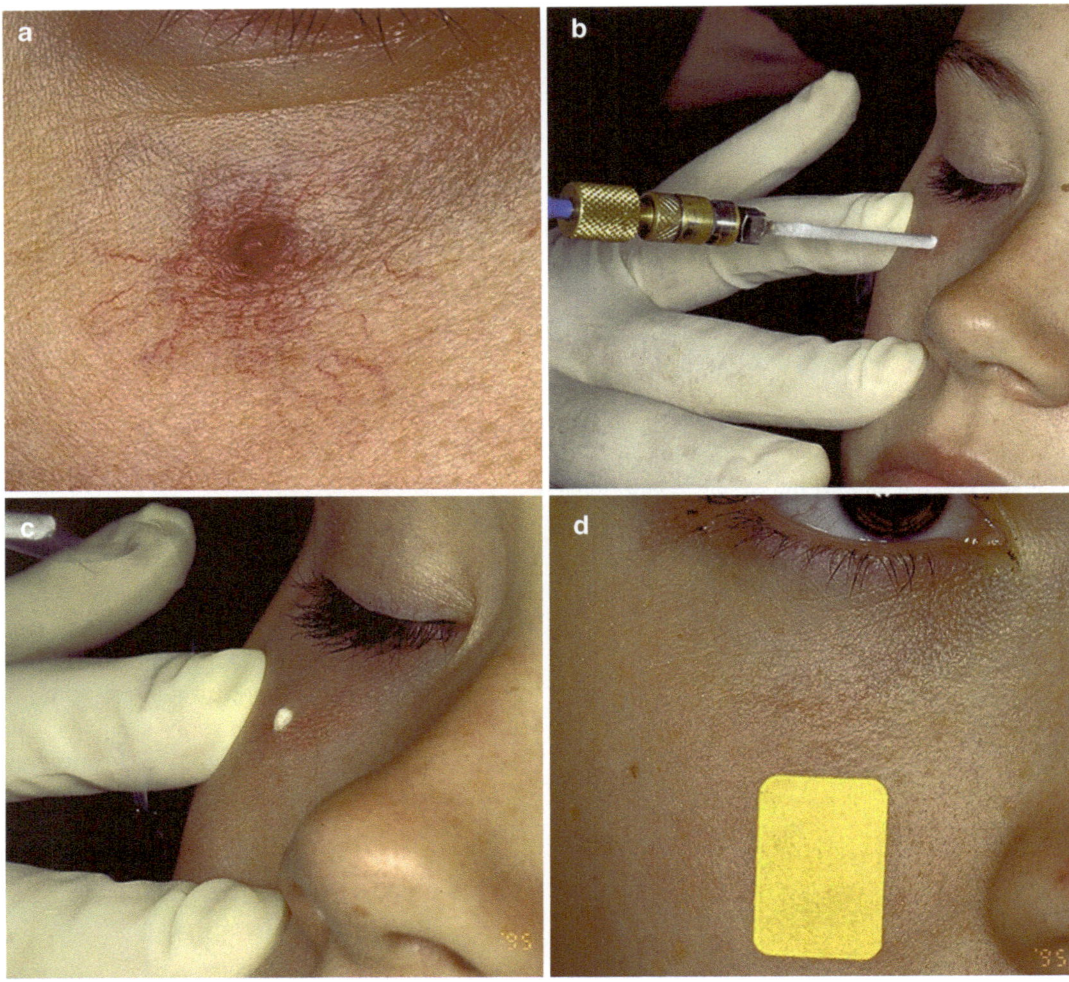

Fig. 11.12 Treatment of a spider telangiectasia with a single close (probe) freeze-thaw cycle of a few seconds

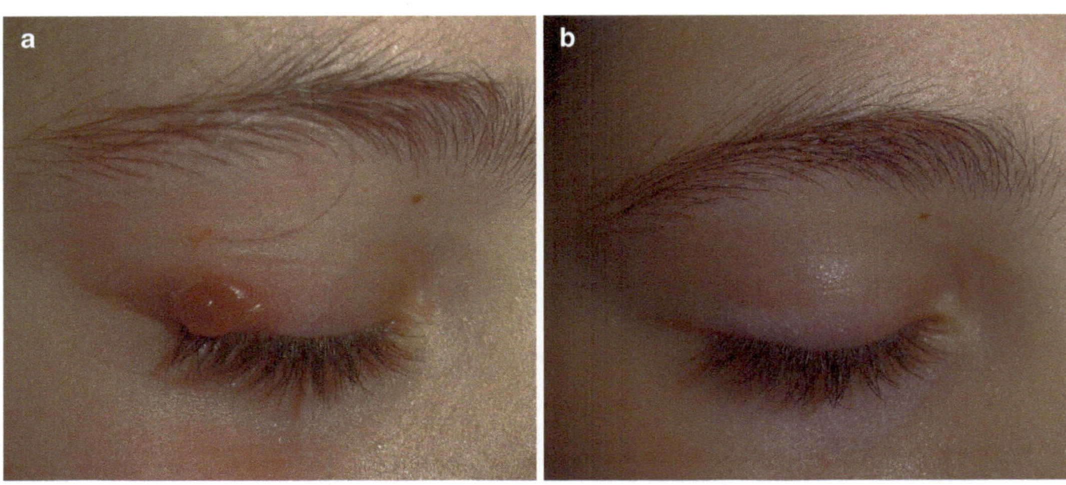

Fig. 11.13 (**a**, **b**) Pyogenic granuloma of the upper eyelid treated with a cryotweezer. One single cycle. Before and after treatment

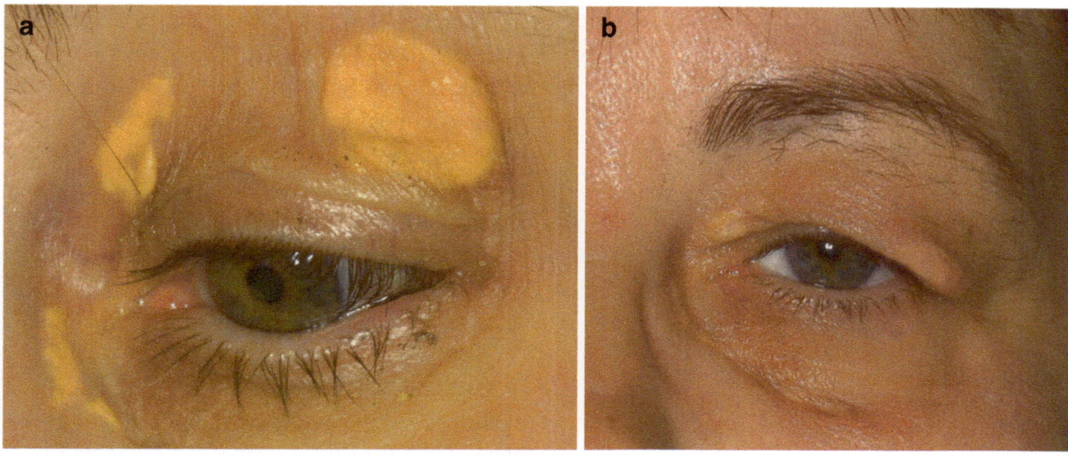

Fig. 11.14 (**a**, **b**) Xantelasma in the upper and lower eyelid. Open (spray) technique, applied slightly, one freeze-thaw cycle. Three treatments carried out at monthly intervals. Before and after treatment

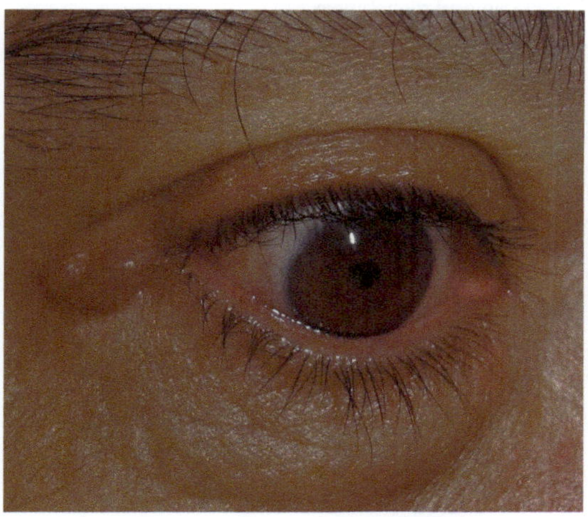

Fig. 11.15 Eccrine hidrocystoma on the outer angle of the eye

Open (spray) technique [6, 7] applied slightly and with caution over the area for 5–10 s is sufficient. There is no need to include a margin of healthy skin. One treatment is usually not enough, and freezing should be repeated two to three times (with 1 month intervals) (Fig. 11.14a, b).

11.3.6 Eyelid Cystic Lesions Simulating Neoplasms

11.3.6.1 Eyelid Eccrine and Apocrine Hidrocystoma

Eccrine hidrocystomas are cystic lesions of the eyelid that spare the eyelid margins, the lower half of the upper eyelid pretarsal skin, or the pretarsal lower eyelid skin (Fig. 11.15). Apocrine glands instead are restricted to the eyelid margins and canthi where the cysts were located [8]. They are clear, fluid-filled tumors, mostly solitary, but occasionally are multiple. They are best treated by emptying via a needle puncture and then contact probe with pressure for a few seconds leaving a 1–2 mm margin. Successful results have been observed in domestic animals as well [9].

11.3.7 Eyelid Inflammatory Lesions Simulating Neoplasms

11.3.7.1 Eyelid Molluscum Contagiosum Infection

Immunosuppressed patients, elderly people, and very young children can occasionally present with these viral lesions (Fig. 11.16). Spray or contact method can be used with good outcome. One single slight freezing is sufficient. Cryotweezers can also be an optional treatment.

11.3.8 Others: Lid Margin (Hair Structure)

11.3.8.1 Trichiasis/Distichiasis (Fig. 11.17)

Trichiasis refers to the abnormal position of eyelashes that grow back toward the eye. This can cause irritation of the conjunctiva or cornea.

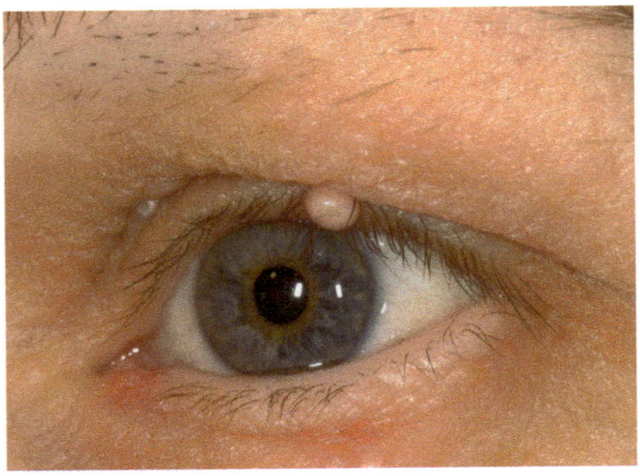

Fig. 11.16 Eyelid molluscum contagiosum

Cryosurgery stands as one of the best treatment options [10–12] (Fig. 11.18). Contact or spray techniques can be used. The lower lid tends to respond better; treating a single or a few eyelashes is better than treating the whole area. For a single eyelash or a few eyelashes, point probes are the best. For large areas, spray technique is indicated. Freezing must be deep, with two freeze-thaw cycles. Once done, it is better to remove the eyelashes with high-quality forceps (Fig. 11.19).

Distichiasis is instead the abnormal growth of eyelashes on the posterior lamella of the tarsal plate. They tend to be softer eyelashes, but they still can cause irritation and lacrimation. Although

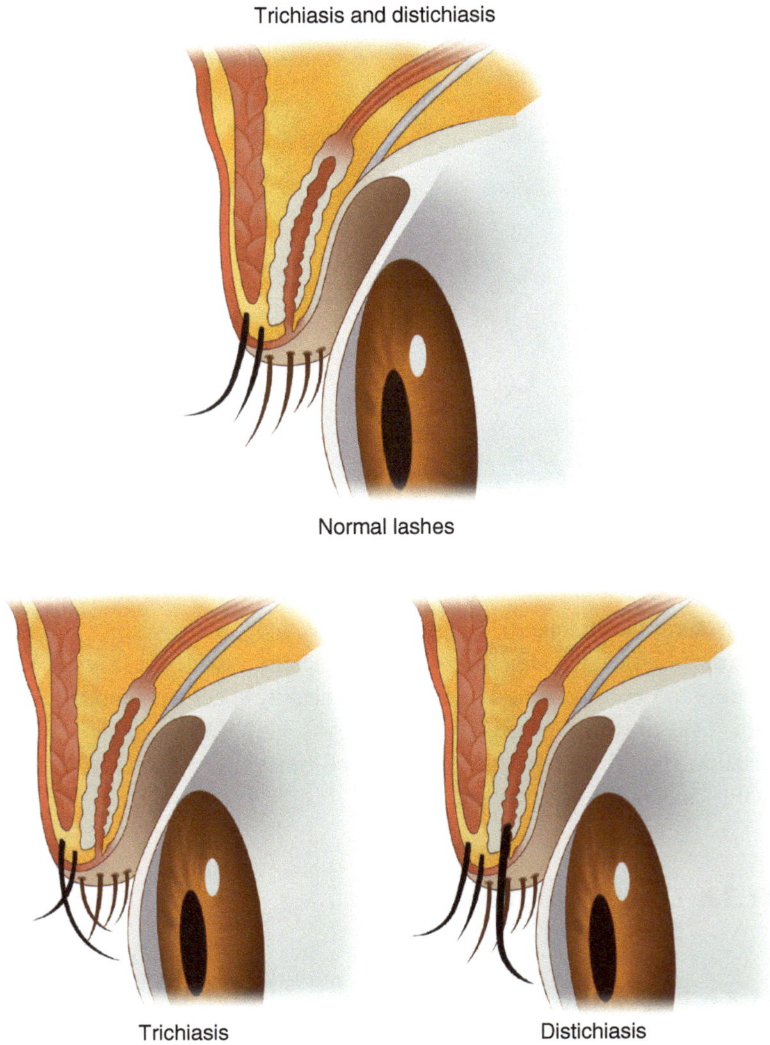

Fig. 11.17 Differences between trichiasis and distichiasis. In trichiasis, eyelashes grow back toward the eye. In distichiasis, the abnormal growth of eyelashes occurs on the posterior lamella of the tarsal plate

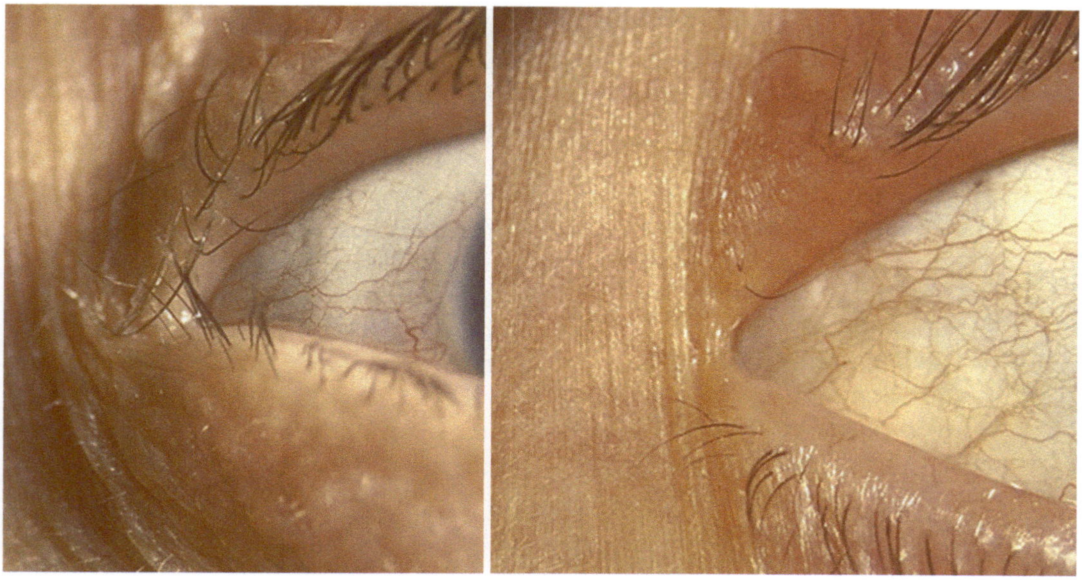

Fig. 11.18 Trichiasis treated with double freeze-thaw cycle open (spray) technique, on the upper and lower lid margin

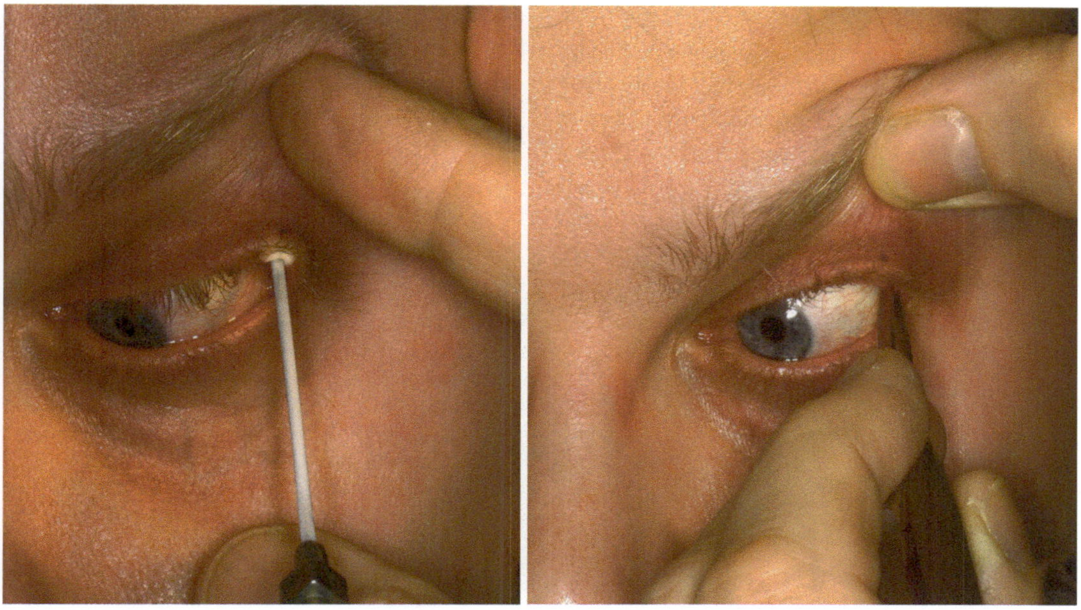

Fig. 11.19 Trichiasis treated with close (probe) technique with removal of the eyelashes after treatment with a high-quality forceps

surgery is preferred, cryosurgery stands as an excellent alternative [13] in older people because it is a low-risk alternative.

11.3.9 Vascular Tumors and Related Lesions of the Conjunctiva

11.3.9.1 Conjunctival Capillary Hemangioma and Conjunctival Pyogenic Granuloma

These vascular tumors are both amenable to close-contact treatment similar to their counterparts in the eyelids. Treatment is best done with warm probes, fixing them in position, and one cycle with the freezing front reaching just to the bottom of the lesion; no extra margin is needed.

11.4 Side Effects

Postoperative care and expected secondary effects are no different than in other areas. Daily washing with water and baby shampoo are best to avoid secondary infections and irritations. Edema is usually present from the beginning but lasts just a couple of days and has no pain associated with it. Defective protection may lead to temporary pain if LN droplets touch the surface epithelium. Subcutaneous insufflation can occur if the lesion had been previously debulked prior to spray freezing.

Essential Tidbits

- Protect the eye with nonconductive material shields such as plastic.
- Previous eye drops of oxybuprocaine or tetracaine are needed to anesthetize the conjunctival surface.
- Make sure the patient is in a comfortable position. The patient should avoid sudden movements in order to avoid accidental injuries.

Conclusions

Cryosurgery stands as the treatment of choice for many of the previously mentioned lesions. It is a technique used by ophthalmologists for many other conditions besides those mentioned in this chapter [14, 15]. It is a bloodless procedure that usually does not require local anesthesia. It is cost-effective, and no assistant is needed. The operator must be familiar with the anatomical area, and precautions must be taken to avoid accidental damage to the eye.

Glossary

Distichiasis Abnormal growth of lashes from the orifices of the meibomian glands on the posterior lamella of the tarsal plate. It is not common.

Trichiasis Abnormally positioned eyelashes that grow back toward the eye. It is a relatively common condition.

References

1. Fraunfelder FT, Farris Jr HE, Wallace TR. Cryosurgery for ocular and periocular lesions. J Dermatol Surg Oncol. 1977;3(4):422–7.
2. Suhonen RE, Kuflik EG. Cryosurgical methods for eyelid lesions. J Dermatolog Treat. 2001;12(3):135–9.
3. Shields JA, Shields CL. Eyelid, conjunctival, and orbital tumors: an atlas and text. 2nd ed. Philadelphia: Lippincott Wiliams & Wilkins; 2008.
4. Suhonen R. Multipurpose skin microscope-an aid to the assessment of treatment efficacy of skin disorders. J Dermatol Treat. 1993;4:131.4.
5. Tronina SA, Bobrova NF, Khrinenko VP. Combined surgical method of orbital and periorbital hemangioma treatment in infants. Orbit. 2008;27(4):249–57.
6. Blume U, Zouboulis CC, Pineda Fernandez MS. New indications in cryosurgery. Dermatol Monatschr. 1993;179:265–9.
7. Dewan SP, Kaur A, Gupta RK. Effectiveness of cryosurgery in xanthelasma palpebrarum. Indian J Dermatol Venereol Leprol. 1995;61(1):4–7.
8. Jakobiec FA, Zakka FR. A reappraisal of eyelid eccrine and apocrine hidrocystomas: microanatomic and immunohistochemical studies of 40 lesions. Am J Ophthalmol. 2011;151(2):358–74.
9. Sivagurunathan A, Goodhead AD, Du Plessis EC. Multiple eyelid apocrine hidrocystoma in a domestic short-haired cat. J S Afr Vet Assoc. 2010; 81(1):65–8.

10. Matthaus W, Matthes R. Technik und Langzeitergebnisse del Kryoepilation bei trichiasis und Distichiasis. Klin Monatsbl Augenheilkd. 1990:196(2):59–61.
11. Fraunfelder FT, Petursson GJ. The use of liquid nitrogen cryospray for treatment of trichiasis. Ophthalmic Surg. 1979;10:42–6.
12. Elder MJ, Bernauer W. Cryotherapy for trichiasis in ocular cicatricial pemphigoid. Br J Ophthalmol. 1994;78:769–71.
13. Sarkar S, Bagchi K, Mukherjee G. Congenital distichiasis treated by a time-based cryosurgical technique–a case report. J Indian Med Assoc. 2012; 110(10):747–8.
14. Fraunfelder FW. Cryotherapy for pterygia. Ophthalmology. 2008;115(12):2314–e2.
15. Fraunfelder F. Liquid nitrogen cryotherapy for surface eye disease (an AOS thesis). Trans Am Opthalmol Soc. 2008;106:301–24.

Cryosurgery for Vascular Lesions 12

Paola Pasquali and Mildred J. Gutiérrez

Contents

P. Pasquali, MD (✉)
Department of Dermatology, Pius Hospital de Valls, 43800 Tarragona, Spain
e-mail: pasqualipaola@gmail.com

M.J. Gutiérrez, MD
Department of Dermatology, Hospital Central Universitario Dr. Antonio María Pineda, Barquisimeto, Venezuela
e-mail: mildredgutierre@yahoo.com

Key Points

- Cryosurgery stands as a treatment option for vascular lesions.
- Correct selection of vascular lesions is essential to guarantee the best therapeutic and cosmetic results.
- Contact technique is the best alternative, although spraying and tweezers can be used for selected lesions.
- Imaging techniques such as dermoscopy, high-frequency ultrasound, and nuclear magnetic resonance with or without contrast provide essential information to help make the correct therapeutic decision.

12.1 Introduction

Vascular tissue is susceptible to temperatures. High temperatures cause vasodilation, and low temperatures cause vasoconstriction. Cryosurgical destruction of a vascular nest is possible as long as the tumor is correctly selected regarding location, growth, depth, and tumor histology.

Despite the advent of several ablative procedures such as radiofrequency or laser therapy, cryosurgery continues to occupy a very important position in the therapeutic armamentarium of a dermatologist. Cryotherapy is a simple, safe, and inexpensive office procedure for the treatment of various

P. Pasquali (ed.), *Cryosurgery: A Practical Manual*,
DOI 10.1007/978-3-662-43939-5_12, © Springer-Verlag Berlin Heidelberg 2015

benign, premalignant, and well-circumscribed malignant tumors. It provides satisfactory cosmetic results with minimal complications as long as patients are correctly selected and treatment is undertaken by a trained and experienced dermatologist [1, 2].

12.2 The Why, Where, When, and How of Vascular Tumor Cryosurgery

12.2.1 Why

Vascular lesions are particularly susceptible to cryosurgical destruction. The first effect of cold on vessels is vasoconstriction and, with sufficient low temperature, stasis. At −15 and −40 °C, there will be endothelial damage. With thawing, microthrombi will form inside the vessels, and the subsequent edema and hyperemia will bring about tissue necrosis [3].

The size of the vessel and the speed of blood flow are crucial. Smaller blood vessels, with slow blood flow, are ideal for cryosurgical treatment and are relatively easy to be destroyed by subzero temperatures of −15 and −20 °C.

Once a vascular tumor is frozen, there will be a direct damage with cell necrosis that will occur mostly at the center of the lesion where the lower temperatures are achieved. Indirect cell damage occurs after cryoablation due to damage on blood vessels. A later cryosurgical event is thrombosis which is observed in all capillaries, arterioles and venules. Platelets become activated causing thrombus formation and subsequent ischemia. The vascular stasis results in further tissue damage post-cryoablation [4].

12.2.2 Where

12.2.2.1 Tumor Selection

Treatment of benign vascular neoplasms like hemangiomas has been a matter of controversies. The most common vascular lesions amenable to cryosurgical treatment are summarized in Table 12.1.

Table 12.1 Most common vascular lesions amenable to cryosurgical treatment

Type of tumor		Preferred type
Benign neoplasia	Infantile hemangioma	Superficial or mixed hemangiomas
		Recent appearance, rapid growing, with no signs of involution
	Cherry or senile angiomas	Any
Malformations	Hypertrophic capillary malformation	Nodular lesions
		For symptomatic and/or cosmetic purpose
	Venous malformations	In conjunction with other treatment modalities (surgery, ligation, embolization)
	Lymphatic or hemolymphatic malformations	In conjunction with other treatment modalities (surgery, ligation, embolization)
		In superficial lesions
		For symptomatic and/or cosmetic purpose
	Combined vascular malformations	In conjunction with other treatment modalities (surgery, ligation, embolization)
Hyperplasia	Pyogenic granulomas	Any location
Dilation of preexisting vessels	Venous lakes	Depending on vessel size and local blood flow
	Spider angioma	Any
	Angiokeratomas	Any

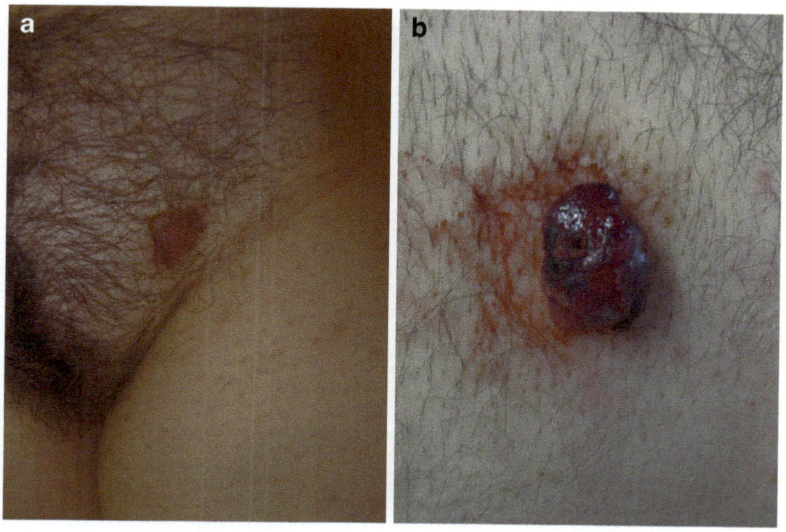

Fig. 12.1 (**a**) A pyogenic granuloma. (**b**) A malignant melanoma

In general, cryosurgery is best suited for patients with light skin and for treatment of lesions in non-hair-bearing areas of the body. Among the advantages, one can identify the following: (a) no need of injecting local anesthesia, (b) fast and safe, (c) low cost, and (d) no incision/no suture.

It is a treatment that can be repeated when necessary, and the postoperative care is relatively simple.

12.2.3 When

When dealing with vascular tumors, there are multiple noninvasive techniques that will help diagnose and decide which one is the most suitable technique [5]. The first important consideration is to have a diagnostic certainty. For instance, a nasal glioma mimicking a hemangioma [6] or a malignant melanoma can be mistaken for a pyogenic granuloma (Fig. 12.1a, b).

12.2.3.1 Dermoscopy

Dermoscopy can be used for diagnostic purposes [7] as well as a follow-up to cryosurgical treatment. A dermoscopic picture of the lesion can be compared to the postsurgical image in order to determine the improvement by verifying the reduction in lesion or in vessels (Fig. 12.2).

12.2.3.2 Temperature Control

The surface temperature of a vascular lesion is usually higher by several degrees than body temperature. By measuring the tumor's surface temperature before and after treatment, one can register improvement. After treatment, there should be fewer vessels present and therefore a lower temperature. An infrared technology or a temple touch thermometer will be sufficient to monitor the tissue temperature (Fig. 12.3).

12.2.3.3 High-Frequency Ultrasound/Doppler

Ultrasound (US), especially with a high-resolution transducer, has been advocated as useful in examining small and superficial soft tissue masses that are suggestive of hemangiomas or vascular malformations. Vascular tumor ultrasound stands as one of the easier and more universally practiced noninvasive techniques [8] that give information about size, shape, depth, and, more importantly, vascularity [9]. In addition, US will help differentiate between a cystic and a solid lesion. Doppler US will give information about the presence or absence of flow and the degree of vascularization (Fig. 12.4). The Doppler characteristics of vascular malformations are helpful in differentiating low- from high-flow vascular malformations [10]. The sonographic depiction of abundant low-flow vascular channels can be a predictor of the potential success of percutaneous sclerosis. In addition, US can be used to guide

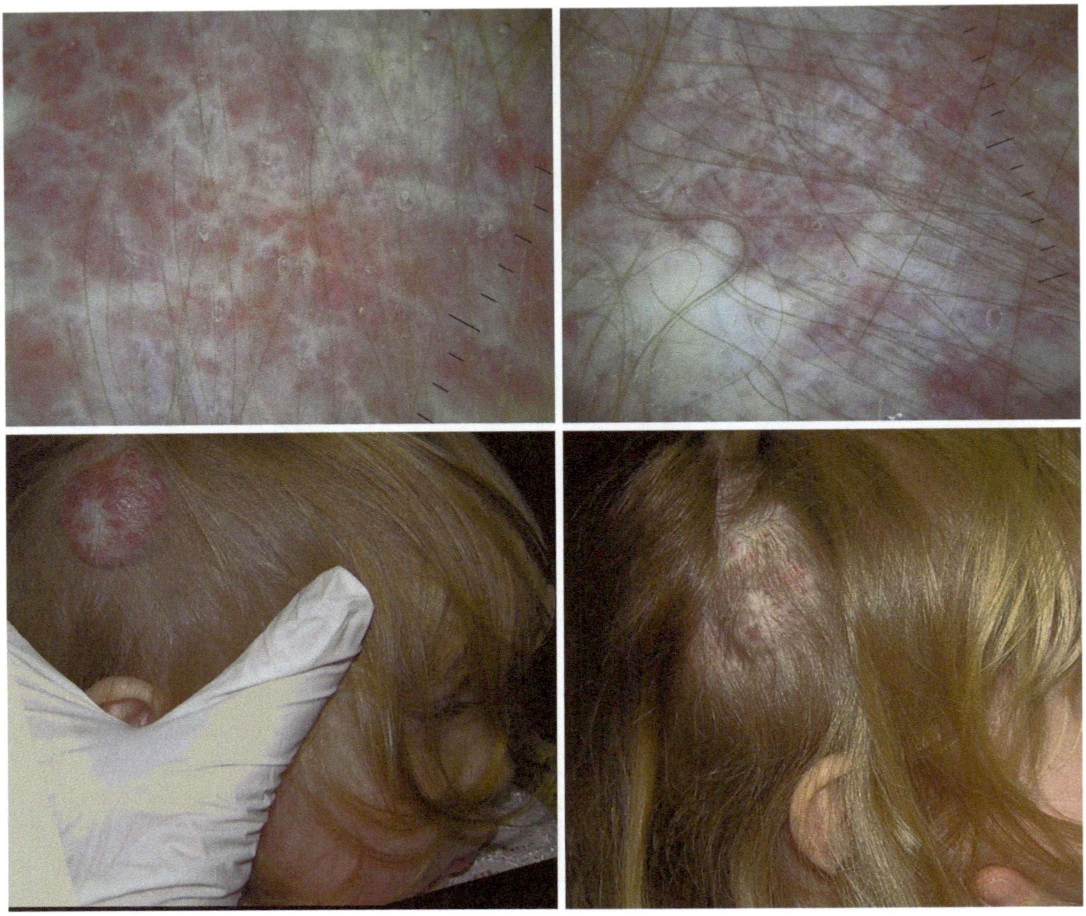

Fig. 12.2 A dermoscopic image of a capillary hemangioma taken before treatment (*left column*) and at control evaluation 1 month later. It puts into evidence the areas with fibrous tissue, the diminished number of capillaries, and the color difference

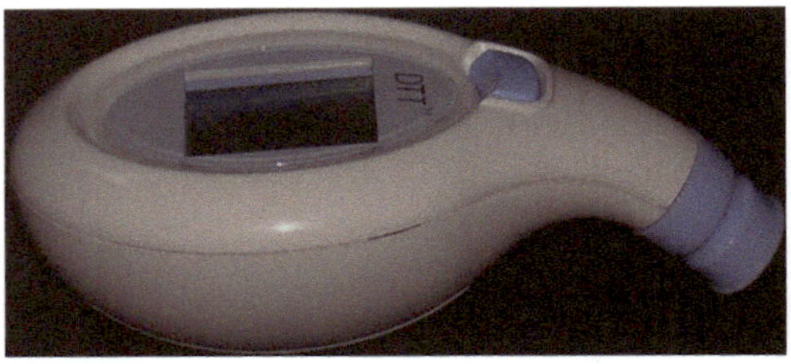

Fig. 12.3 A temple touch thermometer used to measure superficial temperature in capillary hemangiomas (Courtesy of and Copyright © 2014 Medline Industries, Inc.)

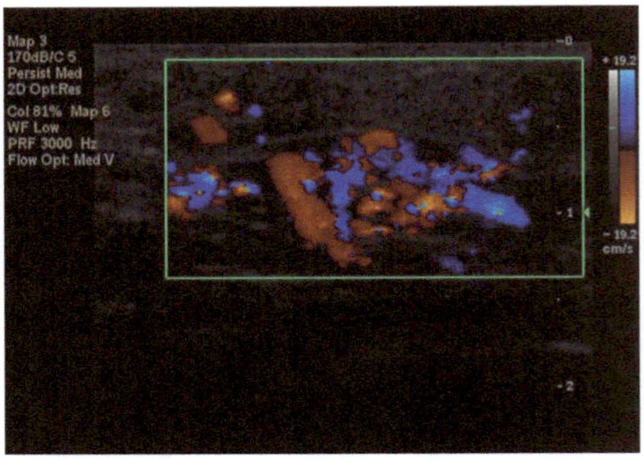

Fig. 12.4 Color Doppler analysis of the vascular mapping of a vascular malformation in the abdomen of a child

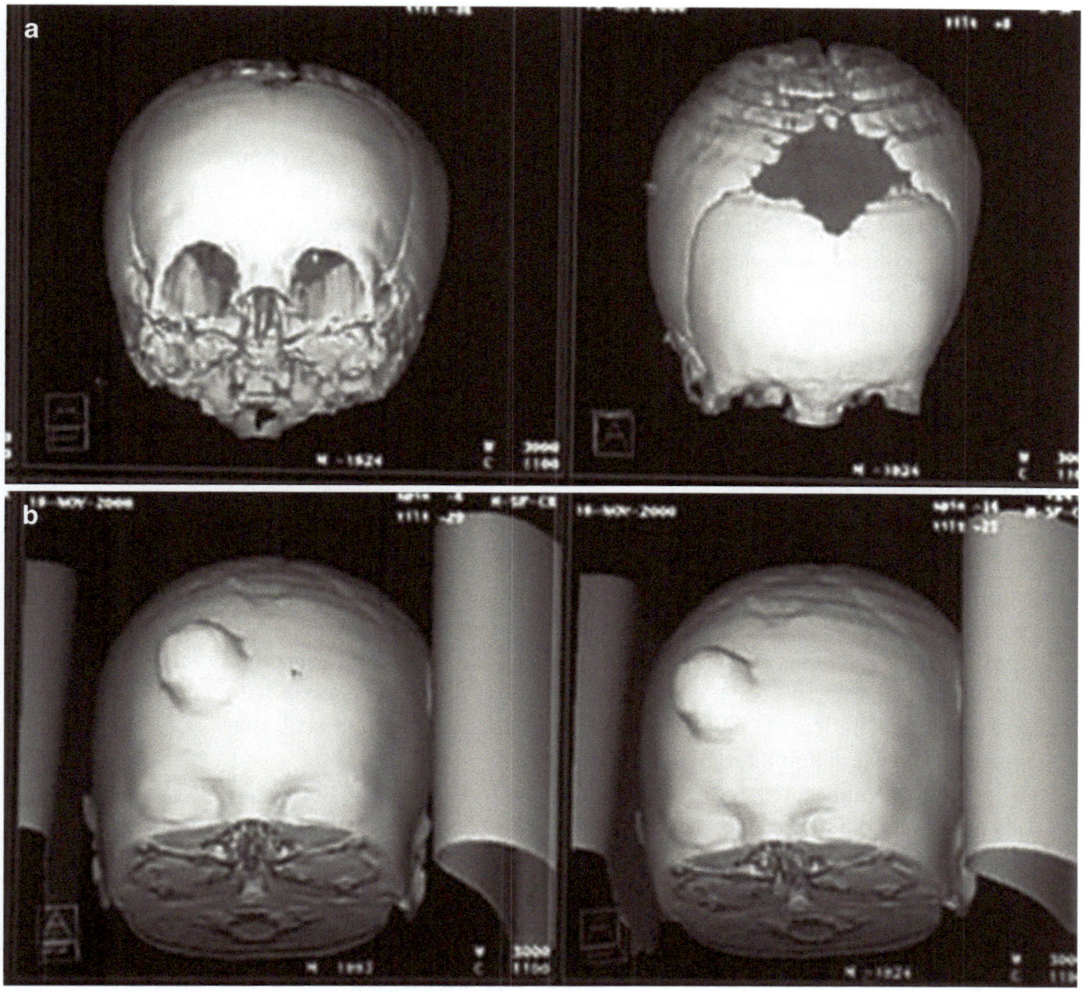

Fig. 12.5 3D reconstruction of a CT scan done on a mixed capillary hemangioma in the frontal area of the same patient in Fig. 12.6

needle placement during percutaneous sclerosis in a combination treatment approach (cryosurgery plus infiltration).

12.2.3.4 CT Scan Angiography and Nuclear Magnetic Resonance Imaging

CT scan angiography is an imaging technique that combines a CT scan with an injection of contrast material to produce a picture of the vasculature of a tumor. It can help differentiate between a hemangioma and a vascular malformation [11]. A 3D reconstruction displays the total volume of the lesion as well as the thickness and number of vessels (Fig. 12.5). MR imaging with gadolinium contrast is the diagnostic modality of choice for large and deep lesions or for those where US has not been diagnostic [8]. Intravenous gadolinium helps differentiate between cystic or solid tumors and between venous and lymphatic malformations [12], allowing the determining of lesion size and number and size of vessels involved [13]. This information is necessary to determine the feasibility of cryosurgical treatment or the need to combine treatment modalities.

12.2.3.5 Other Noninvasive Imaging Techniques: Reflectance Confocal Microscopy (RCM)

Confocal microscopy might be helpful in characterizing vascular lesions in vivo before cryosurgical treatment. There is good correlation between RCM morphology and established histopathology criteria for common vascular lesions such as pyogenic granuloma, capillary vascular malformations, and venous lakes [14].

12.2.4 How

12.2.4.1 The Rule of the 4 Ps

As a general rule for most vascular lesions, cryosurgical treatment is performed with probe or close technique, although there are conditions where spraying or tweezers can work as well. When using probes, there is a simple rule to follow called the 4P rule (probe, pressure, previously frozen probe, patience):

Probe: Blood is a warm liquid (around 38 °C) that has a slightly higher temperature than the body. If a superficial freezing is performed, there will only be destruction of the most superficial skin structures, leaving the rest of the vessels untreated. Blood present in deeply seated vessels will keep the area warm. Therefore, the ideal treatment of vascular lesions is with probes (contact or close cryosurgery). Probes will freeze deeper at a constant low temperature. Metal probes limit the "heat sink" effect.

Pressure: Vascular tumors tend to be non-painful renitent tumors. They can be pressed, squeezing out some of the blood inside them. By doing so, the lesion's temperature goes down (less blood, less temperature). Pressure minimizes blood flow. As the blood flow is reduced, local temperature will be lower and cryosurgical treatment more effective.

Previously frozen probe: A previously frozen probe sticks less to the surface. When treating vascular tumors, it is best to have the possibility of removing it fast from the skin surface. The reasons are (a) a sudden movement while doing the procedure from the patient or surgeon's part could cause an accidental breaking of the vascular tissue and a profuse undesired bleeding (this is especially true when dealing with small children). (b) Once freezing has been completed, the probe has to be removed as soon as possible to avoid further freezing that could leave an undesired scar. In vascular tumors, there is no need to freeze margins above 1 mm.

Patience: Despite all precautions such as drying the surface and previously freezing the probe, probes can occasionally get stuck to the surface. Be patient: the need to remove the probe from the site should not tempt the surgeon to force it out because this will simply break the tissue. In the case of a vascular lesion, bleeding can become a real issue. If, in spite of these precautions, the probe cannot be removed, allowing some warm water to run over the probe will rapidly release it from the surface. Keep a cup with warm water at hand as a precaution at all times.

12.3 Capillary Hemangiomas

Capillary hemangiomas, also called strawberry or infantile hemangiomas, are sometimes classified as benign neoplasms or vascular hyperplasias. They are the most frequent benign tumors of infancy and are composed of proliferating endothelial-like cells. Clinically, they can present themselves as superficial, deep, or mixed hemangioma (Fig. 12.6a, b), with regard to the depth of the vascular nest within the skin. Superficial hemangioma are bright red and sometimes called strawberry tumors. Deep lesions are violaceous tumors covered with normal skin, and mixed lesions have the bright and granulous surface but tend to be elevated. Histopathologically, hemangiomas can present as well-circumscribed, densely packed endothelial cells and small vascular spaces. These tumors usually appear after 1–2 weeks of birth and begin a rapid process of growth that can last up to 6 months. They sometimes ulcerate in the process of growing. After the growth period, they begin a very slow involution period that can last up to 6–7 years. During this

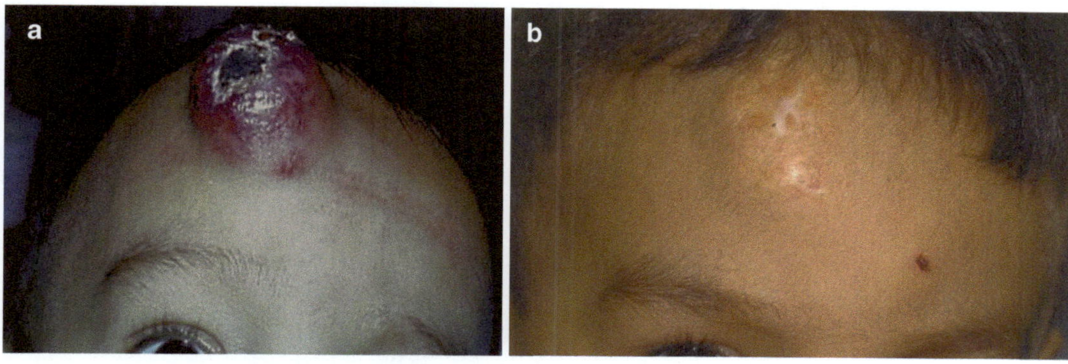

Fig. 12.6 (**a**) A large frontal mixed capillary hemangioma ulcerated in the center. A combined treatment with steroid infiltration for the deep part of the lesion and close (probe) technique on the ulcerated superficial and medial part of the tumor. (**b**) A control image 3 years after treatment

period, certain hemangiomas ulcerate. Therefore, ulceration can be a sign of both rapid growth or involution [15].

According to the American Academy of Dermatology, the goals in the management of hemangiomas are to prevent or reverse the complication of alarming hemangiomas, prevent permanent disfigurement, minimize psychosocial stress for patients and relatives, avoid aggressive and potentially unsightly procedures, and prevent or adequately treat ulceration, thereby minimizing scarring, infections, and pain [16].

Possible interventions are left for those rapidly growing hemangiomas, especially those in areas that put the child in danger, such as:

- Tumors close to airways that can limit breathing capacity.
- Bleeding tumors.
- Tumors around eyelids that can cause occlusion amblyopia. This in turn can degenerate to irreversible loss of vision due to damage to ocular dominance columns during the critical period (first 2 years of life).
- Large tumors which are causing irreversible damage.
- Tumors in visible areas capable of affecting the social and emotional well-being of the child.
- Tumors in genital areas that get easily irritated/ulcerated and cause discomfort.

Correct selection for lesions is indispensable [17]. Lesions that have begun spontaneous involution and are not putting the child in any risk are best left to regress spontaneously.

Hemangiomas involve a therapeutic challenge for dermatologists. About 10–20 % of these require active treatment due to functional interference and/or significant disfigurement [18]; cryosurgery today is still an alternative [19, 20] and often the method of choice [21–24]. Smaller lesions yield better results than larger ones [25]; genital and mucosal lesions yield excellent results from cryosurgical treatment [26].

Although there are many options available nowadays to treat hemangiomas, cryosurgery stands as an alternative [27] for its excellent results, simplicity of the procedure, quick application, and low cost [28, 29]. Each case should be studied carefully, and the best therapeutic alternative available should be offered.

Once decided that a hemangioma will be treated with cryosurgery, one suggestion is to have the caretaker bring the child in very hungry, with no recent meal in the stomach in order to avoid the possibility of having the child regurgitate during the procedure. Most important is the fact that babies feel comforted if fed immediately after the procedure and seem to forget about the stressful or uncomfortable surgical situation they have just been put through.

Local anesthesia (EMLA) can help, but make sure to remove and dry the surface very well before attempting to apply the probe; otherwise, there is a risk that it will get stuck to the skin. One cycle, with a previously frozen probe, applied with pressure for a few seconds (until the tumors turn completely white) is sufficient

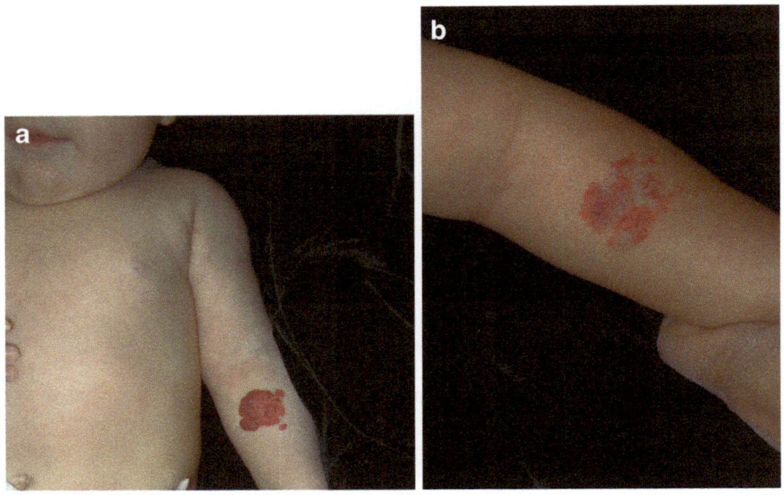

Fig. 12.7 (**a**) A superficial hemangioma on the left arm. (**b**) One single freeze-thaw cycle with close (probe) technique, with a precooled probe applied with pressure for few seconds

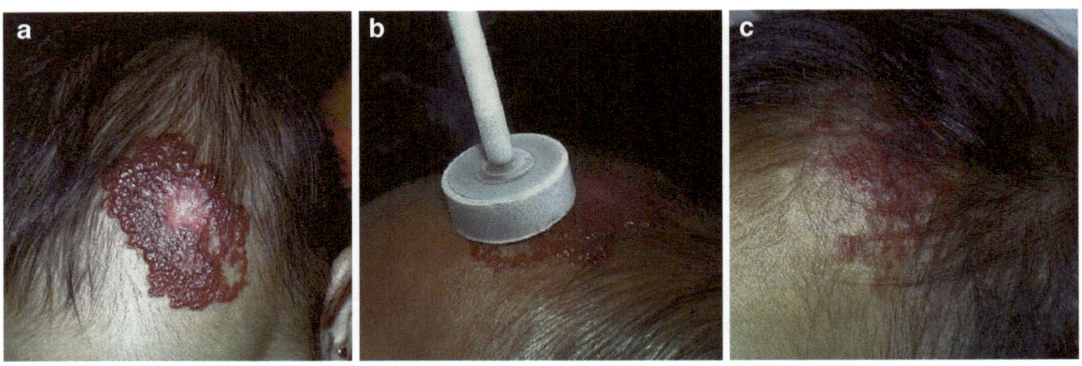

Fig. 12.8 (**a**) Large capillary hemangioma on the head of a child. (**b**) The lesion was treated with a precooled 2 cm flat probe, applied with pressure for a few seconds with one freeze-thaw cycle. (**c**) One month after treatment

to destroy most superficial hemangioma vessels (Fig. 12.7a, b). Treat superficial capillary hemangiomas with one freeze-thaw cycle with a 1-mm margin with a precooled (previously frozen) probe (Fig. 12.8a–c). A mixed hemangioma will require combination treatments with cryosurgery and local infiltrations of depot steroid, and the freezing period will be longer. Extensively deep hemangioma should not be treated with cryosurgery.

12.4 Cherry or Senile Angiomas

Cherry nevi need to be treated as infantile hemangiomas. Apply a precooled (previously frozen) probe with pressure. The probe has to match in size or be slightly smaller than the lesion. A few seconds are sufficient, and the freezing front should not expand more than 1 mm over the external lesion margin (Fig. 12.9a, b). Large lesions might require a second freeze cycle. For protruding lesions, cryotweezers can be an optional treatment (Fig. 12.10).

12.5 Vascular Malformations

The most common congenital vascular lesions are vascular malformations (VMs). These lesions are the outcome of errors in vascular formation during embryonic life. VMs do not proliferate. Nevertheless, the dilated blood vessels that build up these lesions gradually enlarge. VMs can be

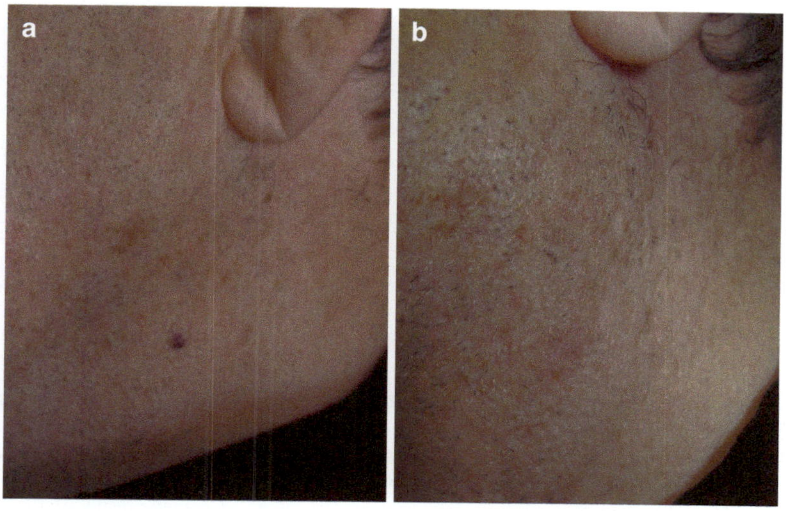

Fig. 12.9 (**a**) A small cherry angioma treated with a 2 mm precooled flat probe with one freeze-thaw cycle. (**b**) One month post treatment

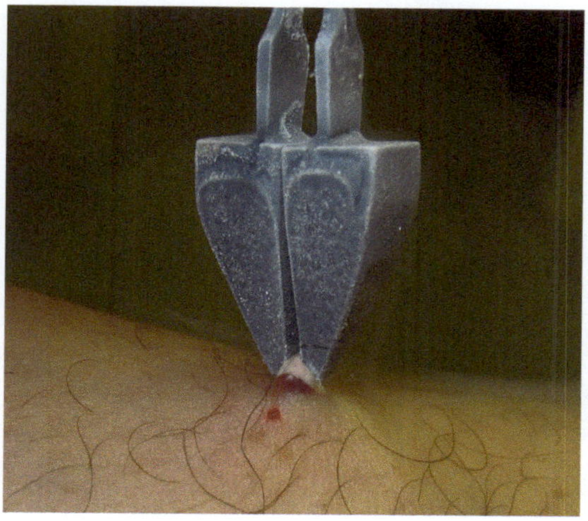

Fig. 12.10 A cherry angioma grasped with a cryotweezer. The freezing front will be allowed to reach just to the skin surface

classified, based on the type of blood flow, into slow-flow (capillary, venous, lymphatic) lesions, high-flow (arterial) lesions, and combined slow-/fast-flow lesions (Fig. 12.11a, b). Based on the size of the lymph lumens, these lesions can be divided into microcystic lesions (previously termed lymphangiomas), macrocystic lesions (previously termed cystic hygromas), and a combined form [30].

Hypertrophic capillary malformations can present large vascular "nodular" areas that can be treated as venous lakes (1–2 freeze-thaw cycle, previously frozen probe). For protruding lesions, cryotweezers can be an option (Fig. 12.12a, b).

Large areas of hypertrophic tissue are of cosmetic concern to some patients. The result of dye laser treatment is usually unsatisfactory due to the thickness of the involved tissue. Large flat probes or door knob probes can be used to diminish such thickness in chosen areas of major concern.

Lymphangiomas and hemolymphangiomas as well as hypertrophic capillary malformations are suitable for cryosurgical treatment. Mucous lymphangiomas respond well to probe cryosurgery. In the skin, the presence of a moderate fibrous element makes them less responsive to treatment. Two or more treatments might be required (Fig. 12.13a, b). A combined excisional and cryosurgical approach is sometimes useful.

12.6 Pyogenic Granulomas

Pyogenic granulomas are very common lesions present at the site of superficial traumatisms in pregnant women and in small children, and it is considered by some as an excess growth of granulation tissue [31]. Some have a thrombosis of small superficial vessels that make it mandatory to rule out a nodular malignant melanoma.

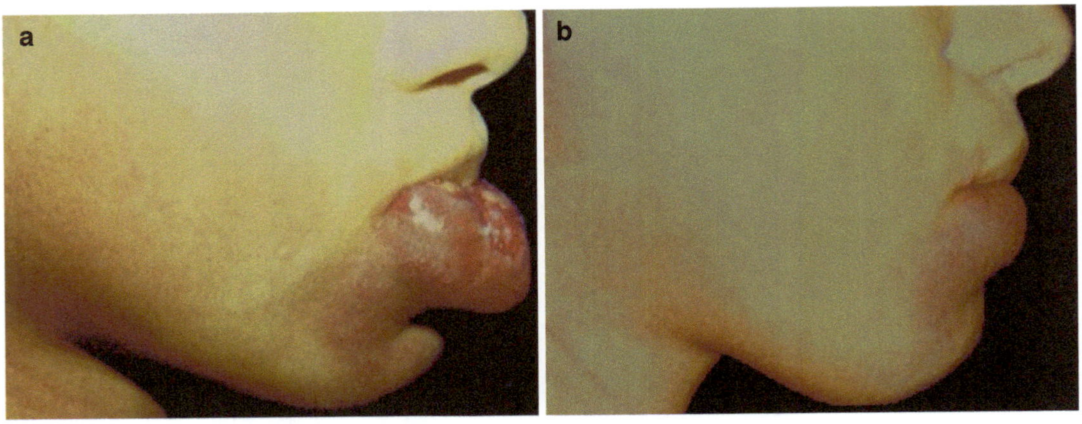

Fig. 12.11 (**a**) A mixed vascular malformation (capillary, venous, and arterial) in a type 3 skin patient. Treatment was done by a multidisciplinary team (vascular surgeons ligated the large feeding blood vessels, cryosurgeons froze the tumoral mass in the inner mucosa). (**b**) Cosmetic result after 6 months of treatments

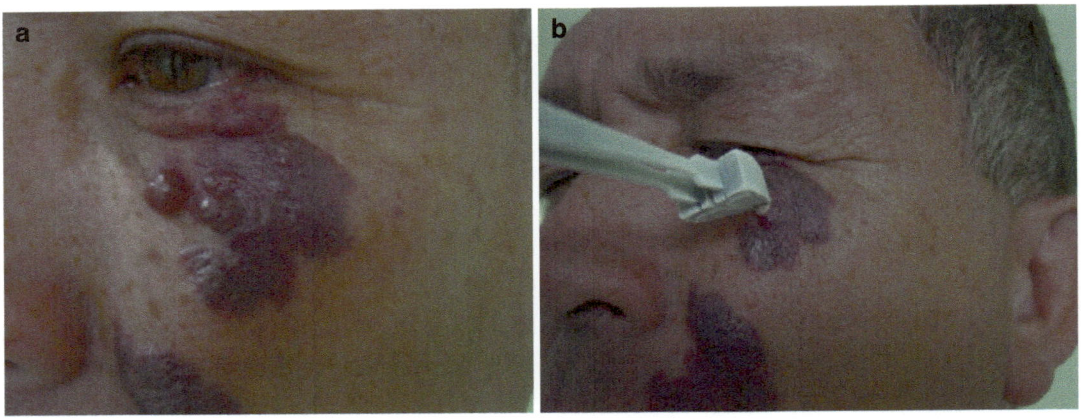

Fig. 12.12 (**a**) Hypertrophic capillary malformation in the face. (**b**) Cryotweezer treatment of nodular A component

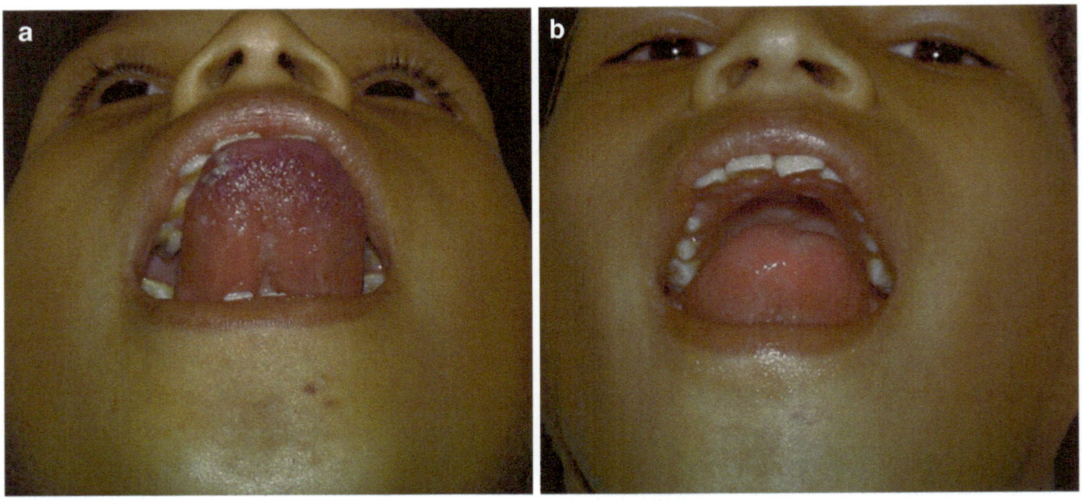

Fig. 12.13 (**a**) Hemolymphangioma of the tongue. Multiple one freeze-thaw cycle separated into 4 week intervals. (**b**) Result after 4 sessions

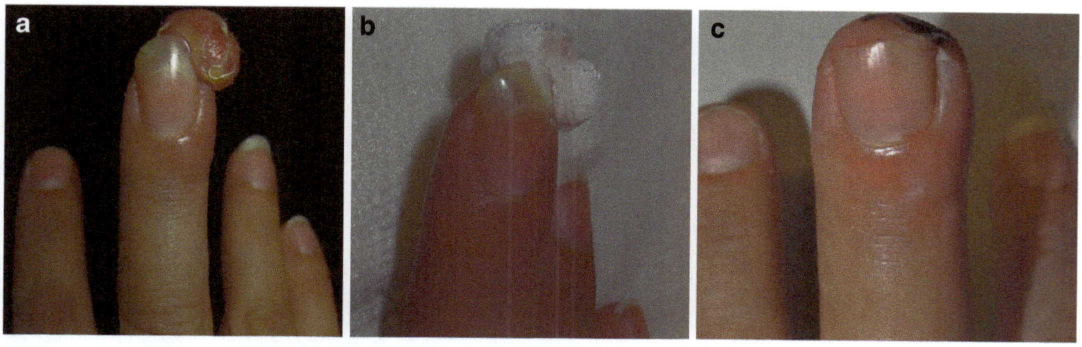

Fig. 12.14 (**a**) Large pyogenic granuloma on the finger tip. The lesion bled easily, and the patient was afraid to cut her fingernail. (**b**) One freeze-thaw cycle with open (spraying) technique from the center, allowing the freezing front to advance slowly until it reached the skin surface. (**c**) Shaving of the tumor while it was still frozen with no bleeding. A hemostatic solution was applied as thawing set in

Cryosurgery has been proven effective for treating pyogenic granulomas [32, 33]. Freezing has to include the whole lesion and extend up to 1 mm at the base. Treatment can be performed using a concave probe, ideal for large raised lesions of a size that fits the probe. One cycle is sufficient.

For small lesions, one cycle with a previously frozen probe or even a cryotweezer will do. For very large lesions, an excellent option is spray freezing from the center, allowing the freezing front to advance slowly down to the base. Once completely frozen, shaving can be done and the specimen can be sent for histologic examination. Before complete thawing, freeze the base where the feeding vessel emerges or apply a hemostatic solution. Make sure that, once complete thawing has occurred, there is no bleeding before covering the lesion (Fig. 12.14a–c).

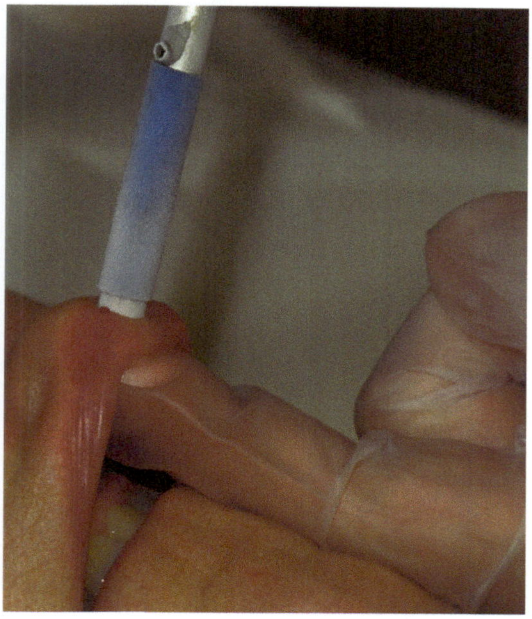

Fig. 12.15 Probe technique for venous lakes. The probe was precooled and applied with pressure. The finger was placed under the lesion and helped to keep the probe in place, assisted in pressuring the tumor toward the probe, and allowed for sensing that the freezing front was reaching the mucosa ("tattoo" formation)

12.7 Venous Lakes

These lesions are superficial varicose veins that are present in actinically damaged skin. They are very frequent in older people and mostly present in the lips, oral mucosa, earlobes, and face. They are easily depressed, a sign that helps to confirm the diagnosis.

When lesions are 2–5 mm, they are easily treated by cryosurgery. For small lesions (2.3 mm), no local anesthesia is required. In larger ones, local anesthesia is an option. One cycle using a previously frozen probe of the correct size applied with pressure will be sufficient (approximately 10 s freezing) (Fig. 12.15).

12.8 Spider Angiomas

These common vascular lesions are basically formed by a central arteriole that arises vertically from the dermis with many horizontal small branches.

Cryosurgery can be applied with a pointed probe. Some prefer to apply it without previously

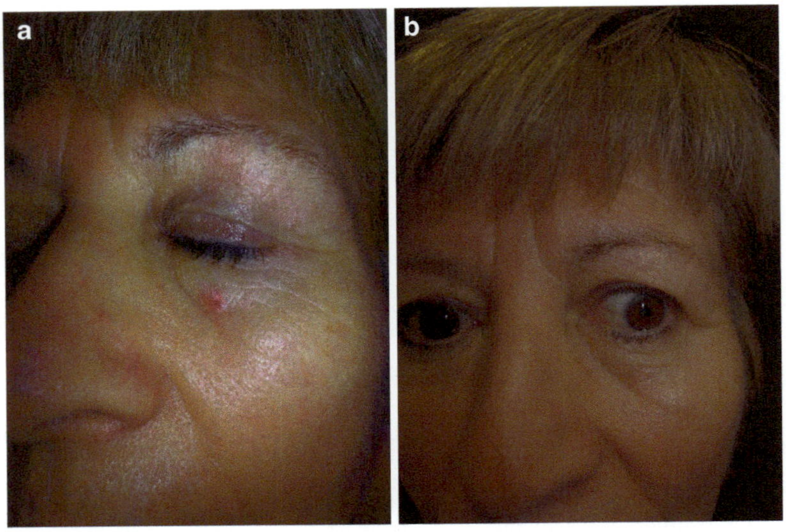

Fig. 12.16 (**a**) Spider telangiectasia in the lower eyelid. Treatment was performed with a sharp pointed probe, not precooled (in order to position it more precisely over the "head" of the telangiectasia), and applied with pressure for a few seconds. (**b**) One month posttreatment

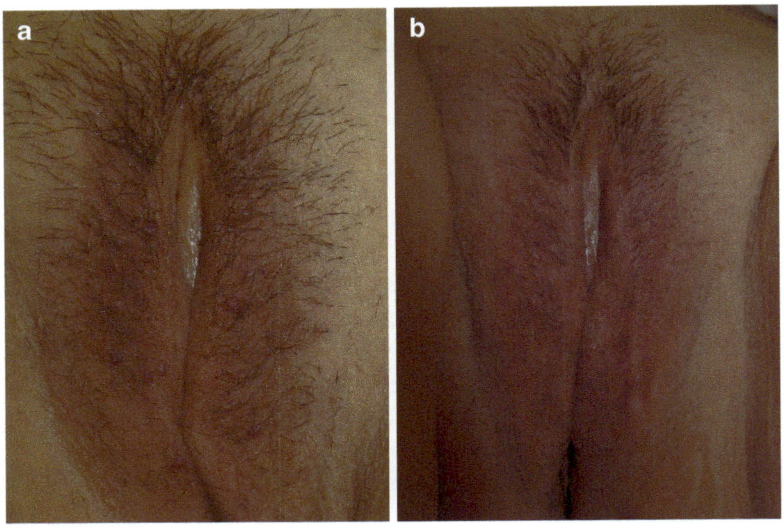

Fig. 12.17 (**a**) Multiple small angiokeratomas on the labia majora. (**b**) Two months after a one session treatment with a precooled probe (2 mm) applied with pressure. No topical or local anesthesia required

freezing the probe in order to be more precise in locating the fine point right in the central vessels. One cycle is sufficient (Fig. 12.16a, b). In recurrence, the procedure can be repeated.

12.9 Angiokeratomas (AK)

For the four clinical types of acquired angiokeratomas (solitary or sporadic, of Fordyce, of Mibelli, corporis diffusum) [28] described, cryosurgery can be an option for the first three types. Angiokeratomas have in common dilated vessels located in the upper dermis and hyperkeratotic epidermis. In individual lesions, local thrombosis can give a black appearance that can mimic a malignant melanoma or vice versa. A confirmation of the diagnosis is mandatory.

A double freeze-thaw cycle with a previously frozen probe, fitting the lesion and applied with pressure, should be sufficient. For residual lesions, the procedure can be repeated (Fig. 12.17a, b). No local anesthesia is required.

12.10 Other Vascular Lesions

12.10.1 HIV-Related Kaposi Sarcoma

These lesions can be treated by performing two 30 s freeze-thaw cycles with 3-mm margins every 4 weeks. It is a treatment that should be reserved for unaesthetic lesions that persist after antiretroviral treatment, preferably in the upper part of the trunk, the arms, or the face. It can be done by spraying or probe; in the latter, protect the probe with a protective cover for ultrasound transducers or a "finger" cut out from a latex glove.

12.11 Postoperative Considerations

Once a vascular lesion has been treated with cryosurgery, the follow-up is relatively simple. Daily cleaning with water and soap is sufficient. For large tumors, it is recommended that you cover it right after cleaning because oozing can be copious. The only important consideration is concerning crust formation. The crust should never be removed after vascular tumor cryosurgery in order to avoid exposing vessels that could result in bleeding. Once the crust starts forming, the patient has to apply antibiotic ointment daily. For small children, it is convenient to keep the lesion covered in order to avoid accidental removal or infection.

Essential Tidbits

- For vascular lesion treatment, abide by the 4P rule: probe, pressure, previously frozen probe, patience.
- For probes stuck on the skin or mucosa, never use force. Let the thaw begin and remove gently. If necessary to unstick to avoid excessive freezing, let some warm water run over the probe until it thaws and detaches.
- During postoperative care, never remove the crust. Let it fall off when dry.

Conclusions

Cryosurgery is an excellent alternative treatment in the management of the most common vascular tumors. Although many alternatives exist – lasers, surgery, topical and oral medication, and infiltration – some cases respond with just one single modality treatment, others require multiple sessions, and still others long periods of oral medication. In addition, combined vascular malformations tend to be difficult to treat and require a multidisciplinary approach.

In small superficial hemangiomas, cryosurgery stands as a fast, convenient, and inexpensive treatment that provides excellent results, with good medical and cosmetic outcomes, even with mild, superficial cryosurgery [22]. For pyogenic granulomas and spider angiomas, one single session is usually sufficient, while venous lakes can recur if a large feeding vessel is present.

Besides the expected edema, healing is fast and cosmetic results excellent. The speed of the procedure and the low cost are additional advantages.

References

1. Sharma VK, Khandpur S. Guidelines for cryotherapy. Indian J Dermatol Venereol Leprol. 2009;75:90–100.
2. Andrews MD. Cryosurgery for common skin conditions. Am Fam Physician. 2004;69:2365–72.
3. Zhang A, Xu LX, Sandison GA, Cheng S. Morphological study of endothelial cells during freezing. Phys Med Biol. 2006;51(23):6047–60.
4. Baust JG, Gage AA. The molecular basis of cryosurgery. BJU Int. 2005;95:1187–91.
5. Burrows PE, Laor T, Paltiel H, Robertson RL. Diagnostic imaging in the evaluation of vascular birthmarks. Dermatol Clin. 1998;16(3):455–88.
6. Gamboa A, Pasquali P, Trujillo B, González LA. Glioma nasal: Presentación de un caso tratado con criocirugía y revisión de la literatura. Dermatología Venezolana. 2005;43(1):34–6.
7. Miyake M, Oiso N, Kawada A. Dermoscopic Appearances in the Superficial and Deep Type of Infantile Hemangioma. J Cosmet Dermatol Sci Appl. 2012;2:212–3.

8. Paltiel HL, Burrows PE, Mulliken JB. Color Doppler ultrasound of soft tissue vascular anomalies. Radiology. 1994;193:292–5.
9. Whittle P, Baldassare G. Ultrasonografia de piel y anexos. Rev Chil Radiol [online]. 2004;10:81–8.
10. Navarro OM. Soft tissue masses in children. Radiol Clin North Am. 2011;49(6):1235–59, vi–vii.
11. Chen H, Lin X, Jin Y, Fan X, Li W, Ma G, Hu X. Deep infantile hemangiomas and early venous malformations: differential diagnosis by 3D CT angiography. Ann Plast Surg. 2010;64(6):755–8.
12. Navarro OM, Laffan EE, Ngan BY. Pediatric soft tissue tumours and pseudotumors: MR Imaging with pathologic correlation. Part 1. Imaging approach, pseudotumors, vascular lesions and adipocytic tumors. Radiographics. 2009;29:887–906.
13. Tan KT, Kirby J, Rajan DK, Hayeems E, Beecroft JR, Simons ME. Percutaneous sodium tetradecyl sulfate sclerotherapy for peripheral venous vascular malformations: a single-center experience. J Vasc Interv Radiol. 2007;18(3):343–51.
14. Astner S, González S, Cuevas J, Röwert-Huber J, Sterry W, Stockfleth E, Ulrich M. Preliminary evaluation of benign vascular lesions using in vivo reflectance confocal microscopy. Dermatol Surg. 2010;36(7): 1099–110.
15. De Kok E, Martin R, Pasquali P, Trujillo B. Hemangiomas en la infancia. Dematol Venez. 2005;43(1):16–8.
16. Frieden IJ, Eichenfield LF, Esterly NB, Geronemus R, Mallory S. Guidelines of care for hemangiomas of infancy. American Academy of Dermatology Guidelines/ Outcomes Committee. J Am Acad Dermatol. 1997;37: 631–7.
17. Serra AM, Soares FM, Cunha Júnior AG, Costa IM. Therapeutic management of skin hemangiomas in children. An Bras Dermatol [serial on the Internet]. 2010;85(3):307–17. [Cited 2014 Jan 19].
18. Ohtsuka H, Shioyan N, Tanake S. Cryosurgery for hemangiomas of the body surface and oral cavity. Ann Plast Surg. 1980;4:462–8.
19. Momotov AG, Polischuk SM, Gruminsk VS. Cryosurgical method of therapy for congenital vascular lesion in children. Klin Khir. 2002;6:44–7.
20. Vozmediano JF, Echeverría C, Armario JC. Cryosurgery for the treatment of hemangiomas Foliadermatol. Perú. 2004;15(2):111–4.
21. Moreno M, Cortez F, Rodrìguez S. Eficacia y seguridad en el tratamiento de hemangiomas infantiles de alto riesgo en lactantes menores tras sedación con solución de hidrato de cloral al 10 %. Dermatol Peruana. 2008;18(3):284–94.
22. Reynoso J, Abreu R, Marte T, Isa M, Almeida M, Nuñez A, Marte A. Críocirugía en el tratamiento de los hemangiomas. Revisión estadística en el Instituto Dermatológico y Cirugía de la Piel"Dr. Humberto Bogaert Díaz". Enero-Diciembre 2008. Rev Domin Dermatol. 2011;38(1):1–4.
23. Bassukas ID, Abuzahra F, Hundeiker M. Regression phase as therapeutic goal of cryosurgical treatment of growing capillary infantile hemangiomas. Treatment decision, treatment strategy and results of an open clinical study. Hautarzt. 2000;51(4):231–8. [Article in German].
24. Zouboulis OC. Cryosurgery in dermatology. Eur J Dermatol. 1998;8:466–74.
25. Reischle S, Schuller-Petrovic S. Treatment of capillary hemangiomas of early childhood with a new method of cryosurgery. J Am Acad Dermatol. 2000;42:809–13.
26. Dachow-Siwiéc E. Treatment of cryosurgery in the premalignant and bening lesions of the skin. In: Breittbat EW, Dachów-Siwiéc E, editors. Advances in cryosurgery, Clinics dermatology. New York: Elsevier; 1990. p. 74–5.
27. Michel S, Wlotzke U, Hohenleutner U, Landthaler M. Laser and cryotherapy of hemangioma in infants in a direct comparison. Hautarzt. 1998;49(3):192–6. [Article in German].
28. Della Nina BI, Oliveira ZN, Machado MC, Macea JM. Apresentação, evolução e tratamento dos hemangiomas cutâneos - Experiência do Ambulatório de Dermatologia Infantil do Hospital das Clínicas da Faculdade de Medicina da Universidade de São Paulo. An Bras Dermatol. 2006;81:323–7.
29. Gadelha AR, Costa IMC. Cirurgia Dermatológica em Consultório. In: Souza JJ, editor. Criocirurgia de lesões benignas e pré-malignas. São Paulo: Ed. Atheneu; 2003. p. 361–6.
30. Greene AK. Vascular anomalies: current overview of the field. Clin Plast Surg. 2011;38(1):1–5.
31. Requena L. Tumores cutáneos de partes blandas. Aula Médica; 2012.
32. Mirshams M, Daneshpazhooh M, Mirshekari A, Taheri A, Mansoori P, Hekmat S. Cryotherapy in the treatment of pyogenic granuloma. J Eur Acad Dermatol Venereol. 2006;20:788–90.
33. Ghodsi SZ, Raziei M, Taheri A, Karami M, Mansoori P, Farnaghi F. Comparison of cryotherapy and curettage for the treatment of pyogenic granuloma: a randomized trial. Br J Dermatol. 2006;154(4):671–5.

Part III

Non-invasive Imaging Techniques

High-Frequency Ultrasound (HFUS) in the Management of Skin Cancer Treated with Cryosurgery

13

Paola Pasquali

Contents

Key Points

- High-frequency ultrasound (22 MHz) of skin malignancies gives information on volume and shape to help select the best treatment.
- HFUS identifies BCC with more than one histologic subtype, especially when there is a need to identify nodular elements within a clinically superficial tumor.
- Multiple BCC patients will benefit from a previous HFUS of all lesions before deciding treatment upon an approach or cryosurgical technique.
- Trans-cryosurgical HFUS enables visualization of the depth obtained by the freezing front.

13.1 Introduction

Until a few decades ago, dermatologists had based, and in some cases still base, most of their diagnoses on simple clinical evaluations. Fortunately, techniques and digital imaging have become available in user-friendly formats. Compact, less expensive equipment has come to market, and less invasive technologies have been developed. Today, imaging is used in diagnosis, treatment evaluation, and post-therapeutic control. In malignant tumor management, it is not feasible to biopsy every single lesion, particularly in those patients with

P. Pasquali, MD
Department of Dermatology, Pius Hospital de Valls, 43800 Tarragona, Spain
e-mail: pasqualipaola@gmail.com

P. Pasquali (ed.), *Cryosurgery: A Practical Manual*,
DOI 10.1007/978-3-662-43939-5_13, © Springer-Verlag Berlin Heidelberg 2015

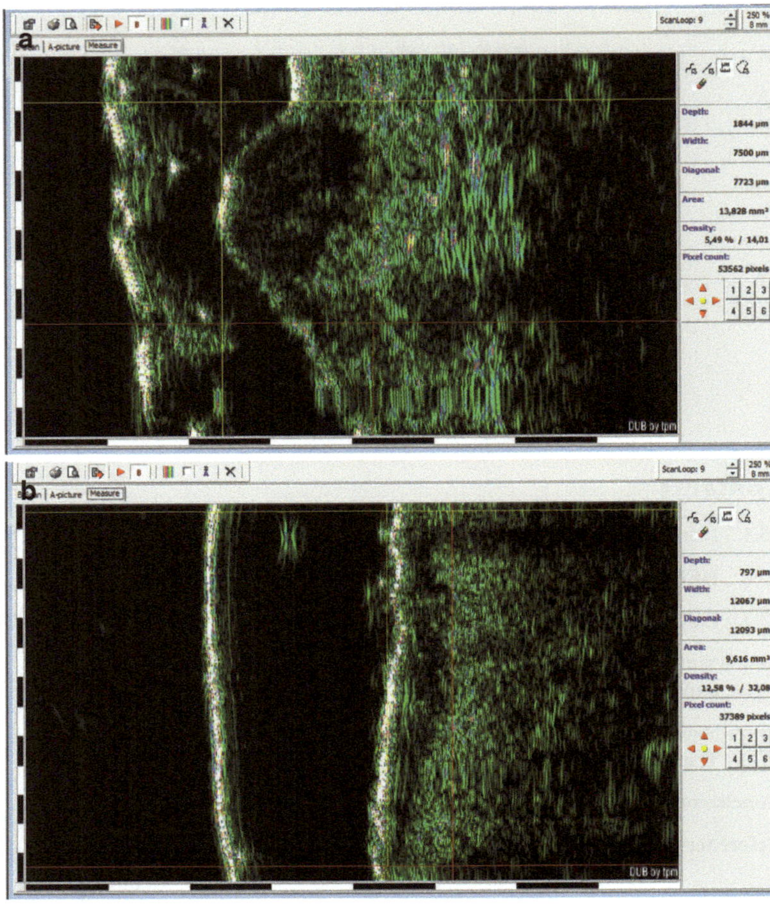

Fig. 13.1 (**a**) HFUS of a nodular BCC (size: 1,844 mm depth × 7,500 mm width; (**b**) HFUS of a superficial BCC (0,797 mm depth × 12,067 mm width

multiple lesions (such as basal cell carcinomas); therefore, clinical evaluation will necessarily support itself with imaging technology in order to obtain the correct diagnosis [1].

Dermoscopy has become immensely popular and stands as an indispensable tool to uncover clinically invisible morphological aspects of skin lesions. On the other end of the spectrum of the noninvasive tools for diagnosing skin lesions one finds reflectance confocal microscopy which will identify cellular structures to a resolution similar to histology. It still has not gained the place it deserves in daily practice probably due to its high cost and need for formal training to interpret its images.

In the middle of this spectrum stands high-frequency ultrasound (HFUS). It is a noninvasive technique capable of complementing tumor information not obtainable by the aforementioned methods [2, 3]. It is a small, portable piece of equipment, easy to carry and use. Its cost is intermediate, between dermoscopy and confocal microscopy; it requires training for image interpretation.

HFUS allows visualizing shape as well as measuring the length, depth, and width of skin tumors (Fig. 13.1a, b). The 22–50 MHz applicators are the most commonly used in dermatology and ideal for those lesions less than 12 mm in length and 6–8 mm in depth.

It seems inconceivable today to examine the skin without the aid of a dermoscope; soon, high-frequency ultrasound (HFUS/HRUS, high-resolution ultrasound, high-resolution echography) should be included in the indispensable armamentarium of those actively working on skin cancer. For some, this has been a common practice for many years [4]. Combining noninvasive techniques (dermoscopy, HFUS, confocal) will save time and money as well as unnecessary biopsies.

The more information is available on a particular tumor, the better treatment can be provided. Clinical evaluation and dermoscopy will give information on the superficial morphologic aspects, HFUS will provide information on shape and volume [5, 6], and confocal microscopy will provide information on cellular aspects [7] (Fig. 13.2a–d).

There is an excellent correlation between dermoscopy and HFUS dimensions [5]. This means that the dimensions obtained by dermoscopy correspond to the HFUS length of the tumor. Therefore, the dermoscopy image corresponds to the real size of the tumor; however, only through HFUS one will know the actual depth and shape of the tumor.

Some tumor characteristics that can be better understood by HFUS evaluation are:

- *Volume/Shape*. The shape and size of a tumor can provide information of the type of tumor. Most BCC are anechoic and have a roughly elliptical shape; occasionally, they are elongated anechoic and have a collar necklace or rosary pattern (Fig. 13.3). SCC are also hypoechoic, but a thick superficial crust needs to be removed before visualization [4]. They are usually thick lesions with irregular "iceberg" shapes. HFUS imaging will be of great help in choosing the proper site for biopsy or selecting the best method for tumor removal. In addition, some tumors have an iceberg shape: they appear small at the surface while the length underneath the surface is larger. This could be the cause of positive margins after surgery.
- *Depth*. The knowledge of the depth of tumors helps in deciding the correct surgical technique. For example, superficial BCC lesions can be diagnosed by clinical/dermoscopy [8] examination. Treatment options include cryosurgery, topical immunomodulators like imiquimod, photodynamic therapy (PDT), and curettage/electrocoagulation, among others. There is no need for costly, lengthy, expensive, and invasive techniques like Mohs micrographic surgery on a superficial carcinoma. Although this seems logical, the out-of-proportion use of Mohs surgery (1 out of every 4 tumors are treated with MMS [9]) suggests that this technique is being used for treating many superficial lesions. The HFUS image of a superficial BCC shows a hypoechoic elliptical area(s) of less than 1 mm of depth. Individually, each island of tumor measures 1–1.2 mm in depth. Lengthwise, they can be small (1–2 mm) but can also be quite large, requiring a segmental HFUS evaluation in order to cover the whole area. HFUS allows the determination as to whether BCC is only superficial or it has a deeper component within the tumor. Apparently "superficial BCC" can "hide" nodular or even morpheaform elements (admixture tumor), as is the case in roughly one-third of all BCC [10, 11] (Fig. 13.4a, b). The latter is a common cause of treatment failure and recurrence (Fig. 13.5). Sometimes this reoccurrence is many years later. The tumor's depth has to be determined throughout the whole tumor area using HFUS readings. The deep margin evaluation by HFUS is limited to tumors under 8 mm in depth. Proper selection of the biopsy site is of utmost importance [12]; therefore, HFUS-guided biopsy could be another possible indication.
- *Length*. The longitudinal/width margin evaluation by HFUS is limited to tumors under 12 mm. For large lesions, HFUS might need to be performed by sectors.

13.2 HFUS and Cryosurgery

The combination of HFUS and cryosurgery has the following advantages:

1. This combination gives the surgeon information regarding the volume, depth, and length of the tumor.
2. This combination allows for visualization of the depth of the freezing front.

13.3 HFUS Volume and Cryosurgery

Cancer cells need a temperature of at least – 50 °C to be destroyed. That temperature must be reached throughout the entire tumor including the safety margin of 4 mm. The temperature at

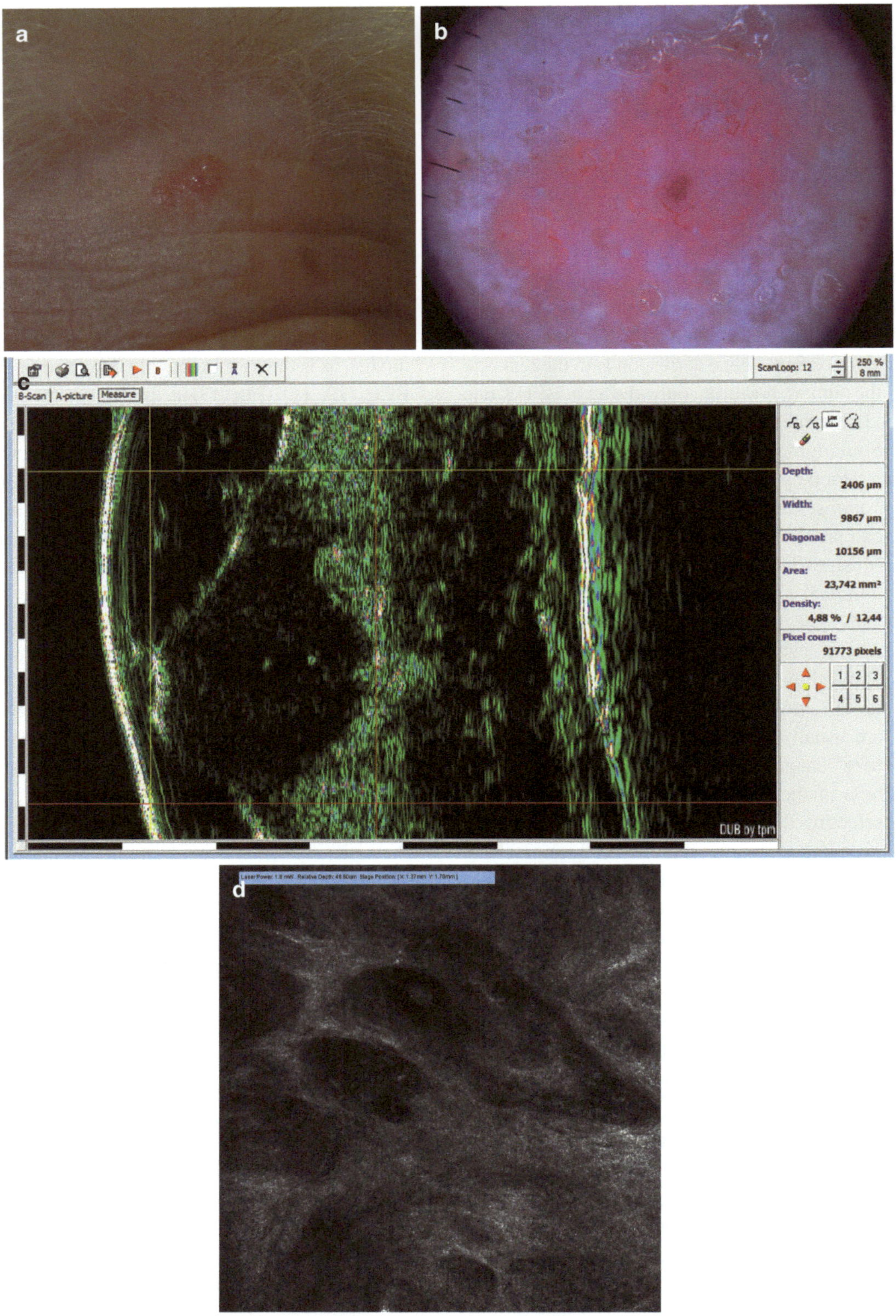

Fig. 13.2 (**a–d**) Four ways of looking at a nodular BCC: (**a**) clinical photograph, (**b**) dermoscopic image, (**c**) HFUS, (**d**) confocal microcopy (**d**: Courtesy of Rainer Hofmann-Wellenhof, MD)

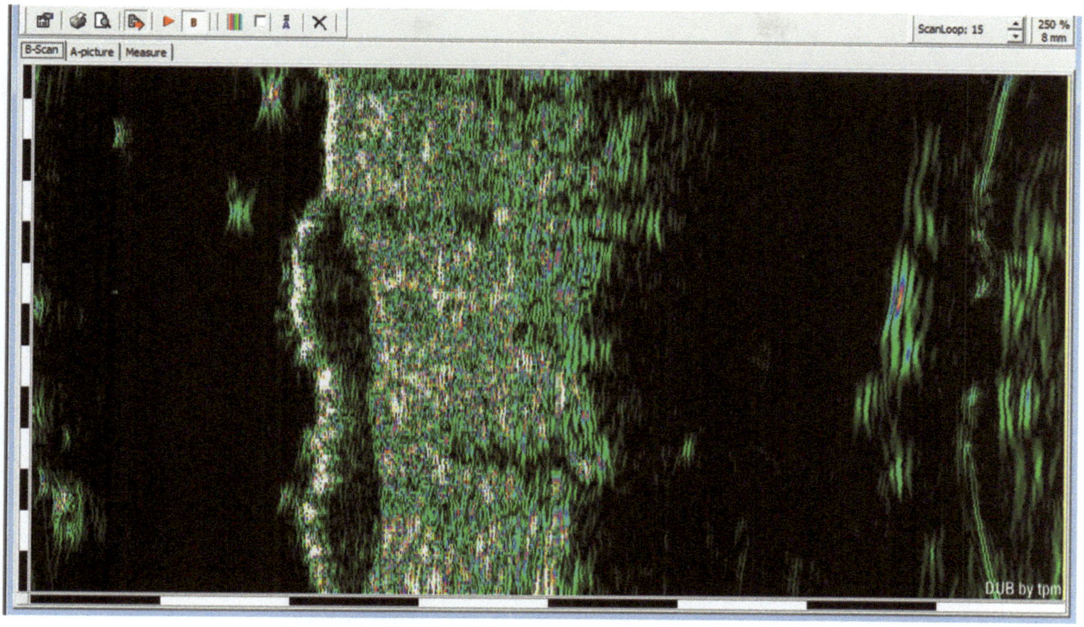

Fig. 13.3 Collar necklace HFUS image of a superficial BCC

the center of the freezing ball is the first to achieve the optimal killing temperatures. The concern is at the periphery of the tumor where suboptimal freezing temperatures might leave undestroyed malignant cells. Therefore, temperature needs to be measured at the periphery. Following the isotherm, the temperature at the depth of the tumor can be inferred (Fig. 13.6).

Deep tumors are best treated with close (probe) or chamber technique because a greater depth is reached (Fig. 13.7). In general, the length/depth ratio is 6 × 1 (for nodular BCC the ratio is 4 × 1) [5]. Superficial/shallow tumors can be treated both by open (spray) or close (probe) technique.

13.4 Multiple BCC Management and HFUS

Management of syndromic and non-syndromic multiple BCC represents a real challenge. No one treatment alternative is sufficient, and multidisciplinary approach/combination treatments are usually required. One of the problems is

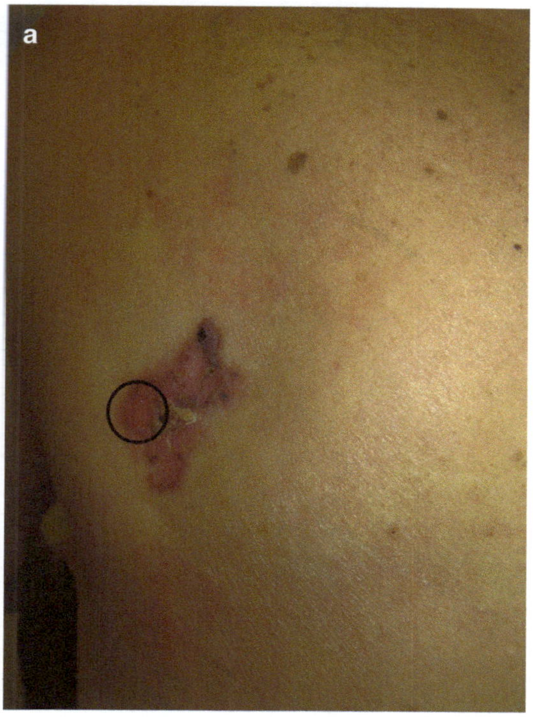

Fig. 13.4 (**a**, **b**) A very large pigmented BCC on the back. (**a**) Clinical evaluation and dermoscopy showed a superficial BCC with an ulcerated area (*circle*). (**b**) HFUS showed a nodular area

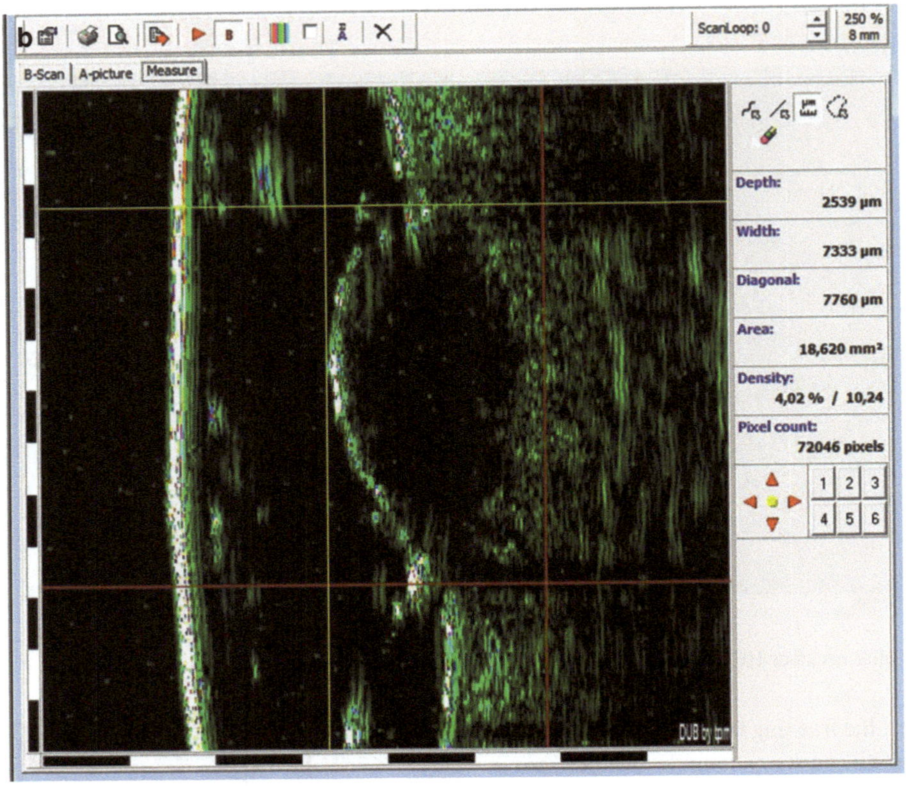

Fig. 13.4 (continued)

that the complete genetics involved in the genesis of these tumors is still not fully understood, especially in non-syndromic cases [13]. Genetically induced BCC includes conditions like Gorlin, Bazex-Dupré-Christol, and Rombo syndrome as well as xeroderma pigmentosum. Other disorders that can be associated with multiple early onset skin malignancies include those with defects in DNA replication/repair functions, genodermatoses affecting folliculosebaceous unit, immune response, and melanin biosynthesis [14].

Many treatment modalities have been proposed that range from topical and oral treatments, PDT, surgical excision, cryosurgery, Mohs micrographic surgery (MMS), to ablative lasers. It is advisable to excise aggressive lesions and reserve skin preserving alternatives for the rest [15]. For multiple BCC patients, an algorithm suggests the workup recommended (Fig. 13.8), indicating the most common skin-sparing modalities [16] and deep tumor removal modalities (Table 13.1).

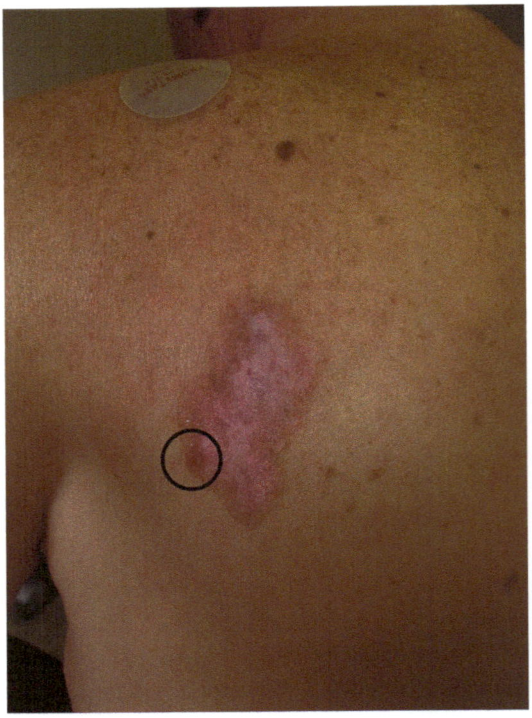

Fig. 13.5 Same patient as in Fig. 13.4. BCC was treated with topical imiquimod treatment. After healing from the imiquimod treatment, there was residual tumor (corresponding to the nodular part). This residual tumor was later treated with cryosurgery (close technique)

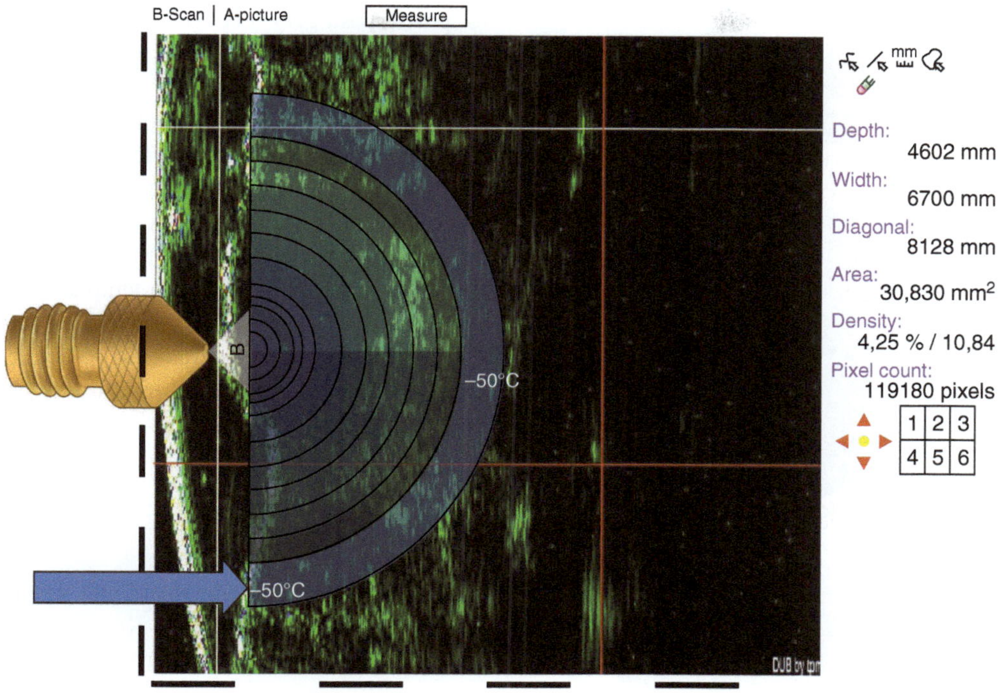

Fig. 13.6 The ice ball expands in a roughly hemispherical shape. The temperature decreases from the center out in isotherm. The lateral spread from the edge of a probe is approximately equal to the depth of the freeze. The temperatures at the base and at the lateral margin are the same

In multiple BCC patients, a previous HFUS map of the lesions should be performed to choose the best treatment option (Fig. 13.9).

Cryosurgery can be the treatment of choice for both superficial or deep tumors. In both cases, the following concepts are of utmost importance:

- *Temperature*. Keep always in mind the required −50 °C needed to kill a skin cancer cell regardless of tumor depth.
- *Depth*. For deep tumor, it is best to choose the close (probe) technique because the freezing is faster and deeper (covered area of ice ball per minute) as well as more precise (freezing is restrained to the probe or chamber area). For shallow small tumors, open (spray) technique is probably better to reduce damage to deep structures; for deep small tumors, probe cryosurgery is the best but not the sole choice.
- *Spray vs Probe*. Lower temperatures are achieved faster with metal probes. If the correct size probe is available, the close technique will be the best choice.

13.5 Monitoring with HFUS: Trans-cryosurgical HFUS

The distribution of temperature in isothermal areas lets one infer the temperature in hidden parts of the tumor. The combination of HFUS and cryosurgery performed with devices that measure the temperature turns conventional cryosurgery into a non-blinded procedure.

Skin temperature monitoring by infrared sensing spares the use of thermocouple needles. The latter implies invasiveness from needle introduction which was performed mostly blinded (non-US guided).

Once freezing of the tumor has been performed by any chosen cryosurgical technique, the immediate HFUS image is black. This is because US waves are reflected by ice. Once thawing begins (from the surface of the skin down), the superficial part of the tumor becomes evident and, in time (starting from the top down), the whole tumor can be seen (Fig. 13.10a–c).

After the first freezing cycle, the area will be more hypogenic and the tumor larger. This is due

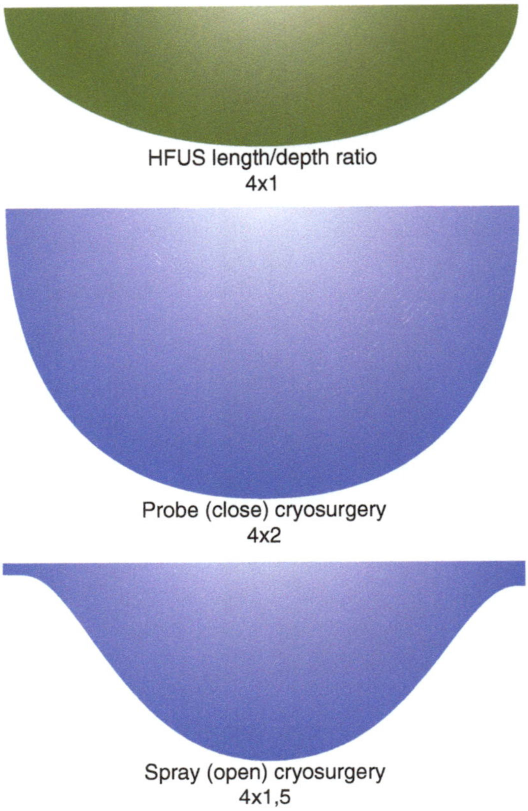

Fig. 13.7 The volume ratio of most nodular BCC measured by HFUS is 4 × 1. The ice ball of a close (probe) cryosurgery is approximately 4 × 2; for spray, cryosurgery has a hat shape, and it is approximately 4 × 1.5 (these last two shapes were obtained from a gelatin model)

to post-cryosurgery edema. After the second freeze-thaw cycle, this edema is even more apparent (Fig. 13.11a–c).

The depth of the freezing front can be visualized with HFUS, and the total thawing time can be measured. The skin temperature at the periphery of the tumor can be measured by infrared technology and the temperature at the bottom of the tumor inferred by isotherm temperature distribution. The previous knowledge of the tumor depth will allow the operator to know if the entirety of the tumor has been frozen at the correct temperature.

Essential Tidbits

- Measure BCC before deciding upon the best treatment option. Knowing the tumor volume will help avoid under- or overtreatment.
- HFUS is ideal for multiple BCC patients.
- Trans-cryosurgery HFUS gives an additional record of thaw time as well as visualizing depth of freezing front.

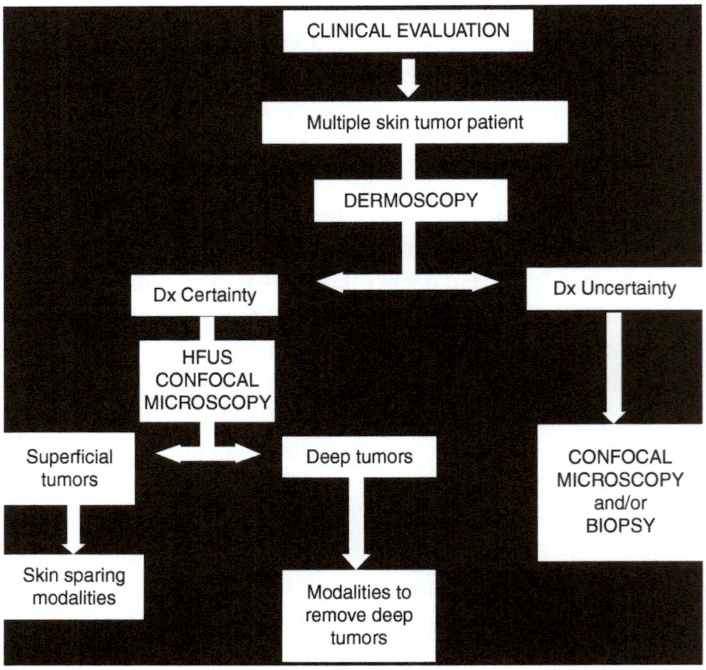

Fig. 13.8 Suggested algorithm for multiple NMSC patients

Conclusions

HFUS gives complementary information to other noninvasive techniques like dermoscopy and confocal microscopy. Further studies will help determine the relationship between shape/volume and histologic type and aid in the development of criteria to diagnose tumor subtypes. Incorporating this noninvasive technique into daily practice will help to select the best treatment modality for each tumor. The appropriateness of selection will reduce the chances of under-treating a tumor (by using a superficial treatment modality on a deep tumor) or overtreating [17] (by using, for instance, MMS in a superficial or small nodular BCC). In both situations (under- and over-treatment), the consequences can be dramatic. With under-treatment, leaving a residual a residual tumor growing under the skin surface freely for years can result in the tumor becoming inoperable or metastatic. Appropriate use criteria will avoid this scenario.

Table 13.1 Most common skin-sparing and deep tumor removal modalitites

Skin-sparing modalities
Topical treatment: imiquimod, 5 FU
PDT
Electrocoagulation/curettage
Shaving
Intralesional agents: 5 FU, methotrexate, bleomycin, IFN alpha (α)-2, IFN α-2a, IFN α-2b
Cryosurgery
Electrochemotherapy
Deep tumor removal modalities
Surgery
Mohs micrographic surgery
Cryosurgery
Electrochemotherapy

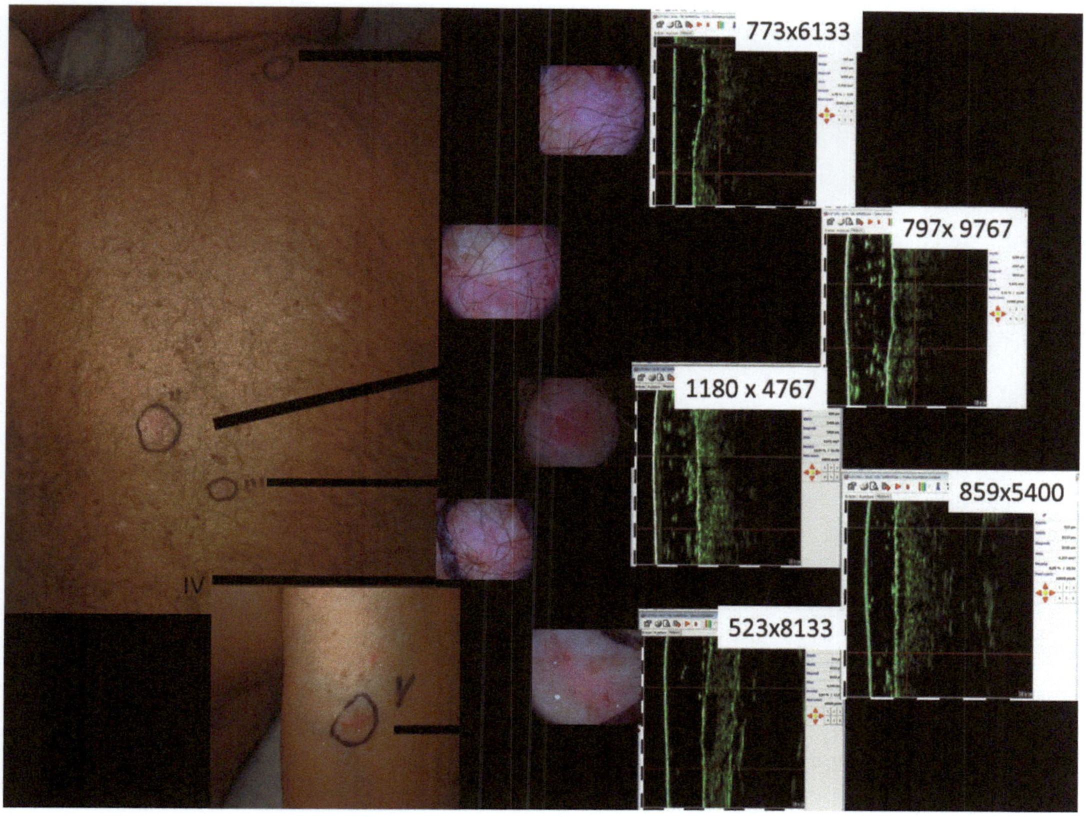

Fig. 13.9 Mapping a patient with multiple BCC. HFUS shows that all lesions are superficial BCC and can be safely treated with skin-sparing modalities

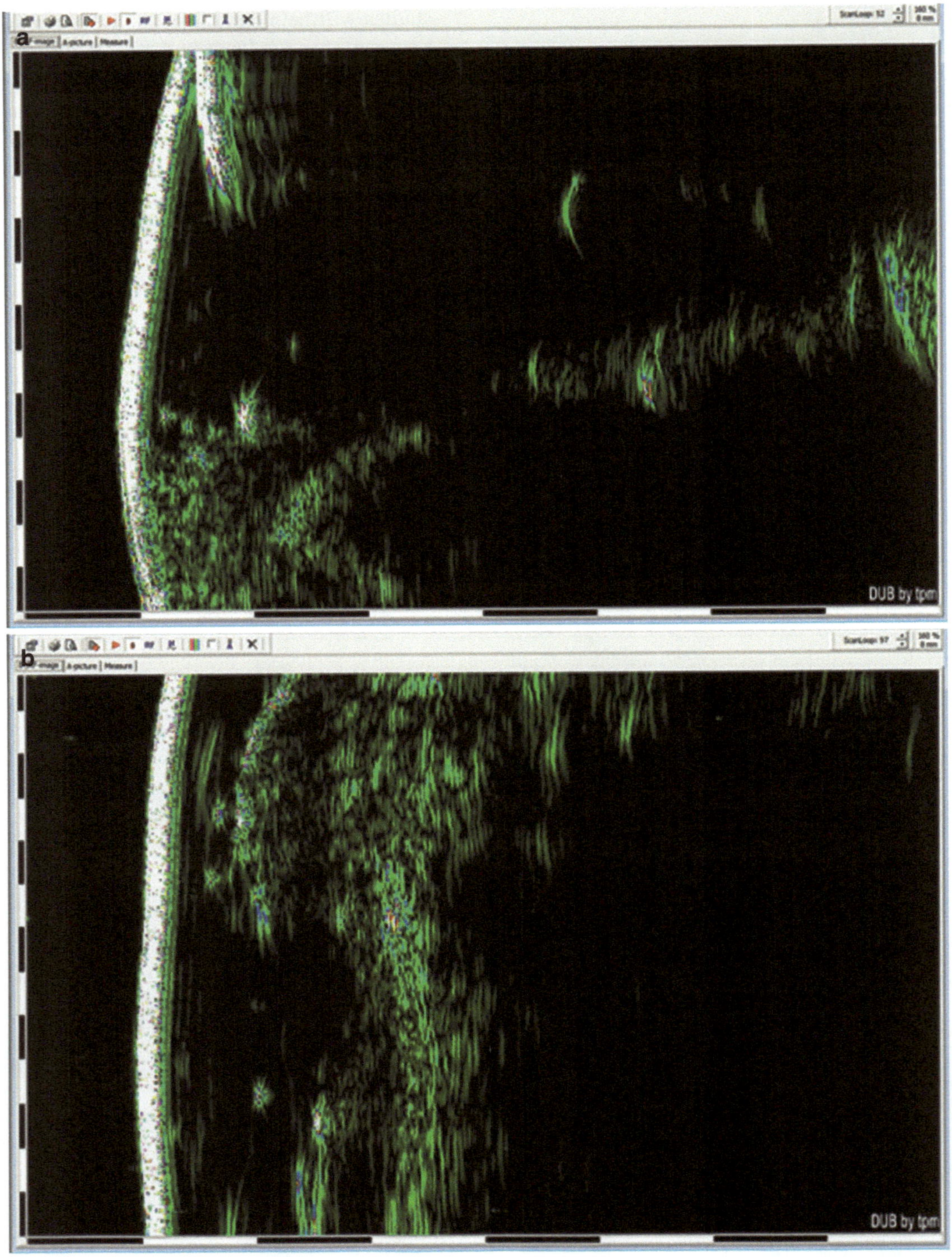

Fig. 13.10 (**a**–**c**) A BCC partially removed by deep shaving and treated with cryosurgery. (**a**) HFUS immediately after freezing showing a black area corresponding to the ice ball; (**b**) As thawing sets in, the superficial part becomes evident first and (**c**) the deeper component becomes apparent with complete thawing

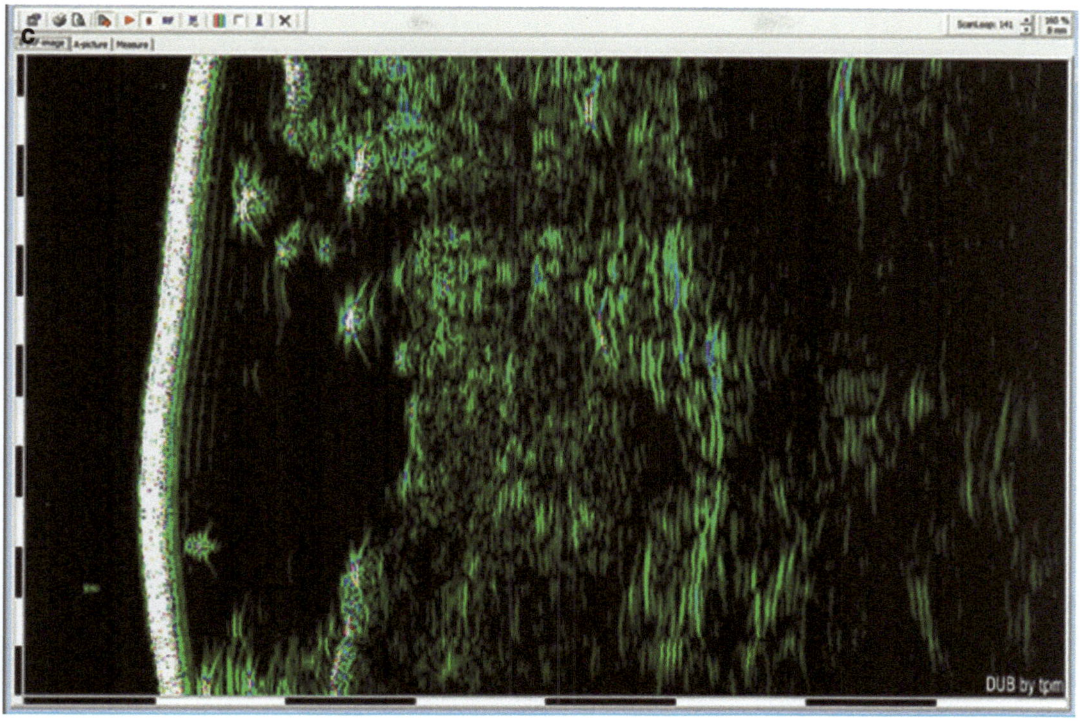

Fig. 13.10 (continued)

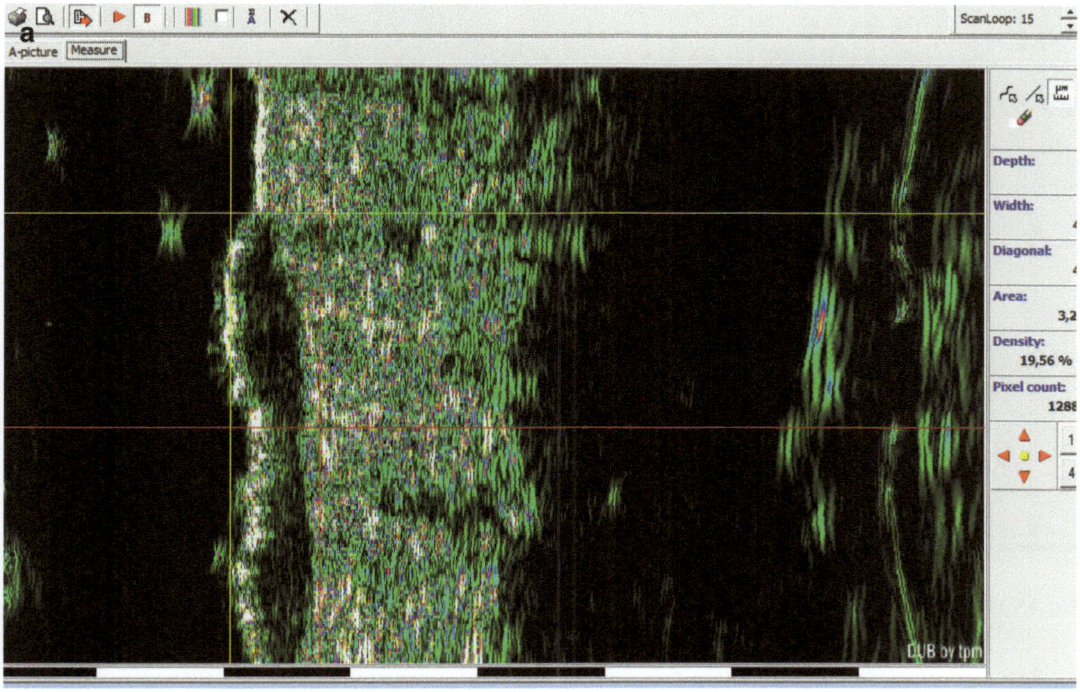

Fig. 13.11 (**a**) Superficial BCC. A small island is measured before treatment (total area: 3,294 mm^2). (**b**) First freeze-thaw cycle showing edematous tissue with slight increase in total area (3,798 mm^2). (**c**) After second freeze-thaw cycle (5,205 mm^2) showing an important local edema

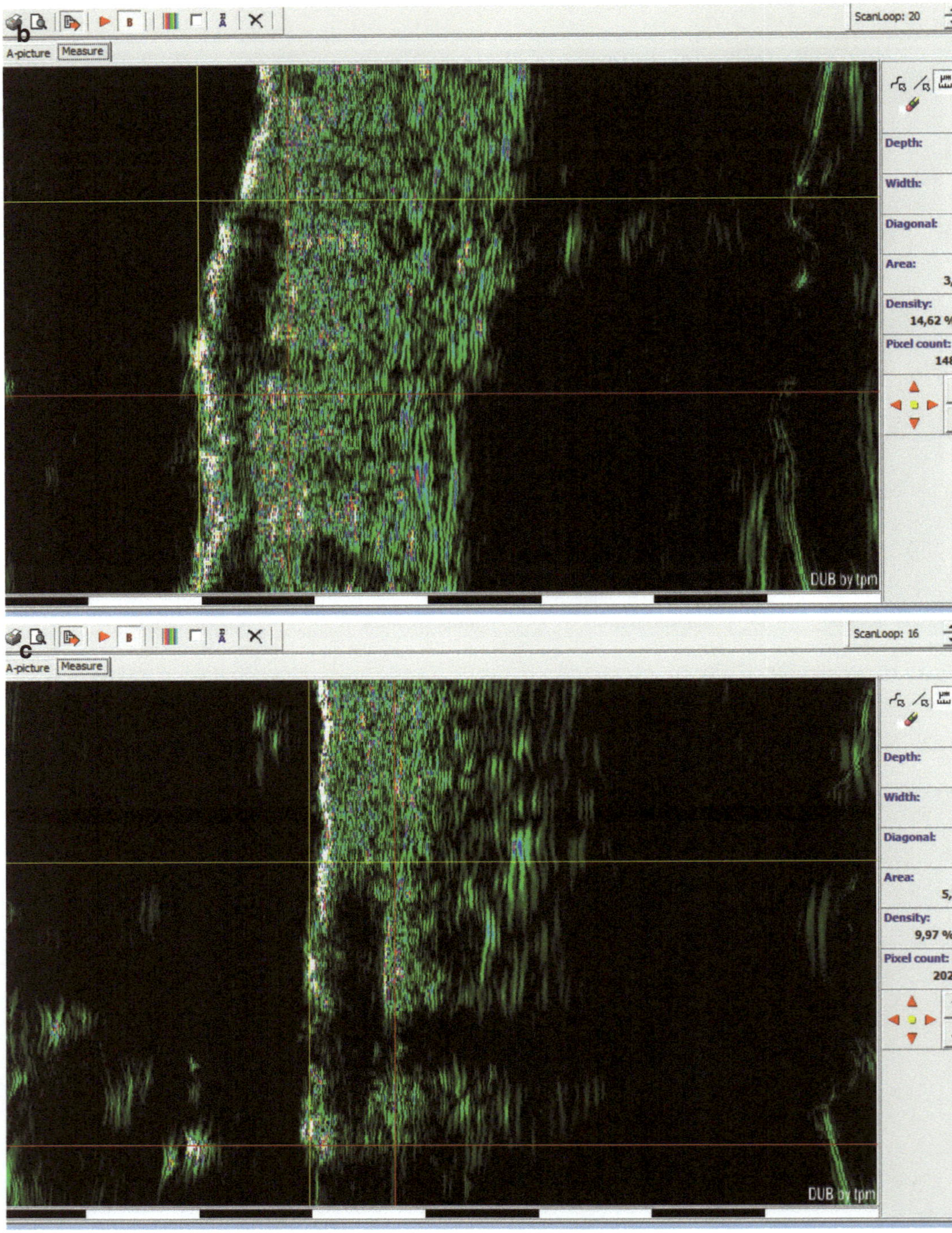

Fig. 13.11 (continued)

Glossary

HFUS	High-frequency ultrasound
MMS	Mohs micrographic surgery
Trans-Cryosurgical HFUS	Consists in doing an HFUS immediately after freezing, with the tissue still frozen

References

1. Wassef C, Rao BK. Uses of non-invasive imaging in the diagnosis of skin cancer: an overview of the currently available modalities. Int J Dermatol. 2013; 52(12):1481–9.
2. Wortsman X. Common applications of dermatologic sonography. J Ultrasound Med. 2012;31:97–111.
3. Wortsman X, Wortsman J. Clinical usefulness of variable-frequency ultrasound in localized lesions of the skin. J Am Acad Dermatol. 2010;62:247–56.
4. Machet L, Ossant F, Bleuzen A, Grégoire JM, Machet MC, Vaillant L. High-resolution ultrasonography: utility in diagnosis, treatment, and monitoring dermatologic diseases. J Radiol. 2006;87(12 Pt 2):1946–61 [Article in French].
5. Pasquali P, Camacho E, Fortuño-Mar A. Use of 22 MHz High-Frequency Ultrasound in the Management of Skin Cancer. In: Baldi A, Pasquali P, Spugnini EP, editors. Skin Cancer A Practical Approach. New York: Humana Press/Springer; 2014. p. 245–56.
6. Hoffmann K, el Gammal S, Matthes U, Altmeyer P. Digital 20 MHz sonography of the skin in preoperative diagnosis. Z Hautkr. 1989;64(10):851. –2, 855–8.
7. Gill M, Longo C, Farnetani F, Cesinaro AM, González S, Pellacani G. Non-invasive in vivo dermatopathology: identification of reflectance confocal microscopic correlates to specific histological features seen in melanocytic neoplasms. J Eur Acad Dermatol Venereol. 2013. doi:10.1111/jdv.12285. [Epub ahead of print].
8. Argenziano G, Giacomel J, Zalaudek I, et al. A clinico-dermoscopic approach for skin cancer screening: recommendations involving a survey of the International Dermoscopy Society. Dermatol Clin. 2013;31(4):525–34.
9. Asgari MM, Olson JM, Alam M. Needs assessment for Mohs micrographic surgery. Dermatol Clin. 2012;30:167–75, x.
10. Sexton M, Jones DB, Maloney ME. Histologic pattern analysis of basal cell carcinoma. J Am Acad Dermatol. 1990;23:1118–26.
11. Crowson AN. Basal cell carcinoma: biology, morphology and clinical implications. Mod Pathol. 2006;19:S127–47.
12. Kamyab-Hesari K, Seirafi H, Naraghi ZS, Shahshahani MM, Rahbar Z, Damavandi MR, Naraghi MM, Rezvani M, Aghazadeh N. Diagnostic accuracy of punch biopsy in subtyping basal cell carcinoma. J Eur Acad Dermatol Venereol. 2012. doi:10.1111/j.1468-3083.2012.04695.x. [Epub ahead of print].
13. Peacock CD, Rudin CM. Skin deep and deeper: multiple pathways in basal cell carcinogenesis. Cancer Prev Res (Phila). 2010;3(10):1213–6.
14. Castori M, Morrone A, Kanitakis J, Grammatico P. Genetic skin diseases predisposing to basal cell carcinoma. Eur J Dermatol. 2012;22(3):299–309.
15. Van der Geer S, Ostertag JU, Krekels GA. Treatment of basal cell carcinomas in patients with nevoid basal cell carcinoma syndrome. J Eur Acad Dermatol Venereol. 2009;23(3):308–13.
16. Chitwood K, Etzkorn J, Cohen G. Topical and intralesional treatment of nonmelanoma skin cancer: efficacy and cost comparisons. Dermatol Surg. 2013; 39(9):1306–16.
17. Ad Hoc Task Force, Connolly SM, Baker DR, Coldiron BM, et al. AAD/ACMS/ASDSA/ASMS 2012 appropriate use criteria for Mohs micrographic surgery: a report of the American Academy of Dermatology, American College of Mohs Surgery, American Society for Dermatologic Surgery Association, and the American Society for Mohs Surgery. J Am Acad Dermatol. 2012;67(4): 531–50.

14 Role of Reflectance Confocal Microscopy in Cryosurgery

Joseph Chao, Rainer Hofmann-Wellenhof, and Clara Curiel-Lewandrowski

Contents

Key Points

- Reflectance confocal microscopy (RCM) is a noninvasive in vivo imaging technique that relays on the natural variation of refractive indices in tissue structures at different depths of the skin to reconstruct the images.
- Melanin has the highest refractive index and appears the brightest on RCM images. Other sources of contrast include keratin, cellular organelles, chromatin, and collagen.
- A clinical breakthrough in RCM has been the capability to bring to the bedside an almost equivalent tool to histological evaluation without the need for invasive diagnostic procedures.
- The RCM technology can be implemented as a diagnostic, surgical margin assessment, and monitoring of therapeutic interventions, such as cryosurgery.

Disclosures Clara Curiel-Lewandrowski: MelaSciences, Inc-Consulting; Medical Directions, Inc-Consulting; DermSpectra LLC-Founder/Member.

Funding Source Supported by a contract (NO1-CN-35158) from the National Cancer Institute, Division of Cancer Prevention, the Arizona Cancer Center Support Grant (CA023074), and Janice and Alan Levine Endowed Chair in Cancer Research, Arizona Cancer Center, University of Arizona.

J. Chao (✉)
Department of Dermatology,
University of Arizona Medical Center,
1501 N. Campbell Avenue, Tucson, AZ 85724, USA
e-mail: jcslater@email.arizona.edu

R. Hofmann-Wellenhof, MD
Department of Dermatology,
Medical University Graz, Auenbruggerplatz 8,
Graz 8036, Austria
e-mail: rainer.hofmann@medunigraz.at

C. Curiel-Lewandrowski, MD (✉)
Section of Dermatology, Department of Medicine,
University of Arizona Cancer Center,
1515 N. Campbell Ave, Tucson 85724, AZ USA
e-mail: ccuriel@email.arizona.edu

P. Pasquali (ed.), *Cryosurgery: A Practical Manual*,
DOI 10.1007/978-3-662-43939-5_14, © Springer-Verlag Berlin Heidelberg 2015

- The aid of RCM in the setting of pigmented lesions include guiding the clinicians to the areas of greater atypia to perform skin biopsies, identification of benign appearing melanocytic lesions, and assessment of lentigo maligna suspected lesions.
- RCM is a highly sensitive and specific imaging modality for the identification and assessment of BCC cases.

14.1 Introduction

Reflectance confocal microscopy (RCM) is a noninvasive in vivo imaging technique intended to help the clinician diagnostically view skin lesions in real time while avoiding trauma or scar formation from surgical biopsies. First described in 1955 by Marvin Minsky [1], it was not until the late 1980s and early 1990s when light and computer technology was advanced enough to image tissue in vivo. In 1995, Rajadhyaksha and colleagues [2] were the first to describe RCM imaging of human skin in vivo, utilizing a laser light source to provide enough illumination and near-infrared wavelengths strong enough to view deeper levels of the skin in high resolution at a cellular level.

RCM's principles rely on the natural variation of refractive indices in tissue structures at different depths of the skin [3]. Of all the molecular structures in the skin, melanin has the highest refractive index and appears the brightest on RCM images [2]. Other sources of contrast include keratin, cellular organelles, chromatin, and collagen (Fig. 14.1).

With the use of a near-infrared diode laser, light projected from the confocal microscope focuses on a specific point in the skin. Reflected light from this point is captured through a pinhole-sized opening by a detector as shown in Fig. 14.2. The use of such a small aperture segregates reflected light from the focal section of interest from other areas of the tissue. The depth of light penetration is dependent on wavelength, laser power, reflectivity of the superficial layers of skin, and scattering properties of the dermis. Of all these factors, only laser power can be changed. At longer wavelengths, deeper penetration is gained at the expense of resolution; therefore, present single-laser confocal microscopes are fixed at 830 nm [2].

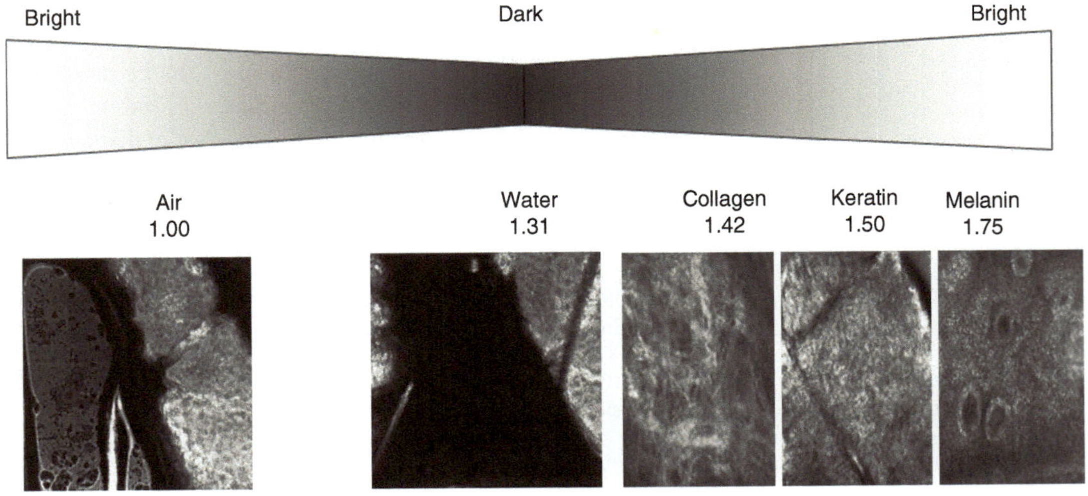

Fig. 14.1 Refractive index. Since the human body contains over 60 % water, this eliminates the need for contrast agent. Therefore, water serves as the standard. The refractive index of water is 1.31. The closer the materials refractive index ratio is to 1.31, the darker the material looks. The further the deviation from this value (+or −), the brighter that material will appear (Reproduced and modified with permission of Caliber I.D. Inc.)

Each section projects as a two-dimensional image (Fig. 14.2) with dimensions of 0.5 mm laterally and 4 mm axially [3] that are oriented parallel (*en face*) to the skin surface. The resolution of each image is comparable to those of histological sections (Fig. 14.3).

The commercially available near-infrared reflectance microscope (VivaScope 1500, Caliber I.D. Henrietta, NY) is equipped with a diode laser with peak emission at 830 nm and has a maximum power of 35 mW. With this system, each image has an effective 500×500 μm field of view and the imaging depth in normal skin is 200–300 μm, i.e., the level of papillary dermis and upper reticular dermis and the spatial resolution in the lateral dimension are 0.5–1.0 μm [4–6]. The new generation of this device (VivaScope 1500, Multilaser) combines reflectance and fluorescence imaging, with available wavelengths of 785 nm (near infrared), 658 nm (red), and 488 nm (blue), which are integrated into a single device amplifying the imaging potentials. These laser wavelengths are applied to the skin, one wavelength at a time, to eliminate the possibility of bleed-through from other fluorophores. The use

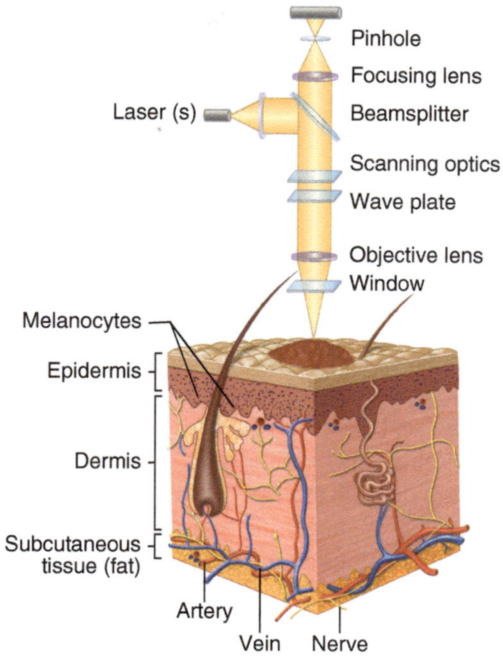

Fig. 14.2 The basis of the technology: refraction. Confocal scanning laser microscopy technology: after emission, light passes through a beam splitter, a scanning and focusing optical lens, and a skin contact device. Cells and their morphology and cytology are clearly resolved. Diagnostic images are captured at relevant depths in the skin (Reproduced and modified with permission of Caliber I.D. Inc.)

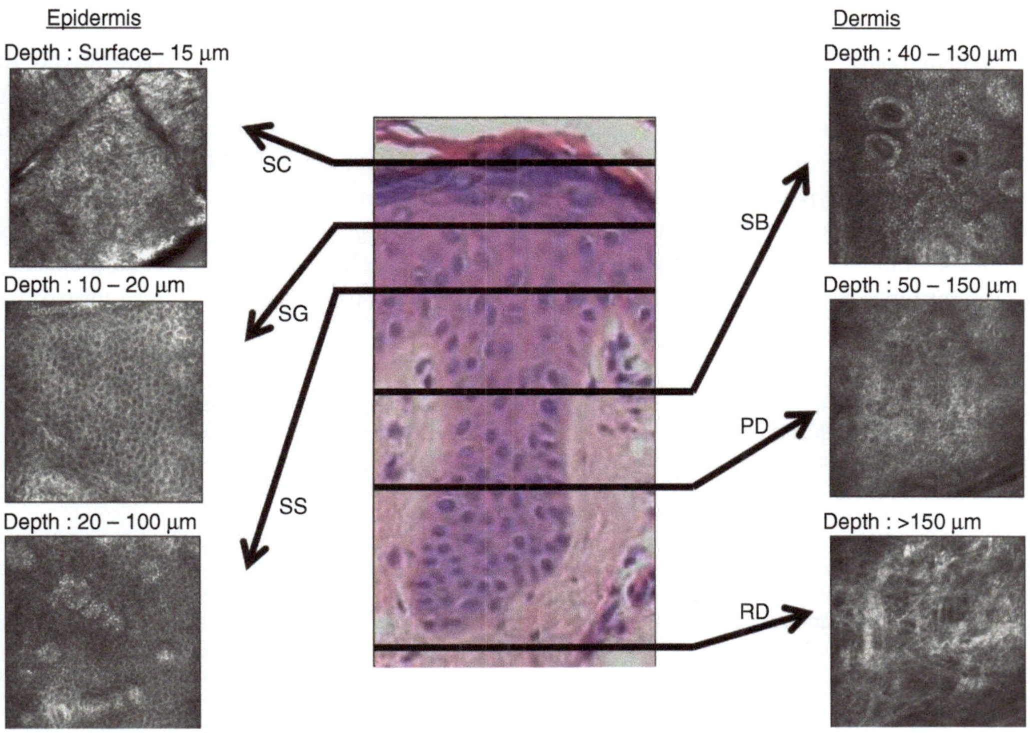

Fig. 14.3 Representative diagram of the skin layers and corresponding RCM images. *SC* Stratum corneum, *SG* Stratum granulosum, *SS* Stratum spinosum, *SB* Stratum basale, *PD* Papillary dermis, *RD* reticular dermis (Reproduced and modified with permission of Caliber I.D. Inc.)

of several fluorescent dyes has been described including the administration of Indocyanine green (ICG) and fluorescein human skin in vivo [7]. The well-defined intercellular staining pattern of ICG in the skin, with a stain duration of almost 48 hours, has allowed the development of automated cell-recognition algorithms currently under investigation. The expanded capabilities of the multilaser microscope allow the implementation of the device not only in studies seeking the assessment of morphological features in the skin (e.g., atypical honeycomb pattern, atypical keratinocytic and melanocytic nest formation, cell pleomorphism, etc.) but also in research studies aiming to develop targeted fluorescence markers in the field of diagnostic and therapeutic biomarkers, as well as drug delivery studies.

14.2 Clinical Application of RCM as a Diagnostic Tool

A clinical breakthrough in RCM has been the capability to bring to the bedside an almost equivalent tool to histological evaluation without the need for invasive diagnostic procedures. In the setting of cryosurgery, RCM has the capability to aid in the diagnostic decision of a lesion prior to undergoing therapy, which has the advantage of avoiding postponing the treatment until the diagnosis is histologically confirmed. The sensitivity and specificity of RCM varies significantly across tumor types, level of training of the operator, and expertise of the individual interpreting the confocal images [8]. The following skin lesions represent clinical examples in which RCM has been evaluated to date with the potential to offer a diagnostic aid in cases considered for cryosurgery intervention.

14.2.1 Pigmented Lesions

Because melanin and melanocytes are the easiest structures to recognize in RCM, much of the research in the field has been focused on the evaluation of pigmented lesions. RCM has been identified as a useful tool in distinguishing melanomas from benign pigmented lesions (Fig. 14.4a–d). Malignant melanoma in situ (MMIS), lentigo maligna (LM) type, shares similar RCM features such as non-edged papillae, round and large pagetoid cells, and nucleated cells in the dermal papillae with other subtypes of malignant melanoma; however, follicular localization of atypical cells has been proposed as a unique finding in LM. A 2013 systematic review examined five cohort studies on RCM diagnostic accuracy for melanoma, LM, and MMIS in clinically equivocal pigmented lesions using various RCM scoring systems and algorithms [9]. The meta-analysis for these RCM studies demonstrated a per-lesion sensitivity of 93 % and specificity of 76 % for melanoma diagnosis. Thus, RCM features of melanoma may be helpful in noninvasively differentiating equivocal pigmented lesions and delineating margins within lesions such as LM.

Overall, the aid of RCM in the setting of pigmented lesions will be in guiding the clinicians to the areas of greater atypia to perform skin biopsies for histological confirmation and exclusion of invasion [10, 11]. In some cases, invasiveness

Fig. 14.4 (**a–d**) RCM features in benign and atypical melanocytic lesions. (**a**) RCM mosaic (4×4 mm) acquired at the suprabasal/epidermal-junctional level, showing a ringed and meshwork pattern in a slightly asymmetrical overall architecture. Also milia-like cysts and comedo-like openings are visible throughout the lesion, whereas atypical cells are lacking. The ringed and meshwork pattern fade off at the border of the lesion. (**b**) Basic image (0.5×0.5 mm) showing mostly edged papillae (*). *Arrow* is showing the milia-like cyst aspect (→). (**c**) RCM mosaic (4×4 mm) of a very asymmetrical lesion, with a mixed pattern (meshwork, ringed, and clod). In the center of the lesion, a nonhomogeneous meshwork pattern is present, with junctional nests, irregular in size and shape. At the periphery, there are junctional and dermal nests (clods). Dense and sparse and a ringed structure shading off at the periphery. (**d**) Basic image (0.5×0.5 mm) of a central area of the atypical nevus showing dishomogeneous and irregular junctional thickenings and nests surrounding non-edged papillae (red → and *). Within dermal papillae dense and dense and sparse nests are seen (*red* *), mixed with inflammatory infiltrate, including plump bright cells (*yellow* *) and small bright spots. Numerous atypical cells are detectable at the DEJ, in single cells or aggregated in nests

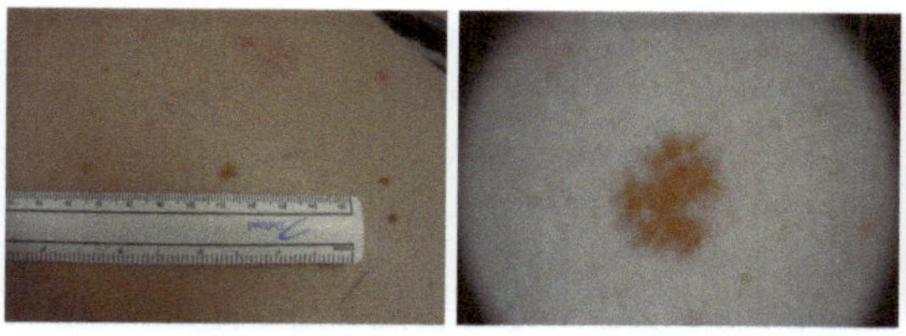

Low-grade Melanocytic neoplasm

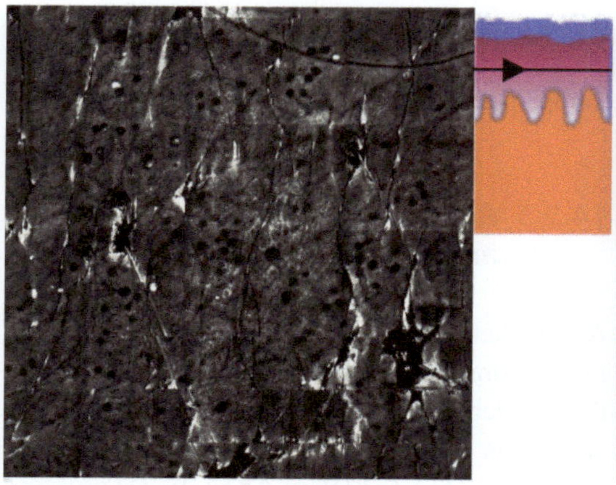

a: RCM mosaic (4 x 4 mm) acquired at the suprabasal/epidermal-junctional level, showing a ringed and meshwork pattern in a slightly asymmetrical overall architecture. Also milia-like cysts and comedo-like openings are visible throughout the lesion, whereas atypical cells are lacking. The ringed and meshwork pattern fade off at the border of the lesion.

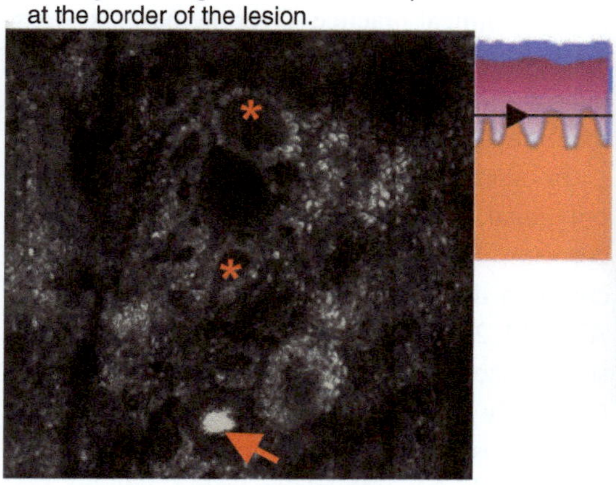

b: Basic image (0,5x0,5 mm) showing mostly edged papillae (*). Arrow is showing the milialike cyst aspect (→).
* Images provided by Curiel and Hofmann

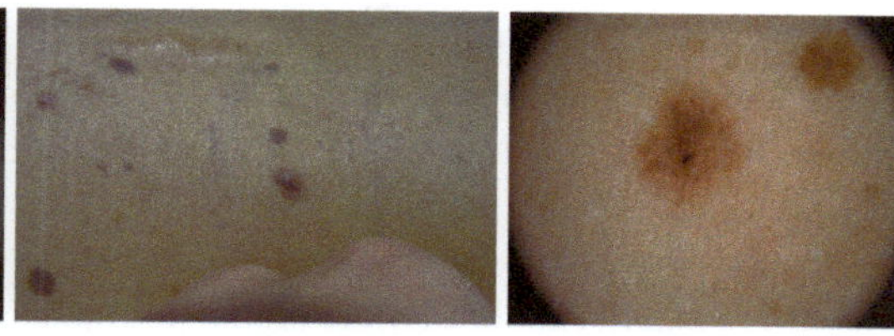

High-grade Melanocytic neoplasm

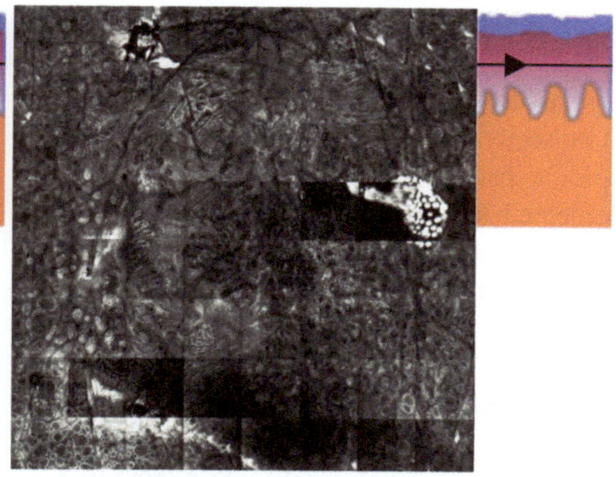

c: RCM mosaic (4 x 4 mm) of a very asymmetrical lesion, with a mixed pattern (meshwork, ringed and clod). In the center of the lesion, a nonhomogeneous meshwork pattern is present, with junctional nests, irregular in size and shape. At the periphery, there are junctional and dermal nests (clods). Dense and sparse, and a ringed structures shading off at the periphery.

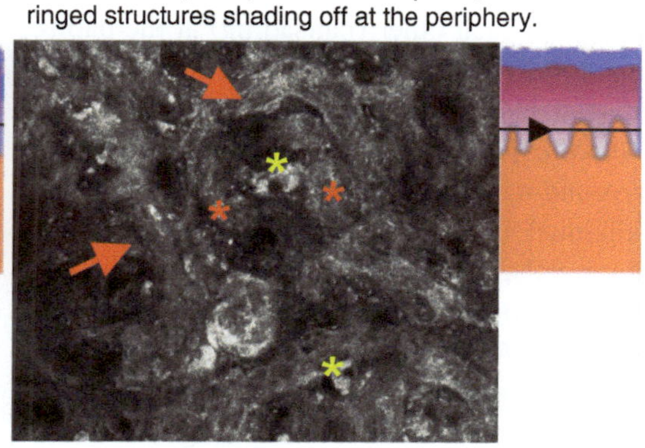

d: Basic image (0,5x0,5 mm) of a central area of the atypical nevus showing dishomogeneous and irregular junctional thickenings and nests surrounding non-edged papillae (red → and *). Within dermal papillae dense and dense&sparse nests are seen (red *), mixed with inflammatory infiltrate, including plump bright cells (yellow *) and small bright spots. Numerous atypical cells are detectable at the DEJ , in single cells or aggregated in nests. * Images provided by Curiel and Hofmann of melanoma can be readily visualized by RCM, which will aid the clinician when making a decision on whether to perform a cryosurgery intervention or not in an atypical pigmented skin lesion. On the other hand, using RCM as a screening modality for borderline pigmented skin lesions of the head and neck can be of value prior to cryosurgery since, not infrequently, lesions with a lower degree of clinical suspicion can demonstrate increasingly concerning features by dermoscopy and RCM evaluation [12]. This scenario is particularly relevant when evaluating pigmented lesions in chronically photoexposed areas such as the head and neck, as well as distal upper extremity areas [13].

14.2.2 Basal Cell Carcinoma

RCM features of basal cell carcinoma (BCC) have been described at two powers of microscopy: mosaic and individual image levels [14, 15]. At the lower magnification of the mosaic grid, tightly packed tumor cells with high refractility (brightness) can been seen oriented parallel to each other (palisading) at the papillary dermis, forming cord-like structures surrounded by hyporefractile darkness (clefting) that corresponds histologically to the mucinous surrounding stroma. At higher magnification of individual images [14], within the individual tumor cells, elongated hyporefractile nuclei are present, producing a polarizing nuclear appearance [14]. Adjacent to tumor cells, dilated and increased vasculature is often seen with leukocytes on the endothelial lining (Fig. 14.5a–h). Small hyperrefractile dendritic cells within and surrounding the islands of tumor cells have also been identified in pigmented BCCs [15, 16]. A 2004 retrospective study showed that the presence of elongated nuclei and polarized nuclei on RCM was 91.6 % sensitive and 97 % specific for BCC [17].

In differentiating between BCC and malignant melanoma (MM), the basaloid cords seen in the papillary dermis are highly specific for BCC [18]. The absence of epidermal honeycomb disarray, papillae (papillae disruption), and cerebriform nests is also useful for diagnosing BCC. Yet, to date, there have been no studies directly comparing pigmented BCCs and MM, and further investigations would be helpful in delineating the RCM features that are unique to each entity. Overall, diagnosis of BCC is one area where RCM holds a high sensitivity and specificity facilitating an RCM diagnostic tool with the potential to spare the need for skin biopsies when interpreted by trained readers.

14.2.3 Actinic Keratosis and Squamous Cell Carcinoma

Actinic keratoses (AK) are one of the most common forms of cutaneous malignancies. While there is debate over whether AK represents a precancerous lesion, studies have shown that without treatment, 0.2–20 % of AKs [19–21] progress to squamous cell carcinomas (SCC). Currently, the diagnostic gold standard for AKs is histopathological examination. While this method represents the most accurate form of identification, it is often time consuming and impractical in daily clinical practice. Over the past six years, a few studies have examined RCM characteristics of clinically diagnosed AK and SCC and their diagnostic value.

In some of these studies, solar elastosis, polygonal, nucleated keratinocytes in the stratum corneum (parakeratosis), scaling, and stratum corneum disruption were seen in a majority of AKs [22, 23]. In particular, certain RCM features seem to be the most reliable in diagnosing AKs. One study noted irregular architecture in the stratum spinosum and stratum granulosum (atypical honeycombing) with pleomorphic cellular features at that level being the most specific and sensitive signs of AK [22]. Another group presented similar findings but also described irregular keratinocyte borders as the main finding seen in images of high power (individual images). In this study, RCM was 93.34 % sensitive and up to 90 % specific for AK when accounting for all of these features [23]. Other features seen in AKs include blood vessel dilation in dermal papillae [24] (Fig. 14.5a–h).

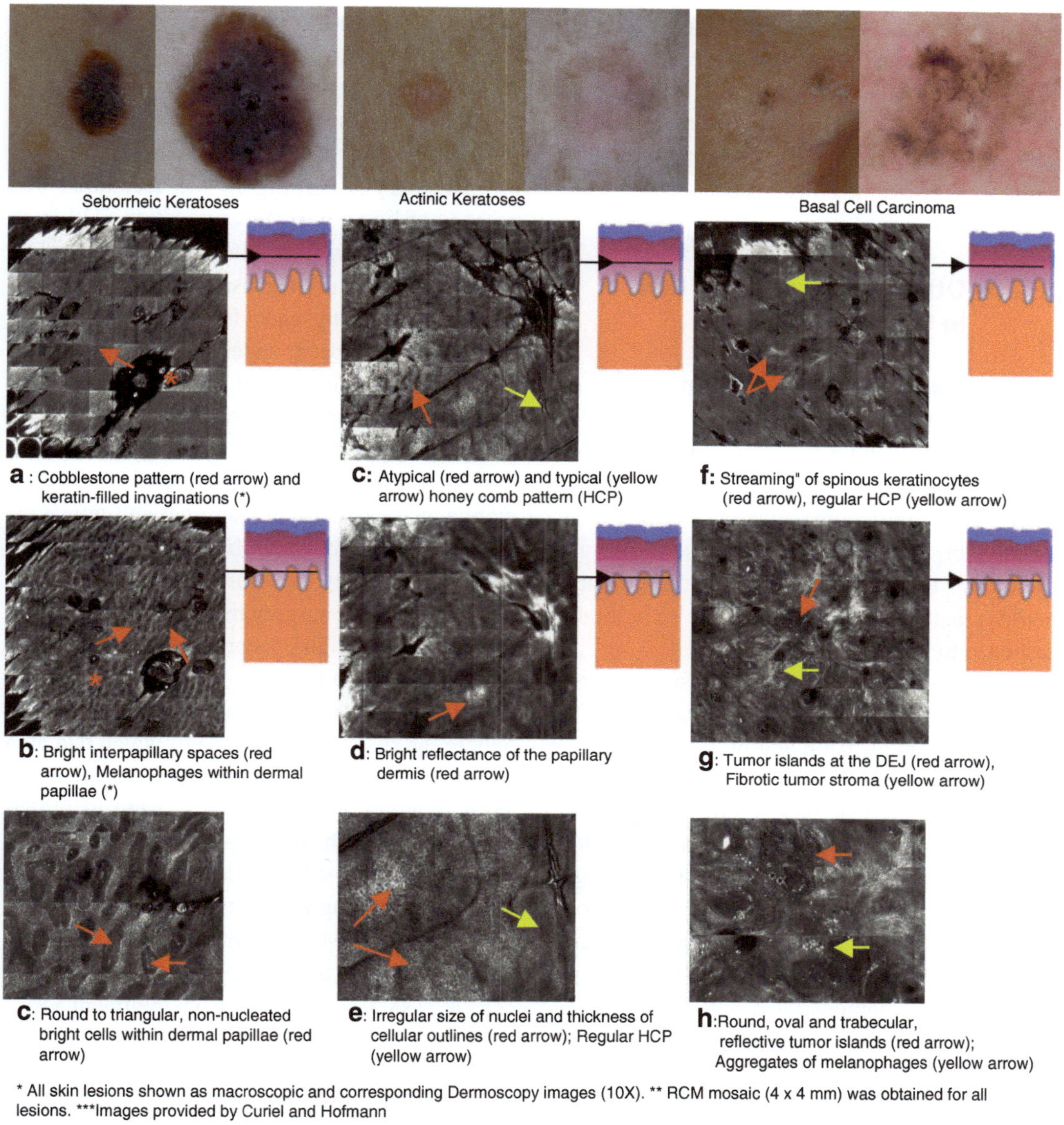

Fig. 14.5 RCM features in benign and atypical keratinocytic neoplasms. (**a**) Cobblestone pattern (*red arrow*) and keratin-filled invaginations (*). (**b**) Bright interpapillary spaces (*red arrow*), melanophages within dermal papillae (*). (**c**) Round to triangular, nonnucleated bright cells within dermal papillae (*red arrow*). Atypical (*red arrow*) and typical (*yellow arrow*) honeycomb pattern (HCP). (**d**) Bright reflectance of the papillary dermis (*red arrow*). (**e**) Irregular size of nuclei and thickness of cellular outlines (*red arrow*); regular HCP (*yellow arrow*). (**f**) "Streaming" of spinous keratinocytes (*red arrow*), regular HCP (*yellow arrow*) pattern. (**g**) Tumor islands at the DEJ (*red arrow*), fibrotic tumor stroma (*yellow arrow*). (**h**) Round, oval and trabecular, reflective tumor islands (*red arrow*); aggregates of melanophages (*yellow arrow*). All skin lesions shown as macroscopic and corresponding dermoscopy images (10×). RCM mosaic (4×4 mm) was obtained for all lesions (Images provided by Curiel and Hofman)

To date, a single study has attempted to compare RCM features of AK to SCC [24]. Although atypical honeycombing was seen in both AKs and SCCs, SCCs showed more extensive atypia in the spinous and granular layers. Similar features in AKs were more focal or displayed milder patterns. Round, bright, nucleated cells seen in the spinous and granular layers corresponding to atypical, dyskeratotic keratinocytes on histopathology were found more frequently in SCCs

(65 %) than AKs (14 %). Dilated blood vessels in the dermal papillae were also more numerous in SCC vs. AK. The findings in this study support the theory that AK, SCCIS, and invasive SCC are not separate entities, but more a continuum in the keratinocytic carcinogenesis process.

14.2.4 Other Applications of RCM in Cryosurgery

14.2.4.1 Noninvasive Determination of Lesion Margins

One of the challenges of cryosurgery and subsequent variability in reported response rates is likely related to the challenge in clinically determining the precise extension of the lesion and, therefore, treatment margins. Such limitation could result in a decreased rate of complete response to therapy.

The current standard for margin assessment is through permanent histological margin evaluation in surgical excision and by staged excisions with frozen histopathological examination used during Mohs microsurgery. RCM has been shown to have good correlation with histopathology in vivo and ex vivo and has demonstrated magnification that is equivocal to the microscopic power used during frozen histopathology examination on Mohs excisions [25]. Fluorescence RCM has also demonstrated high clinical accuracy when studied in Mohs excisions. Karen JK et al. evaluated the accuracy of fluorescence RCM in detecting residual BCC features following surgical excisions. The sensitivity of the instrument was 96.6 % with a specificity of 89.2 %, supporting the potential role of RCM in evaluating surgical margins [26].

In addition to the implementation of RCM in lesions undergoing surgical intervention, the use of RCM prior to cryosurgical application holds the potential to increase the response rate. This approach will be particularly relevant for cutaneous malignancies with ill-defined borders such as AK, superficial BCC, and LM. Future studies assessing the implementation of RCM for margin determination in the cryosurgery setting are needed.

14.2.4.2 Noninvasive Therapy Monitoring

Along with margin identification, response to treatment is essential to cryosurgery. As an operator-dependent treatment, response to therapy can vary according to the technique and potency of liquid nitrogen application. Although a goal temperature is desirable, cryosurgical systems that accurately assess lesion and skin temperature during each freezing and thawing cycle have not been widely implemented into practice. In addition, the system is currently limited to a device by Brymill.

RCM has demonstrated accurate assessment of residual tumor in multiple types of cutaneous malignancies undergoing surgical and nonsurgical treatments. The study by Torres et al. examined the efficacy of imiquimod 5 % as a pre-micrographic surgery treatment for BCC and demonstrated a high concordance between RCM and histological findings [27]. The study by Marra DE et al. reported three patients who had undergone shave biopsies, one of which had also undergone imiquimod treatment. In all three cases, features of residual BCC were identified by RCM in well-healed appearing scars and subsequently confirmed by histological sections during Mohs micrograph surgery [28]. A recent study using RCM to examine superficial BCC (sBCC) response to cryosurgery showed necrotic cells at basal layer after 5 h from treatment application [29]. This was indicative of the higher sensitivity of tumor cells to low temperatures. In a study evaluating the morphological changes of subclinical AKs, RCM identified subclinical AKs at baseline, features of an inflammatory response to imiquimod at 2 weeks and residual atypia in 2 patients after end of treatment without any clinical aspects of AK [30] (Fig. 14.6a–l).

Given the ability of RCM to accurately identify features indicative of different cutaneous malignancies, at a resolution of histological equivalence, the implementation of this imaging tool to monitor NMSC and AK responses is a rational proposition. This will ensure complete tumor clearance in situations where cryosurgery is standard treatment or when it is an appropriate alternative to surgical modalities.

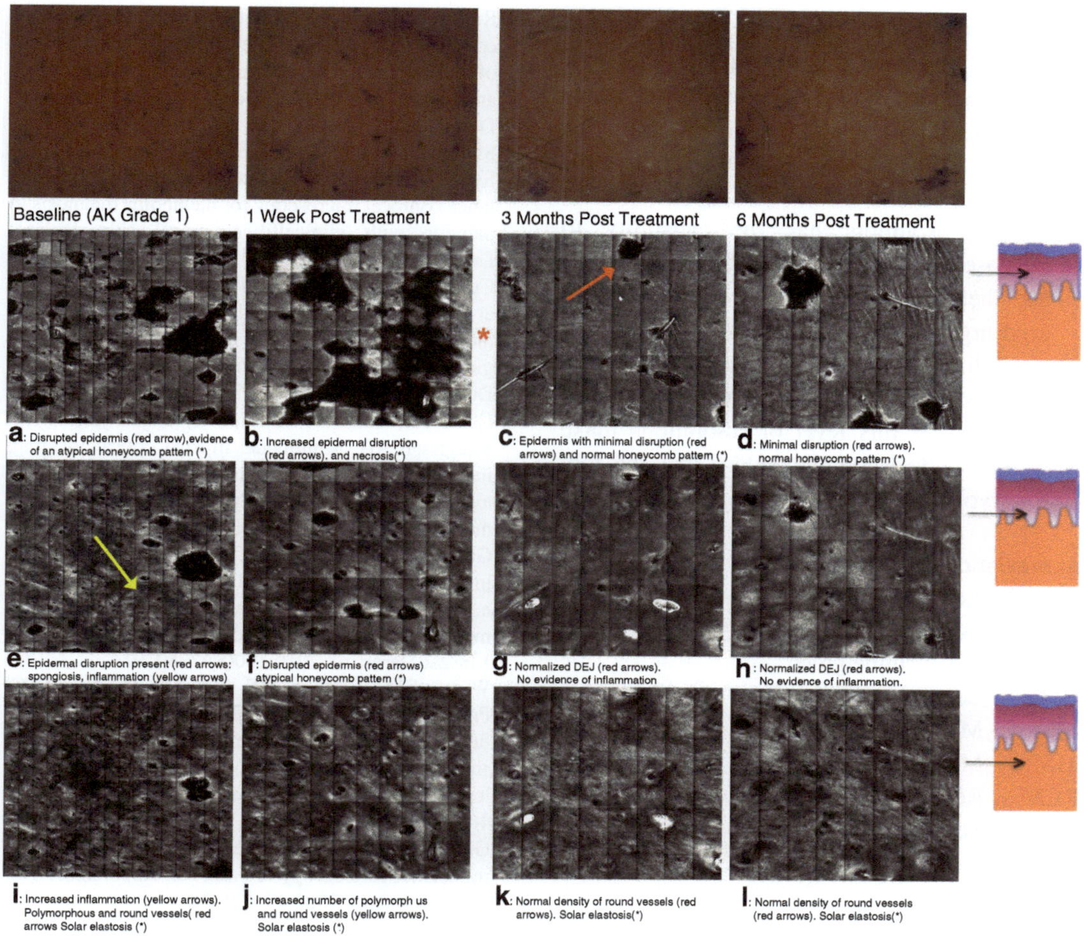

Fig. 14.6 RCM features in actinic keratosis treated with cryosurgery. (**a**) Disrupted epidermis (*red arrow*), evidence of an atypical honeycomb pattern (*). (**b**) Increased epidermal disruption (*red arrows*) and necrosis (*). (**c**) Epidermis with minimal disruption (*red arrows*) and normal honeycomb pattern (*). (**d**) Minimal disruption (*red arrows*). Normal honeycomb pattern (*). (**e**) Epidermal disruption present (*red arrows*), spongiosis, inflammation (*yellow arrows*). (**f**) Disrupted epidermis (*red arrows*) atypical honeycomb pattern (*). (**g**) Normalized DEJ (*red arrows*). No evidence of inflammation. (**h**) Normalized DEJ (*red arrows*). No evidence of inflammation. (**i**) Increased inflammation (*yellow arrows*). Polymorphous and round vessels (*red arrows*). Solar elastosis (*). (**j**) Increased number of polymorphous and round vessels (*yellow arrows*). Solar elastosis (*). (**k**) Normal density of round vessels (*red arrows*). Solar elastosis (*). (**l**) Normal density of round vessels (*red arrows*). Solar elastosis (*)

Essential Tidbits

- RCM will give an almost equivalent information on the tumor's nature without the need for biopsy.
- Confirming a diagnosis of BCC by RCM will help make more accurate treatment decisions.
- In actinic keratosis (AK), confirming diagnoses becomes particularly useful and important due to the relevance of excluding squamous cell carcinoma.
- Regarding cryosurgery, RCM can be used to define lesion margins and measure response to treatment.

Conclusions

As the imaging field continues to evolve at galloping steps, noninvasive imaging tools like RCM are revolutionizing the way we practice. The capacity to visualize and instantaneously document skin findings, at a histological resolution, has the capability to increase the accuracy of our clinical diagnosis and therefore our confidence at the time of cryosurgery interventions. In addition, the capability to noninvasively delineate lesion margins and the opportunity to follow lesions over time at this level of resolutions make RCM an ideal complementary imaging tool for cryosurgery interventions.

Abbreviations

AK	Actinic keratosis
BCC	Basal cell carcinoma
ICG	Indocyanine green
LM	Lentigo maligna
MM	Malignant melanoma
MMIS	Malignant melanoma in situ
RCM	Reflectance confocal microscopy
SCC	Squamous cell carcinoma

References

1. Minsky M. Microscopy apparatus. US Patent 3,013,467. 1957.
2. Rajadhyaksha M, Grossman M, Esterowitz D, et al. In vivo confocal scanning laser microscopy of human skin: melanin provides strong contrast. J Invest Dermatol. 1995;104:946–52.
3. Hofmann-Wellenhof R, et al., editors. Reflectance confocal microscopy for skin diseases. Berlin/Heidelberg: Springer; 2012.
4. Branzan AL, Landthaler M, Szeimies RM. In vivo confocal scanning laser microscopy in dermatology. Lasers Med Sci. 2007;22(2):73–82.
5. Busam KJ, Charles C, Lee G, Halpern AC. Morphologic features of melanocytes, pigmented keratinocytes, and melanophages by in vivo confocal scanning laser microscopy. Mod Pathol. 2001;14(9):862–8.
6. González S, González E, White WM, Rajadhyaksha M, Anderson RR. Allergic contact dermatitis: correlation of in vivo confocal imaging to routine histology. J Am Acad Dermatol. 1999;40(5 Pt 1):708–13.
7. Jonak C, Skvara H, Kunstfeld R, Trautinger F, Schmid JA. Intradermal indocyanine green for in vivo fluorescence laser scanning microscopy of human skin: a pilot study. PLoS One. 2011;6(8):e23972.
8. Rao BK, Mateus R, Wassef C, Pellacani G. In vivo confocal microscopy in clinical practice: comparison of bedside diagnostic accuracy of a trained physician and distant diagnosis of an expert reader. J Am Acad Dermatol. 2013;69(6):e295–300.
9. Stevenson AD, Mickan S, Mallett S, Ayya M. Systematic review of diagnostic accuracy of reflectance confocal microscopy for melanoma diagnosis in patients with clinically equivocal skin lesions. Dermatol Pract Concept. 2013;3(4):5.
10. Curiel-Lewandrowski C, Williams CM, Swindells KJ, et al. Use of in vivo confocal microscopy in malignant melanoma: an aid in diagnosis and assessment of surgical and nonsurgical therapeutic approaches. Arch Dermatol. 2004;140(9):1127–32.
11. Chen CS, Elias M, Busam K, Rajadhyaksha M, Marghoob AA. Multimodal in vivo optical imaging, including confocal microscopy, facilitates presurgical margin mapping for clinically complex lentigo maligna melanoma. Br J Dermatol. 2005;153(5):1031–6.
12. Guitera P, Pellacani G, Crotty KA, et al. The impact of in vivo reflectance confocal microscopy on the diagnostic accuracy of lentigo maligna and equivocal pigmented and nonpigmented macules of the face. J Invest Dermatol. 2010;130(8):2080–91.
13. Wurm EM, Curchin CE, Lambie D, Longo C, Pellacani G, Soyer HP. Confocal features of equivocal facial lesions on severely sun-damaged skin: four case studies with dermatoscopic, confocal, and histopathologic correlation. J Am Acad Dermatol. 2012;66(3):463–73.
14. Gonzalez S, Tannous Z. Real-time, in vivo confocal reflectance microscopy of basal cell carcinoma. J Am Acad Dermatol. 2002;47:869–74.
15. Agero AL, Busam KJ, Benvenuto-Andrade C, et al. Reflectance confocal microscopy of pigmented basal cell carcinoma. J Am Acad Dermatol. 2006;54:638–43.
16. Segura S, Puig S, Carrera C, Palou J, Malvehy J. Dendritic cells in pigmented basal cell carcinoma: a relevant finding by reflectance-mode confocal microscopy. Arch Dermatol. 2007;143:883–6.
17. Nori S, Rius-Diaz F, Cuevas J, et al. Sensitivity and specificity of reflectance-mode confocal microscopy for in vivo diagnosis of basal cell carcinoma: a multicenter study. J Am Acad Dermatol. 2004;51:923–30.
18. Guitera P, Menzies SW, Longo C, Cesinaro AM, Scolyer RA, Pellacani G. In vivo confocal microscopy for diagnosis of melanoma and basal cell carcinoma using a Two-step method: analysis of 710 consecutive clinically equivocal cases. J Invest Dermatol. 2012;132:2386–94.
19. Fuchs A, Marmur E. The kinetics of skin cancer: progression of actinic keratoses to squamous cell carcinoma. Dermatol Surg. 2007;33(9):1099–101.
20. Callen JP, Bickers DR, Moy RL. Actinic keratoses. J Am Acad Dermatol. 1997;36:650–3.
21. Ackerman AB, Mones JM. Solar (actinic) keratosis is squamous cell carcinoma. Br J Dermatol. 2006;155:9–22.

22. Ulrich M, Maltusch A, Rius-Diaz F, et al. Clinical applicability of in vivo reflectance confocal microscopy for the diagnosis of actinic keratoses. Dermatol Surg. 2008;34(5):610–9.
23. Horn M, Gerger A, Ahlgrimm-Siess V, et al. Discrimination of actinic keratoses from normal skin with reflectance mode confocal microscopy. Dermatol Surg. 2008;34(5):620–5.
24. Rishpon A, Kim N, Scope A, et al. Reflectance confocal microscopy criteria for squamous cell carcinomas and actinic keratoses. Arch Dermatol. 2009;145(7):766–72.
25. Patel YG, Nehal KS, Aranda I, et al. Confocal reflectance mosaicing of basal cell carcinomas in Mohs surgical skin excisions. J Biomed Opt. 2007;12:034027.
26. Karen JK, Gareau DS, Dusza SW, et al. Detection of basal cell carcinomas in Mohs excisions with fluorescence confocal mosaicing microscopy. Br J Dermatol. 2009;160:1242–50.
27. Torres A, Niemeyer A, Berkes B, et al. 5% Imiquimod cream and reflectance- mode confocal microscopy as adjunct modalities to Mohs micrographic surgery for treatment of basal cell carcinoma. Dermatol Surg. 2004;30(12 Pt 1):1462–9.
28. Marra DE, Torres A, Schanbacher CF, Gonzalez S. Detection of residual basal cell carcinoma by in vivo confocal microscopy. Dermatol Surg. 2005;31(5):538–41.
29. Ahlgrimm-Siess V, Horn M, Koller S, Ludwig R, Gerger A, Hofmann-Wellenhof R. Monitoring efficacy of cryotherapy for superficial basal cell carcinomas with in vivo reflectance confocal microscopy: a preliminary study. J Dermatol Sci. 2009;53(1):60–4.
30. Ulrich M, Krueger-Corcoran D, Roewert-Huber J, et al. Reflectance confocal microscopy for noninvasive monitoring of therapy and detection of subclinical actinic keratoses. Dermatology. 2010;220:15–24.

Optical Coherence Tomography and Cryosurgery

15

Lotte Themstrup, Christina A. Banzhaf, Gregor Jemec, and Mette Mogensen

Contents

Key Points

- Optical coherence tomography (OCT) is a relatively novel skin imaging technology that enables detecting and estimating keratinocyte carcinoma and actinic keratoses in vivo.
- In cryosurgery-treated AK lesions, OCT imaging has shown subclinical vesicle formation in the lesions within twenty minutes after treatment.
- Studies imply that OCT imaging has a potential as a diagnostic imaging tool in dermatology.

15.1 Optical Coherence Tomography

Optical coherence tomography (OCT) is an imaging tool that provides real-time, cross-sectional skin images to a depth of up to 2 mm. OCT is based on an interferometric technique that detects reflected or backscattered light from tissue, OCT probes the sample with a beam of light and subsequently lets the reflections interfere with a reference beam originating from the same light source. The interference is identified either by time domain (positioning), spectral domain (spectrally separated detectors), or Fourier domain (distributing different optical frequencies onto a detector array). The images produced are composite images (B-scans) based on

L. Themstrup, MD (✉) • C.A. Banzhaf, MD
G. Jemec, MD, DMSc
Department of Dermatology, Roskilde Hospital, Køgevej 7-13, Roskilde 4000, Denmark

Health Sciences Faculty, University of Copenhagen, Copenhagen, Denmark
e-mail: lotte.themstrup@gmail.com; cfrd@regionsjaelland.dk; gbj@regionsjaelland.dk

M. Mogensen, MD, PhD
Health Sciences Faculty, University of Copenhagen, Bispebjerg Bakke 23, 2400 København NV, Copenhagen, Denmark

Department of Dermatology, Bispebjerg Hospital, Copenhagen, Denmark
e-mail: mogensen.mette@gmail.com

P. Pasquali (ed.), *Cryosurgery: A Practical Manual*,
DOI 10.1007/978-3-662-43939-5_15, © Springer-Verlag Berlin Heidelberg 2015

individual A-scans, very similar in appearance to ultrasound scans, albeit at a higher resolution. The axial resolution is dependent on the wavelength used and the lateral resolution of the optics. Commercially available equipment provides lateral resolution of <7.5 μm and axial resolution of 5 μm in the vertical images at up to 2 mm depth and en face images with a resolution of up to 3 μm and up to 1 mm depth.

Generally, skin imaging faces some challenges. Firstly, the skin is easily examined by visual inspection which puts greater demands on the skin imaging tool which has to be both quick and easy, yet provide high quality images. Secondly, skin imaging is challenging due to skin morphology and its unfavorable optical qualities. The skin morphology provides an optical challenge because of the scattering characteristics of the skin. Finally, the abundance of tissue poses a problem in its own right.

OCT therefore has a limited penetration depth, but it provides high-resolution images, which places it in the imaging gap between high-frequency ultrasound (deeper penetration – lower resolution) and confocal microscopy (lower penetration – higher resolution). These features, combined with practical ease of use, strongly suggest that the method may have clinical potential.

15.2 Imaging of Keratinocyte Carcinomas Using Optical Coherence Tomography

The diagnosis of nonmelanoma skin cancer (NMSC) and actinic keratosis (AK), in this chapter referred to as keratinocyte carcinomas, is based on the clinical presentation and a skin biopsy for histological analysis. The clinical diagnosis of keratinocyte carcinoma can be ambiguous, with sensitivity reported around 56–90 pct and the specificity 75–90 pct [1]. A skin biopsy is considered the gold standard for diagnosis of keratinocyte carcinoma, but the biopsy procedure is invasive, sometimes painful, and can lead to scarring. Skin biopsies are therefore not the optimal choice when monitoring a noninvasive treatment.

For destructive treatments with a lower potential for scarring than frank surgery such as cryotherapy, the problem is different. While the potential for scarring is often described as lower, it is not zero, so arguments of non-scarring are less valid. Other practical arguments for cryotherapy can, however, be found elsewhere in this book, and the method is generally used due to speed, efficacy, and cost benefit. It is, however, a destructive method and therefore reliant on pretreatment diagnosis, and here OCT has the potential to provide swift, real-time support of the clinical diagnosis to guide the treatment far better than time-delayed methods. In order to choose the most appropriate therapy, information about the thickness and extent of the lesion is relevant. Traditionally, not only the diagnosis but also the follow-up examination is done by clinical examination and biopsy.

OCT can provide noninvasive imaging of keratinocyte carcinomas. Architectural disarray of the epidermis is an overall characteristic finding in OCT images of these lesions. OCT images of basal cell carcinoma (BCC) often show oval dark areas in the dermis frequently surrounded by a white halo corresponding to BCC islands and surrounding tumor stroma [2–6]. OCT characteristics of AK are focally thickened epidermis with white streaks and dots representing the dysplastic epidermis and possible hyperkeratoses or scale [7] (Fig. 15.1a, b). OCT imaging is to some degree comparable to standard histopathology, and a high correlation between OCT images and histopathology of BCC has been demonstrated [8–11]. Size and delineation of superficial lesions can be estimated using OCT. This potentially makes it a useful tool in the monitoring of noninvasive treatments of keratinocyte carcinomas [12, 13]. However, impaired image quality does in some cases impede identification of a lesion during treatment due to the treatment itself.

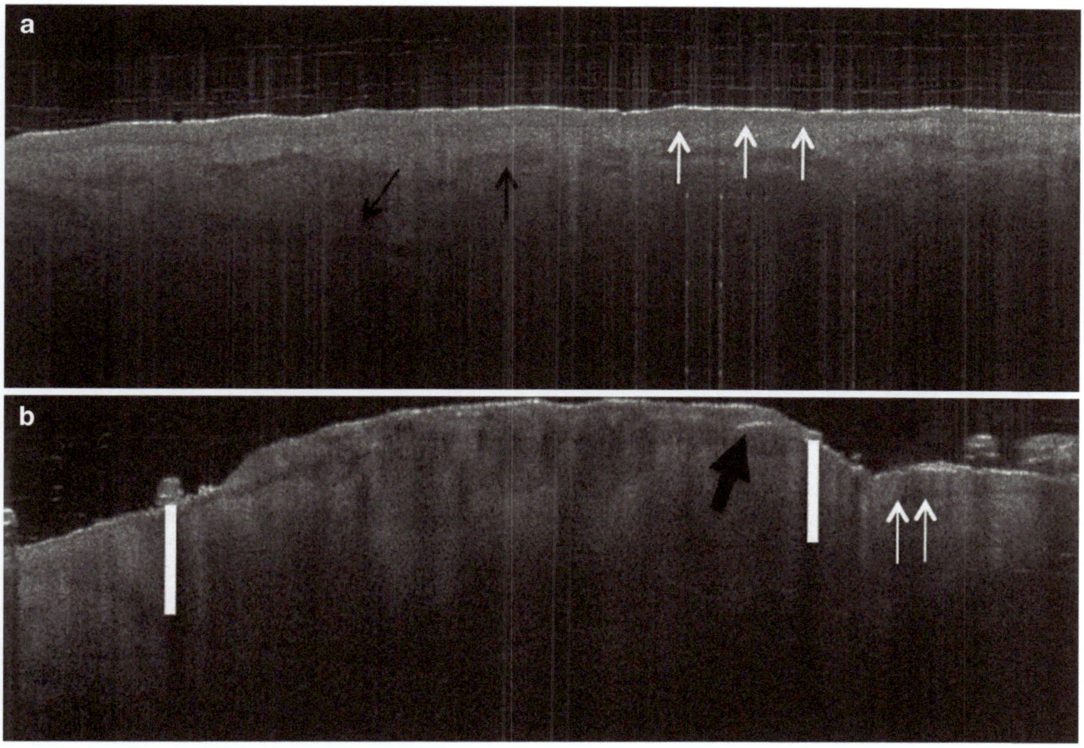

Fig. 15.1 (**a**) Optical coherence tomography (OCT) image of normal skin taken just adjacent to an actinic keratosis (AK) lesion located on the scalp. *White arrows* mark the dermoepidermal junction (DEJ). *Black arrows* mark vessels. (**b**) OCT image of AK lesion located on the scalp. *Vertical white lines* mark disruption of layering. *Thick black arrow* marks characteristic white streak in the epidermis. *White arrows* mark the DEJ

15.3 Optical Coherence Tomography Monitoring of Cryotherapy Treatment

OCT imaging of noninvasive treatment modalities has recently been investigated while OCT imaging in connection with invasive treatments like simple excisions and Mohs surgery has been more extensively studied [12, 14–17]. Cryosurgery of premalignant lesions like AK is traditionally guided clinically by freeze-thaw time and lateral extent of freezing, and therefore, real-time OCT monitoring of cryo treatment has been thought to potentially improve accuracy and efficacy of the procedure. Unfortunately, the immediate effects of cryotherapy impair OCT imaging of the tissue. Cryotherapy induces an opaque iceball in the tissue, which completely prevents visualization of the treated lesion and the freezing depth [18] (Fig. 15.2a–d). The reason for the opacity is that at the OCT wavelength of 1,300 nm, ice is around ten times more absorbing than liquid water. When the tissue freezes the created ice absorbs all of the OCT laser light, and therefore, OCT images of cryotherapy-treated skin only show an impervious frosty white line at the skin surface. Normal OCT imaging depth and resolution reappears in time with the thawing of the tissue. In cryosurgery-treated grade 1 and 2 AK lesions, OCT imaging has showed vesicle formation in the lesions within twenty minutes after treatment [18]. The vesicles were primarily located along the dermoepidermal junction and appeared as dark areas with a maximum height of 0.47 mm (Fig. 15.2a–d). The vesicles were subclinical by the time of the post-cryosurgery

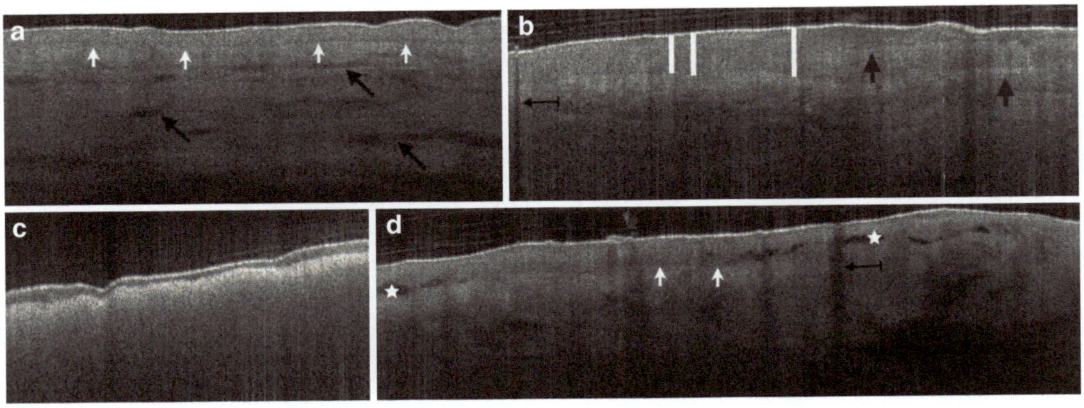

Fig. 15.2 (**a**) Optical coherence tomography (OCT) image of normal skin taken just adjacent to an actinic keratosis (AK) lesion located on the dorsal side of a hand. *White arrows* mark the dermoepidermal junction (DEJ). *Black arrows* mark vessels. (**b**) OCT image of AK lesion before cryo treatment. *Vertical white lines* mark disruption of layering caused by thickening of the epidermis. *Thick black arrows* mark characteristic white streaks in the epidermis. *Thin black arrow* marks a hair casting a shadow. (**c**) OCT image taken seconds after cryosurgery. The treatment produces an opaque iceball. (**d**) OCT image taken 20 min after cryotherapy. *Stars* mark emerging vesicles along the DEJ. *White arrows* mark the DEJ. *Small black arrow* marks a hair casting a shadow

imaging and could thus only be identified using OCT. A vesiculobullous reaction after superficial cryogen application is an indication of successful treatment of superficial epidermal lesions because the separation of epidermis and dermis enables the shedding of the diseased skin [19].

Conclusions

The capability of OCT to identify early tissue changes after cryosurgery of AK lesions implies that OCT could potentially be used as a supplementary tool in assessing the effectiveness of cryosurgery, but specific follow-up studies have not yet been performed. Results from a study on OCT imaging of noninvasive photodynamic therapy of keratinocyte carcinomas and AK indicate that subclinical residual lesions could be identified by OCT at 3 months follow-up [13]. OCT may have the potential to influence patient management by enabling early evaluation of treatment effects. Early detection of complete or partial responses to invasive and noninvasive therapies could make for a better planning of treatment, e.g., reducing treatment area, number of treatments, and thereby reducing pain related to re-treatment. In regard to imaging of the skin and monitoring of treatments, OCT is a relatively novel technology and the cryosurgery and follow-up results are based on studies with small sample sizes. In our view the results are promising and the technology has achieved a level of maturation that makes it possible to explore its clinical use on a larger scale. Additional studies focusing on both the use of OCT as a tool for treatment planning and for follow-up after skin cancer treatments are warranted before OCT can be established as an important tool in the daily clinical practice, but until now more than 15 clinical studies imply that OCT imaging does have a potential as a diagnostic imaging tool in dermatology [8, 20, 21].

Essential Tidbits

- OCT is an imaging tool that provides real-time high-resolution skin images to a depth of up to 2 mm.
- It has been used in monitoring cryosurgery of AK.
- OCT imaging has shown subclinical vesicle formation in the lesions within twenty minutes after cryosurgical AK treatment.
- OCT used in early detection of complete or partial responses to cryosurgery could make for a better planning of treatment.

Glossary

Actinic keratoses (AK) Actinic keratosis (AK) is a UV light–induced premalignant lesion of the skin that may progress to invasive squamous cell carcinoma.

Interferometry An interference pattern is produced by splitting a beam of light into two paths, bouncing the beams back and recombining them. In this way, reflected or backscattered light from the tissue is detected. From the resulting interference signal, one can derive the reflectivity profile along the beam axis.

Keratinocyte carcinomas The most common type of skin cancer including basal cell carcinoma and squamous cell carcinoma.

Mohs surgery A surgical technique. Microscopically controlled surgery used to treat common types of skin cancer like keratinocyte carcinoma.

Optical coherence tomography (OCT) An interferometric imaging technique that detects reflected or backscattered light from the tissue.

Abbreviations

AK	Actinic keratoses
BCC	Basal cell carcinoma
DEJ	Dermoepidermal junction
NMSC	Nonmelanoma skin cancer
OCT	Optical coherence tomography

References

1. Mogensen M, Jemec GB. Diagnosis of nonmelanoma skin cancer/keratinocyte carcinoma: a review of diagnostic accuracy of nonmelanoma skin cancer diagnostic tests and technologies. Dermatol Surg. 2007;33(10):1158–74.
2. Mogensen M, Nurnberg BM, Forman JL, Thomsen JB, Thrane L, Jemec GB. In vivo thickness measurement of basal cell carcinoma and actinic keratosis with optical coherence tomography and 20-MHz ultrasound. Br J Dermatol. 2009;160(5):1026–33.
3. Gambichler T, Orlikov A, Vasa R, Moussa G, Hoffmann K, Stucker M, et al. In vivo optical coherence tomography of basal cell carcinoma. J Dermatol Sci. 2007;45(3):167–73.
4. Forsea AM, Carstea EM, Ghervase L, Giurcaneanu C, Pavelescu G. Clinical application of optical coherence tomography for the imaging of non-melanocytic cutaneous tumors: a pilot multi-modal study. J Med Life. 2010;3(4):381–9.
5. Khandwala M, Penmetsa BR, Dey S, Schofield JB, Jones CA, Podoleanu A. Imaging of periocular basal cell carcinoma using en face optical coherence tomography: a pilot study. Br J Ophthalmol. 2010;94(10):1332–6.
6. Mogensen M, Joergensen TM, Nurnberg BM, Morsy HA, Thomsen JB, Thrane L, et al. Assessment of optical coherence tomography imaging in the diagnosis of non-melanoma skin cancer and benign lesions versus normal skin: observer-blinded evaluation by dermatologists and pathologists. Dermatol Surg. 2009;35(6):965–72.
7. Korde VR, Bonnema GT, Xu W, Krishnamurthy C, Ranger-Moore J, Saboda K, et al. Using optical coherence tomography to evaluate skin sun damage and precancer. Lasers Surg Med. 2007;39(9):687–95.
8. Marschall S, Sander B, Mogensen M, Jorgensen TM, Andersen PE. Optical coherence tomography-current technology and applications in clinical and biomedical research. Anal Bioanal Chem. 2011;400(9):2699–720.
9. Mogensen M, Nurnberg BM, Thrane L, Jorgensen TM, Andersen PE, Jemec GB. How histological features of basal cell carcinomas influence image quality in optical coherence tomography. J Biophotonics. 2011;4(7–8):544–51.
10. Petrova G, Derpalyek E, Gladkova N, et al. Optical coherence tomography using tissue clearing for skin disease diagnosis. Proc Spie. 2003;5140:168–86.
11. Strasswimmer J, Pierce MC, Park BH, Neel V, de Boer JF. Polarization-sensitive optical coherence tomography of invasive basal cell carcinoma. J Biomed Opt. 2004;9(2):292–8.
12. Banzhaf CA, Themstrup L, Ring HC, Mogensen M, Jemec GB. Optical coherence tomography imaging of non-melanoma skin cancer undergoing imiquimod therapy. Skin Res Technol. 2014;20(2):170–6.
13. Themstrup L, Banzhaf CA, Mogensen M, Jemec GB. Optical coherence tomography imaging of Non-melanoma skin cancer undergoing photodynamic therapy reveals subclinical residual lesions. Photodiagnosis Photodyn Ther. 2014;11(1):7–12.
14. Hamdoon Z, Jerjes W, Upile T, Hopper C. Optical coherence tomography-guided photodynamic therapy for skin cancer: case study. Photodiagnosis Photodyn Ther. 2011;8(1):49–52.
15. Cunha D, Richardson T, Sheth N, Orchard G, Coleman A, Mallipeddi R. Comparison of ex vivo optical coherence tomography with conventional frozen-section histology for visualizing basal cell carcinoma during Mohs micrographic surgery. Br J Dermatol. 2011;165(3):576–80.
16. Pomerantz R, Zell D, McKenzie G, Siegel DM. Optical Coherence Tomography Used as a Modality to Delineate Basal Cell Carcinoma prior to Mohs Micrographic Surgery. Case Rep Dermatol. 2011;3(3):212–8.

17. Alawi SA, Kuck M, Wahrlich C, Batz S, McKenzie G, Fluhr JW, et al. Optical coherence tomography for presurgical margin assessment of non-melanoma skin cancer – a practical approach. Exp Dermatol. 2013; 22(8):547–51.
18. Themstrup L, Banzhaf C, Mogensen M, Jemec GB. Cryosurgery treatment of actinic keratoses monitored by optical coherence tomography: a pilot study. Dermatology. 2012;225(3):242–7.
19. Graham GF, Scott CM. Cryosurgery. In: Riegel D, Friedman R, Dzubow LM, editors. Cancer of the skin. 1st ed. Philadelphia: Saunders; 2004. p. 487–97.
20. Sattler E, Kastle R, Welzel J. Optical coherence tomography in dermatology. J Biomed Opt. 2013;18(6): 061224.
21. Gambichler T, Jaedicke V, Terras S. Optical coherence tomography in dermatology: technical and clinical aspects. Arch Dermatol Res. 2011;303(7):457–73.

Part IV

Pre-malignant and Malignant Lesions

Premalignant Lesions: Combination Treatments in Cryosurgery

16

Paola Pasquali

Contents

P. Pasquali, MD
Department of Dermatology, Pius Hospital de Valls, 43800 Tarragona, Spain
e-mail: pasqualipaola@gmail.com

Key Points

- Skin cancerization can be treated with topical or procedural treatments. In both instances, treatments can be directed to individual lesions or to the entire damaged area.
- Cryosurgery is a first-line procedural treatment for individual lesions. Cryopeelings are field treatments not commonly used.
- Combination treatments have used tretinoin, 5FU, diclofenac sodium, and ingenol mebutate. Combining treatments works by adding up different mechanisms and/or potentiate mechanisms, producing an end result that should be better than either option applied individually.

16.1 Introduction

Actinic keratosis (AK) is the third leading cause of dermatological consultations in the United States, [1] and its treatment generates a great economic burden [2, 3]. They are lesions that arise from keratinocytes on sun-exposed areas. They can be predictors and precursors of invasive squamous cell carcinoma [4], although no reliable estimates concerning the frequency of AK developing into invasive carcinoma can be given [5]. The estimated probability of a lesion

P. Pasquali (ed.), *Cryosurgery: A Practical Manual*,
DOI 10.1007/978-3-662-43939-5_16, © Springer-Verlag Berlin Heidelberg 2015

progressing to squamous cell carcinoma ranges from 0.025 to 20 % per lesion per year [6]. AK can: (a) regress, (b) persist, or (c) progress to an in situ or invasive squamous cell carcinoma.

Important risk factors include fair skin, immunosuppression as well as cumulative sun exposure. Face, scalp, dorsal side of hands, and forearms are the most commonly affected areas. Actinic keratoses were seen in the past as isolated or multiple lesions that required punctual treatment. Today, AK is seen as part of the clinical presentation of sun-damaged skin and treatment should include removal of individual lesions combined with field therapies to subside the field damage which includes subclinical and emerging malignancies as well [7].

It is of utmost importance to diagnose AK correctly [8] to avoid sub-treating SCC thinking it was AK. Clinical, dermoscopy, and confocal assessments can aid diagnosis and posttreatment follow-up.

Clinically, AK presents itself as erythematous macules of light or dark pink, red or brown, and sometimes the same color of the skin; they can be a few millimeters up to a few centimeters wide; they can be flat or raised, smooth or scaly. Dermoscopy is an effective method for diagnosis of AK [9], and special features have been described for facial nonpigmented AK [10, 11]. Zalaudek et al. have found that there are significant differences in the dermoscopy pattern of AK, intraepidermal carcinoma, and invasive SCC that can be used to decide proper management [12]. Dermoscopy can also be used for posttreatment assessment.

Treatment options for AK are individual lesion-based or field-directed treatments. Some of these treatments are:

- *Topical individual lesion treatment for single or multiple lesions*: imiquimod, 5-Fluorouracil with 0.5 %, salicylic acid 10 % [13], and ingenol mebutate gel (0.05 and 0.015 %)
- *Topical field treatments*: retinoids [14], 5 Fluorouracil, diclofenac sodium gel 3 % with 2.5 % hyaluronic gel, and ingenol mebutate
- *Procedural individual single or multiple individual therapies*: cryosurgery, electrosurgery, and/or curettage
- *Procedural field treatment*: PDT, cryopeelings

16.2 Cryosurgery in AK

16.2.1 Direct Treatment

Cryosurgery is the most common treatment, with cure rates reported in a wide range from 39 to 83 %, depending on freezing times [15]. Comparison studies have been performed between PDT with cryotherapy [16], showing a 91 % AK clearance in the PDT group vs 68 % in the cryosurgery group; however, in this study, the PDT was repeated after 7 days while cryosurgery was performed only once and without temperature control.

Cryosurgery can be used both as a procedural single/multiple lesion treatment and as field therapy.

Comparison among therapeutic options needs standardization of procedures and treatment of same type of lesions. For cryosurgery, this has not been the case. A breakthrough might have come with the possibility of measuring surface temperature via infrared sensor technology. The first studies have shown that by controlling temperature and treating lesions in a controlled manner, results can be improved [17]. Studies will need to select AK with common clinical, dermoscopy, and confocal criteria in order to guarantee that the treatment is performed on similar lesions and always in the same manner.

Single-lesion treatment is usually performed with open (spraying) technique. An intermediate size tip is usually used, at a constant distance. Freezing has to be at the center of the lesion letting the freezing front advance until reaching approximately 1–2 mm over the external margin of the lesion. One freeze-thaw cycle is sufficient. One of the advantages of cryosurgery is that several lesions can be treated in one session.

Thicker AK will preferably need scraping down since keratin is not a good temperature conductor. In addition, thick keratotic lesions do not allow for a proper dermoscopy evaluation. Once a large crust is removed, dermoscopy finding might indicate if a lesion is a squamous cell carcinoma rather than a KA. Treating SCC believing it is an AK will result in recurrence of an NMSC. A large single lesion in the skin with little skin damage should raise suspicion. Thick, crusty lesions can have SCC at the base.

Hypertrophic AK/SCC can present themselves as cutaneous horns. Cutaneous horns can develop on a keratinocytic base with the histopathology on a spectrum of conditions that include seborrheic keratosis, actinic keratosis, in situ SCC, and invasive SCC. In a study of 163 cutaneous horns, Pyne et al. [18] found 57 % in situ SCC + invasive SCC and 13 % AK; the rest (30 %) were seborrheic keratosis. In a study by Yu [19], almost 39 % of cutaneous horns were malignant or premalignant epidermal lesions. Mantese et al. also found in their series that 59 % out of 222 cutaneous horns studied were premalignant or malignant [20]. Keep in mind that in horny lesions treatment decisions should be made once the base has been evaluated (dermoscopy, confocal, and eventually biopsy) before treating. Hyperkeratotic lesions are more resistant to freezing [21]. These types of lesions will require a deeper freezing than thin lesions. Since keratin is a bad conductor of cold, several approaches are possible: (a) freezing and curettaging of the surface lesion, shaving/cutting the horny part, hemostasia, and then freezing the base either with close technique (probe) as shown in Fig. 16.1a–f or open

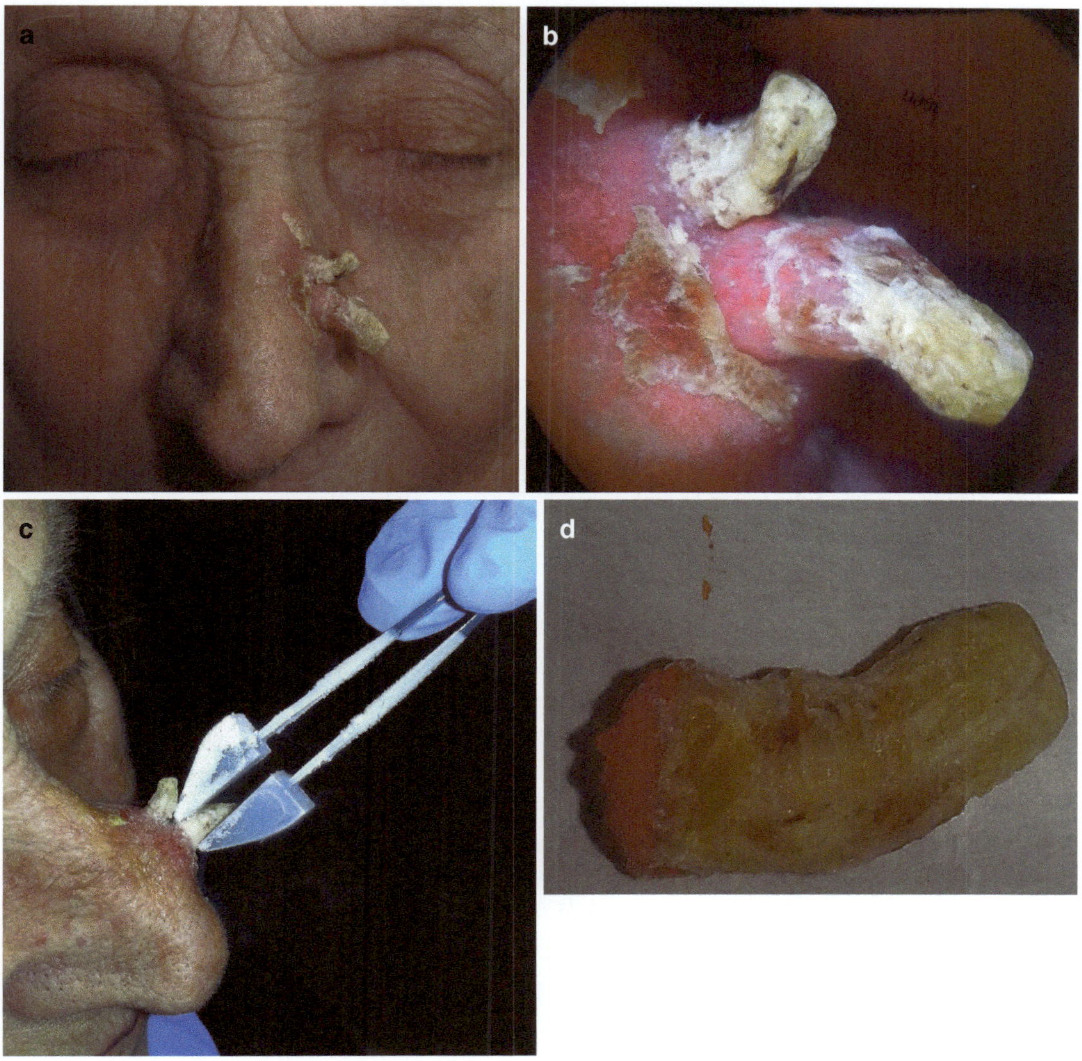

Fig. 16.1 (**a**) Large double cutaneous horn on the nose of 93-year-old patient; (**b**) dermoscopy image of the double cutaneous horn; (**c**) cryotweezer used for freezing the largest lesion down to the base; (**d**) removal by shaving of frozen lesion (histopathology reported a well-differentiated invasive SCC); (**e**) contact freezing with 4 mm probe; the same procedure was performed of the smaller lesion; (**f**) postoperative result after 1 month

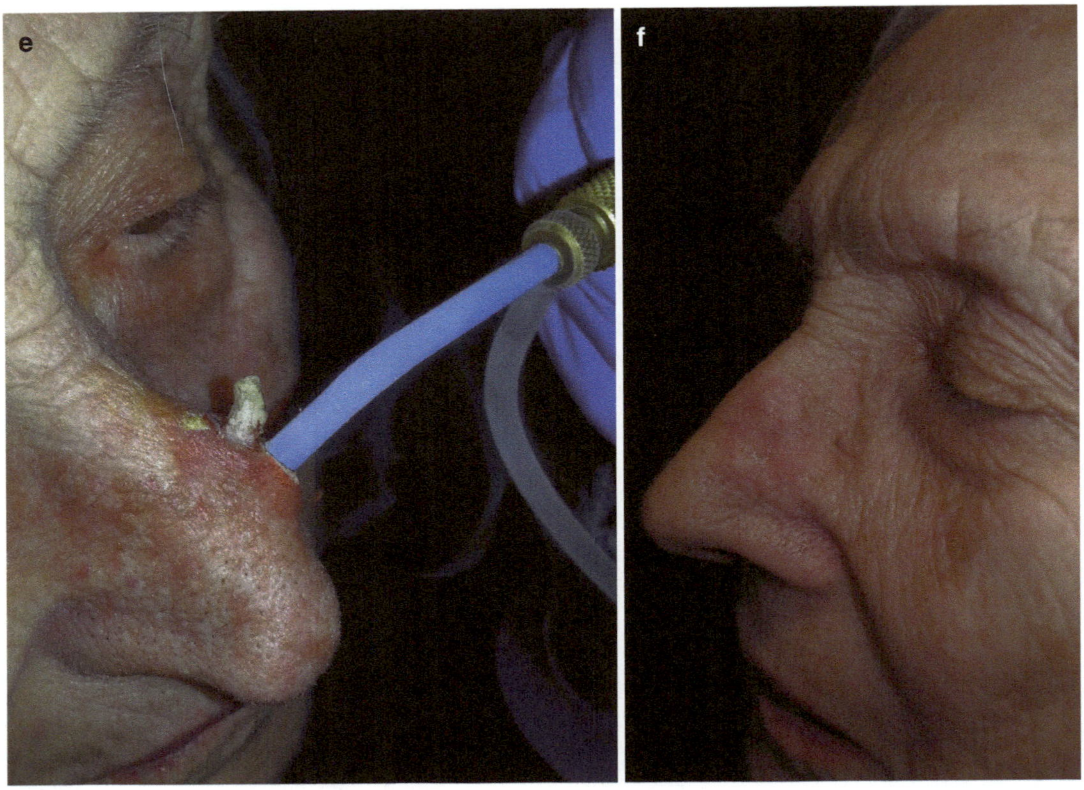

Fig. 16.1 (continued)

technique (spray) (Fig. 16.2a–f and 16.3a, b), (b) previous treatment with retinoid to reduce thickness, and (c) wetting the lesion to make keratin more permeable as done in wart cryosurgical treatment.

16.2.2 Field Treatment

Several therapeutic approaches are available for field treatment. Once applied, patients are the first to notice the improvement: they report softer sensation when touching the treated areas, less scaling, and improved appearance.

Before and after clinical photography aids physicians in confirming such changes. We believe there is the need to develop image change detection algorithms to calculate mathematically such improvement. Changes are easier to detect in infrared photography, which highlights keratin (white) and vessels (black). A simple way to obtain infrared-like images is through image processing [22]. Most photography editing programs have incorporated such a feature.

16.2.3 Cryopeeling

By far, the largest experience of cryopeeling for field cancerization has been reported by Chiarello [23]. In 2000, he published his long-term follow-up results on the use of extensive cryosurgery to treat areas of field cancerization on 373 patients. 34,604 individual AK were treated by open (spraying) technique and the surrounding areas were sprayed at a distance of approximately 5 cm, in a paint brush or circular fashion until the entire area was frozen. For cryopeeling, an acne tip can work very nicely as well (Fig. 16.4) since it allows for feathering the liquid nitrogen in a lineal pattern and covers large areas at once. Chiarello's data show that cryopeeling is twice as effective as 5FU when measured 1–3 years post cryosurgery. The number of SCC recorded over

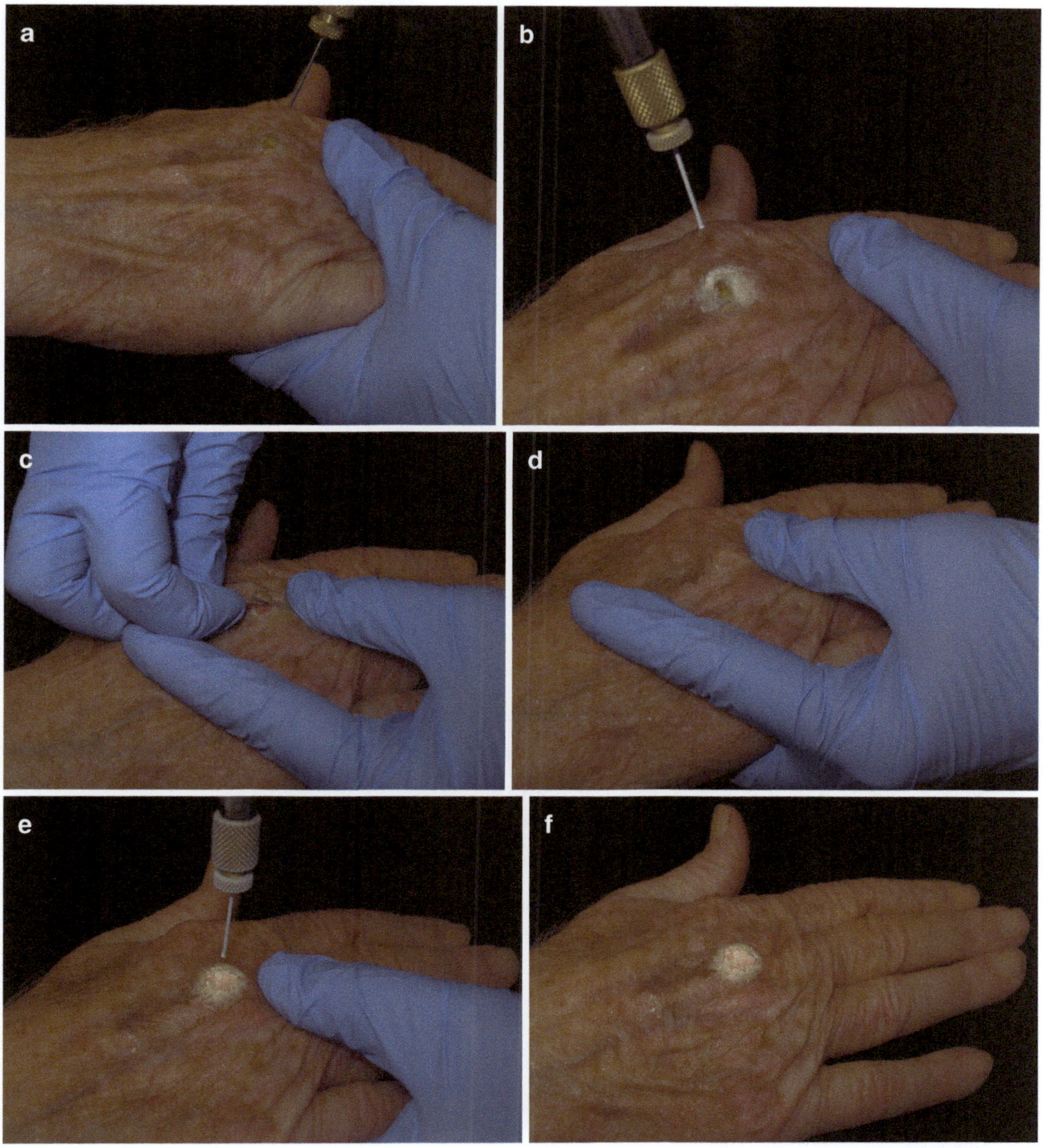

Fig. 16.2 (**a**) Open (spraying) freezing of a hyperkeratotic AK. (**b**) Leaving a 1–2 mm margin. (**c**) Shaving during thawing. (**d**) Hemostasia at the base was followed by (**e**) one spray freeze-thaw cycle with a freezing front that covered the base and 1–2 mm margin (**f**)

5–6 years was 33 with no metastases, a much lower number than predicted if AK had been left untreated [23].

Pain can be an issue when freezing large areas, especially on the head. Chiarello suggests using EMLA or 30 % lidocaine mixed in acid mantle cream vigorously applied after freezing. The immediate post-thawing vasodilation and skin barrier breaking will permit a rapid penetration and relief in seconds; block anesthesia is also an option as well as local injections or "blebs" of 1 or 2 % Xylocaine with epinephrine followed by massage [23].

The results are quite spectacular because most benign lesions are removed as well (seborrheic keratosis, lentigos solaris) (Figs. 16.5a–c,

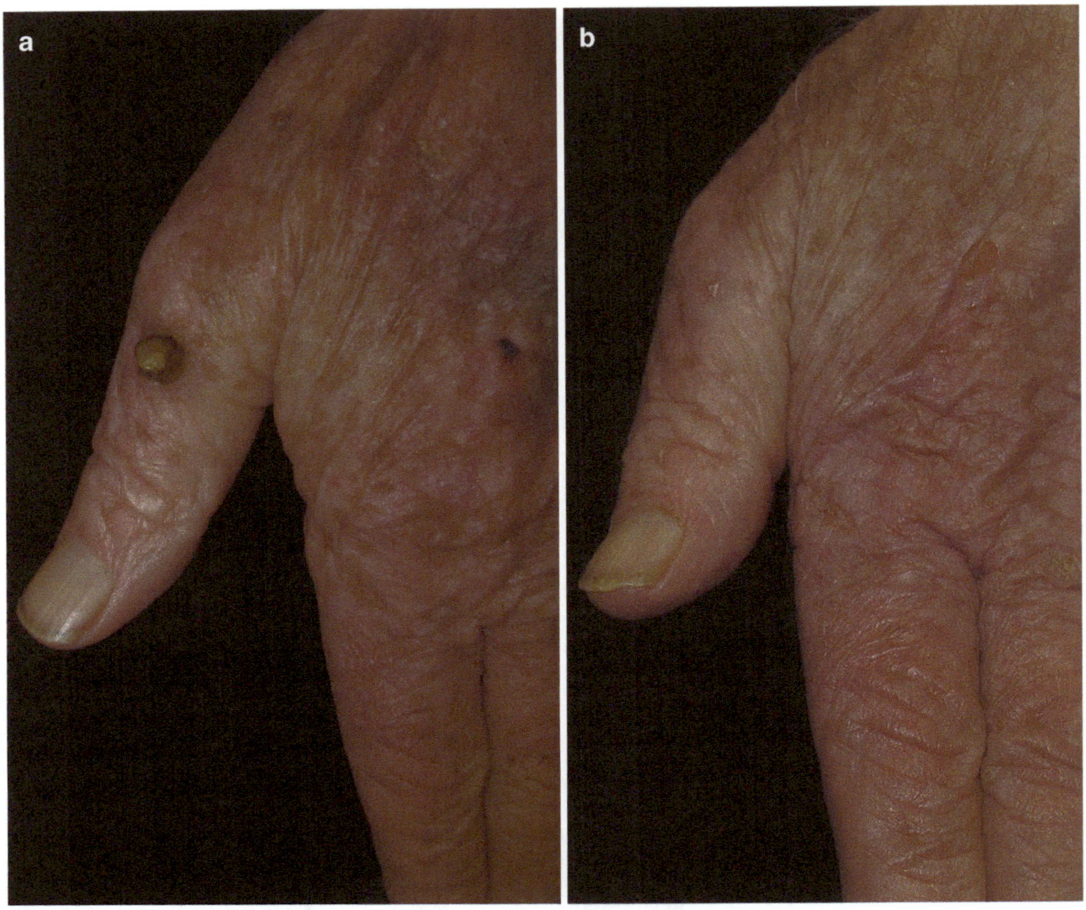

Fig. 16.3 (**a**) A hyperkeratotic lesion on the left hand thumb done with freeze spraying-shaving-hemostasia-freezing at the base and biopsy (which reported an in situ SCC); (**b**) result 4 months later

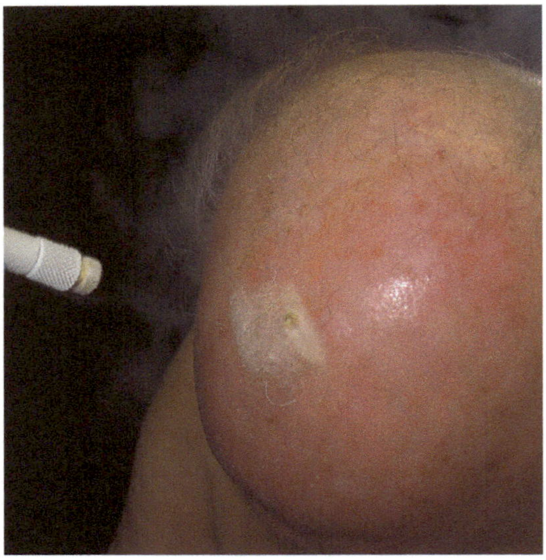

Fig. 16.4 Cryopeeling with acne aperture which feathers LN in a linear pattern

16.6a–c, 16.7a–c, and 16.8a–c). Likewise, make sure the whole field has been carefully examined to avoid peeling away by freezing lesions that needed other treatment procedures.

16.2.4 Combination Treatment

Combining different treatments has two purposes:

- *Summing Up*. Adding up two different mechanisms that run in parallel and that maximize the combined clinical outcome. Such is the case of field plus single-lesion treatment combination. In general, field treatment is best for superficial and also for nonclinical damage but insufficient for thick individual lesions. Individual treatment (topical or procedural) is

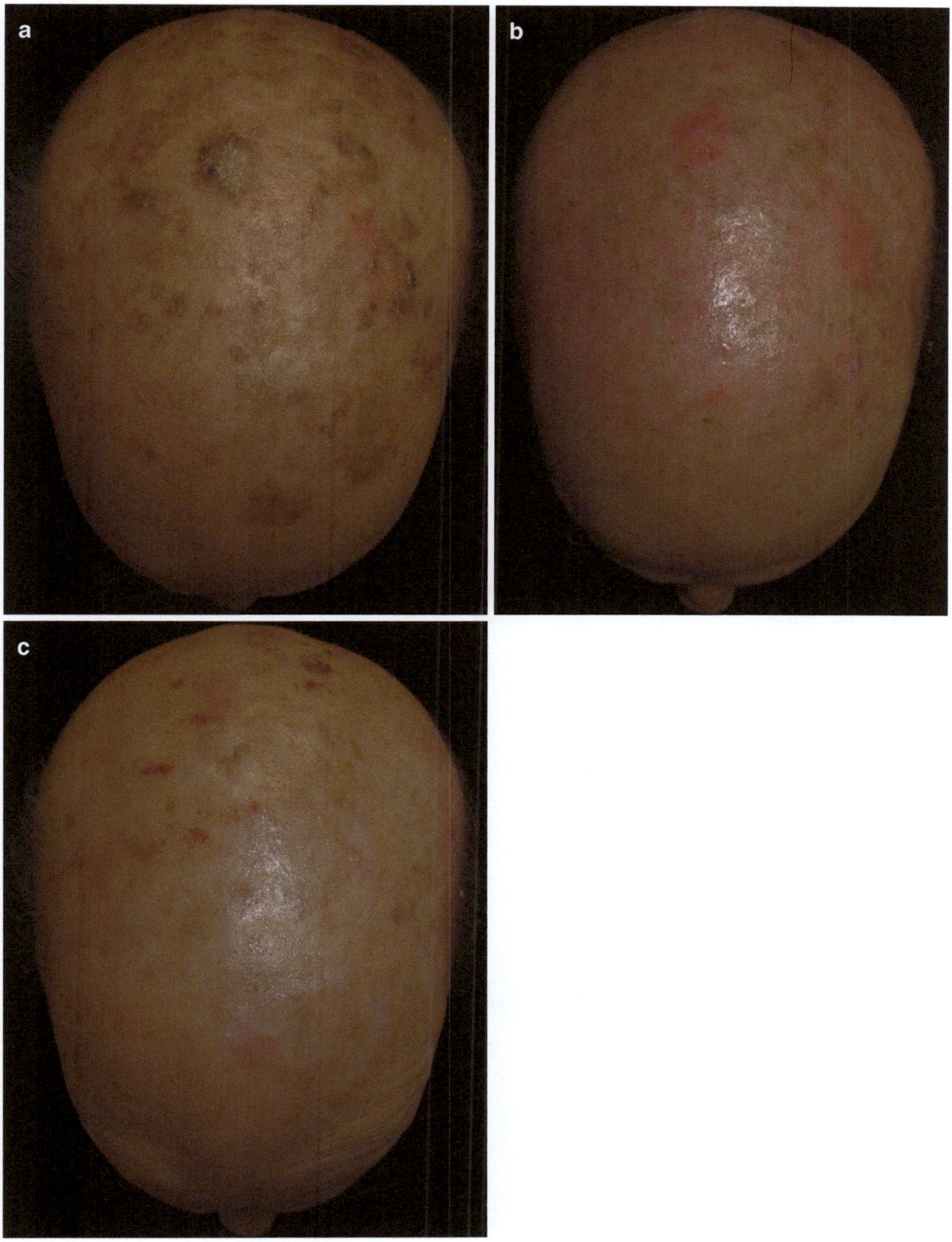

Fig. 16.5 Cryopeeling on sun-damaged scalp. (**a**) Before; (**b**) 3 months after treatment; (**c**) 9 months after treatment

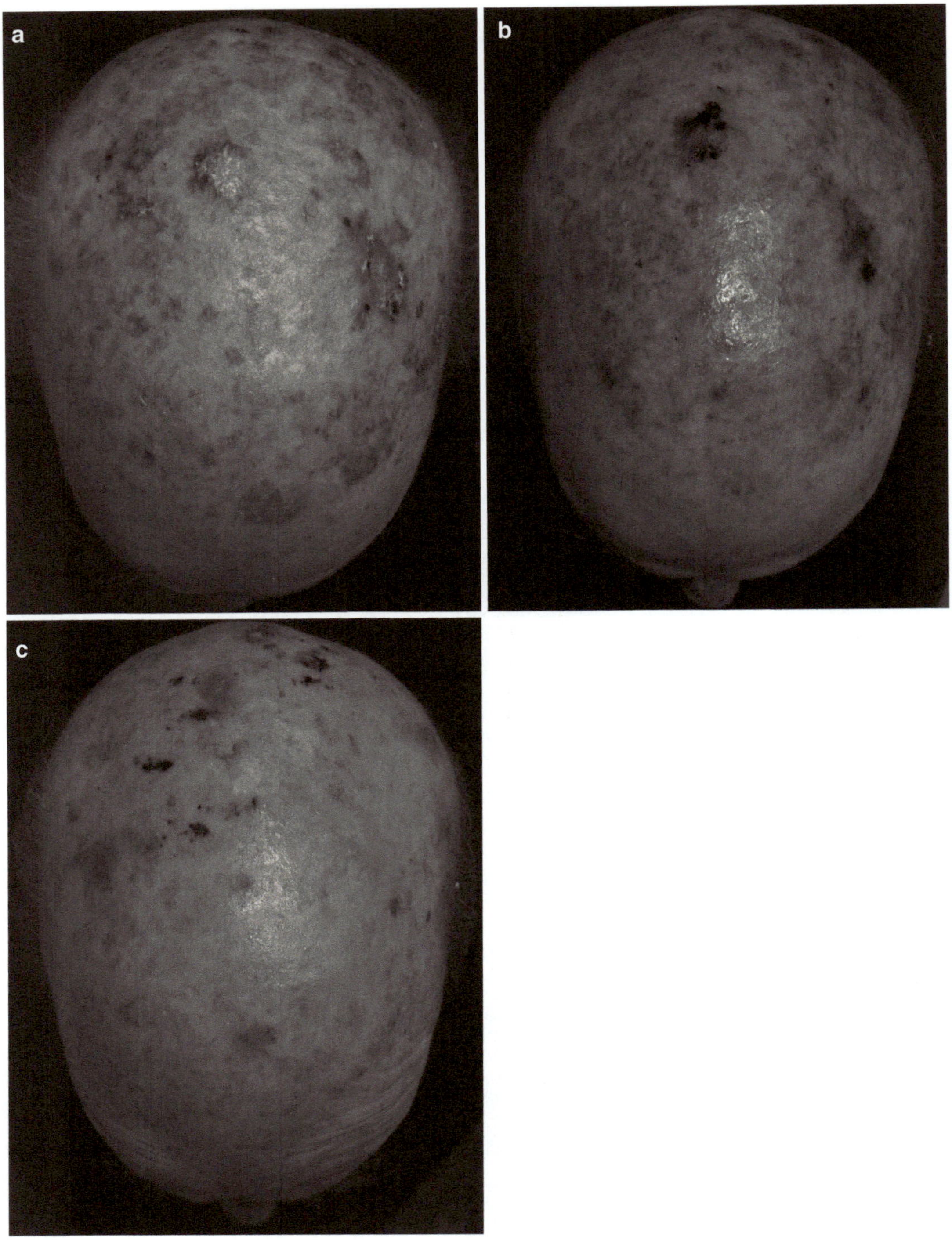

Fig. 16.6 Same patient as in Fig. 16.5 with image processing (infrared) which (**a**) allows to assess the extent of the damage (the hyperkeratotic lesion at 12 looks white due to high content of keratin); (**b**) 3 months post treatment (the hyperkeratotic area at 12 looks black due to redness post cryo, which was deeper in this area because of excess keratin); (**c**) general improvement in the amount of white (keratotic lesions) and black (redness post cryo and redness from sun damage)

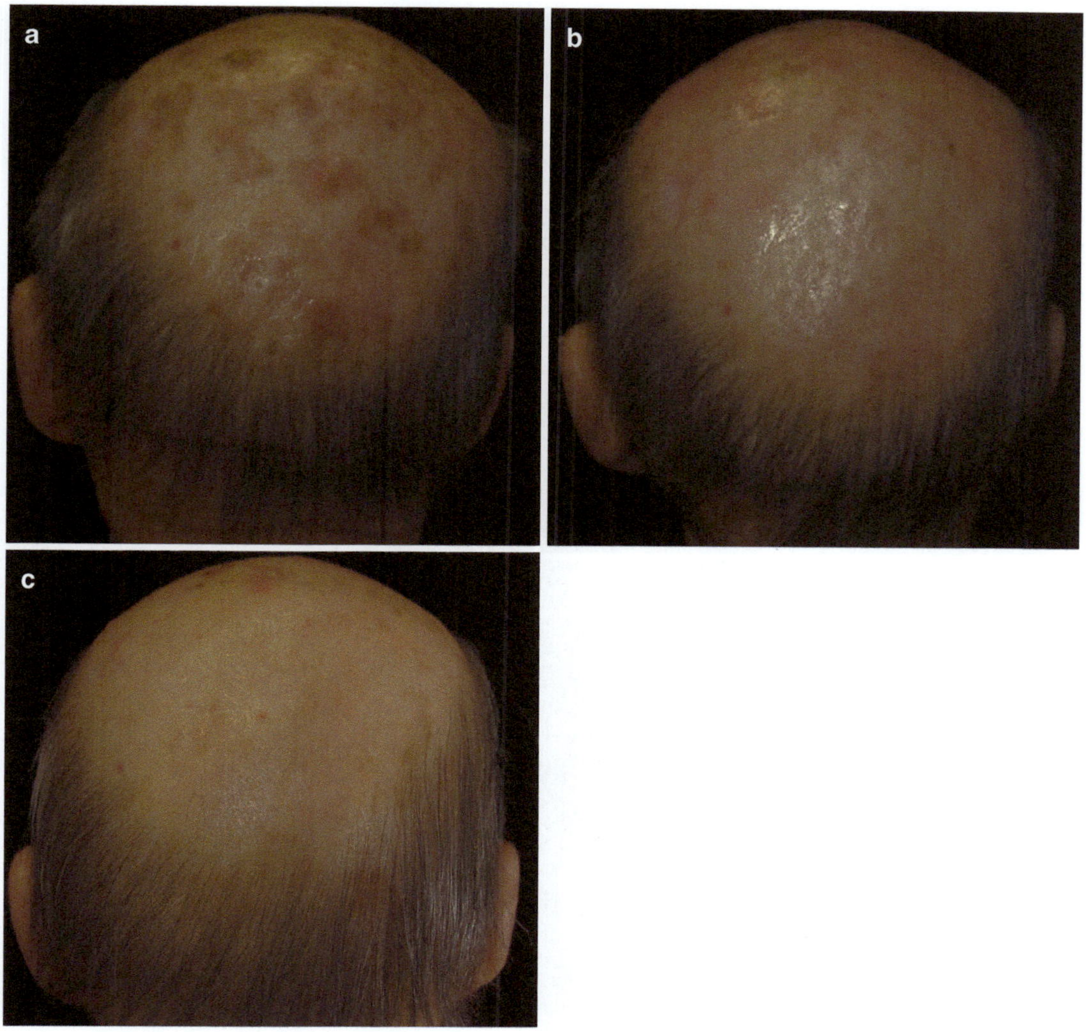

Fig. 16.7 Cryopeeling on sun-damaged area on the occipital area of the scull (**a**) before, (**b**) 3 months, and (**c**) 9 months after treatment

usually more destructive and thus best for thick localized lesions. Some authors have suggested the use of topical or injected substances to augment or assist cryosurgery [24] based on concepts taken from the field of cryopreservation. The concept is valid and additional clinical studies aimed to establish such possibility are warranted.

- *Potentiate*. Two individual treatment options can be maximized by having them work simultaneously or sequentially. The end result should be better than either option applied individually. For example, in the section dealing with keloids, Lopez combines freezing and local corticoid infiltration sequentially. He proposes infiltration of corticosteroid into the fibrous tissue a few minutes (10–15 min) after the last freeze-thaw cycle; keloid tissue edema "softens" the tissue and the injection is greatly facilitated. A higher volume of the drug can be injected into the tissue after the freezing compared with the amount that can be injected without a previous cryosurgery.

In immunocryosurgery, imiquimod is combined with freezing in such a way that the final amount of the topical drug and freezing is less than that used if either approach would be applied separately. The end result is better than with

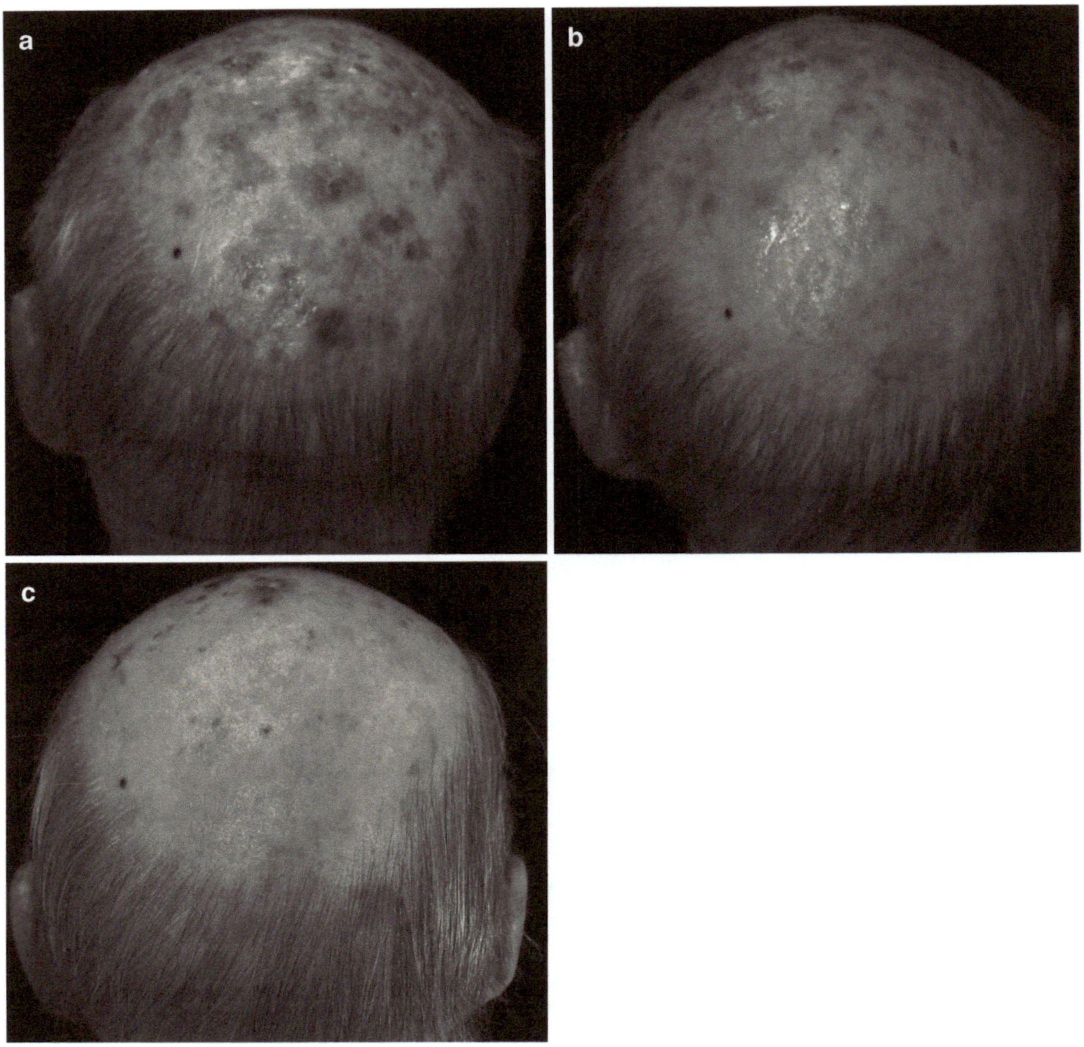

Fig. 16.8 Same patient as in Fig. 16.7 with image processing (infrared) which (**a**) allows assessment of the extent of the damage (redness is seen as black; keratin is seen as white); (**b**) 3 months post treatment; (**c**) 9 months after treatment with almost no black lesions (hypervascularization)

either treatment used separately. This concept (Chap. 3) and its application (Chap. 20) have deserved two entire chapters in this book.

Baust et al. state that since most chemotherapeutic agents initiate apoptosis in cancer cells, subfreezing (which can occur at the periphery of tumors treated with cryosurgery) applied sequentially with low-dose chemotherapy improves cancer cell death in the periphery [25].

In skin cancerization, when a topical treatment is applied before cryosurgery, part of the benefit is related to the loss of the superficial layers of the epidermis. Keratin is a bad conductant of cold; therefore, a desepitelized surface will allow a better and more regular expansion of the freezing front.

When cryosurgery is applied at the start, edema, vasodilation, and also loss of superficial skin layers will allow topical treatments to be absorbed better.

Some authors have suggested that large-diameter lesions (greater than 1 cm) and the presence of pain predict conventional treatment resistance either to topical monotherapy or cryosurgery [26] and require combination treatment.

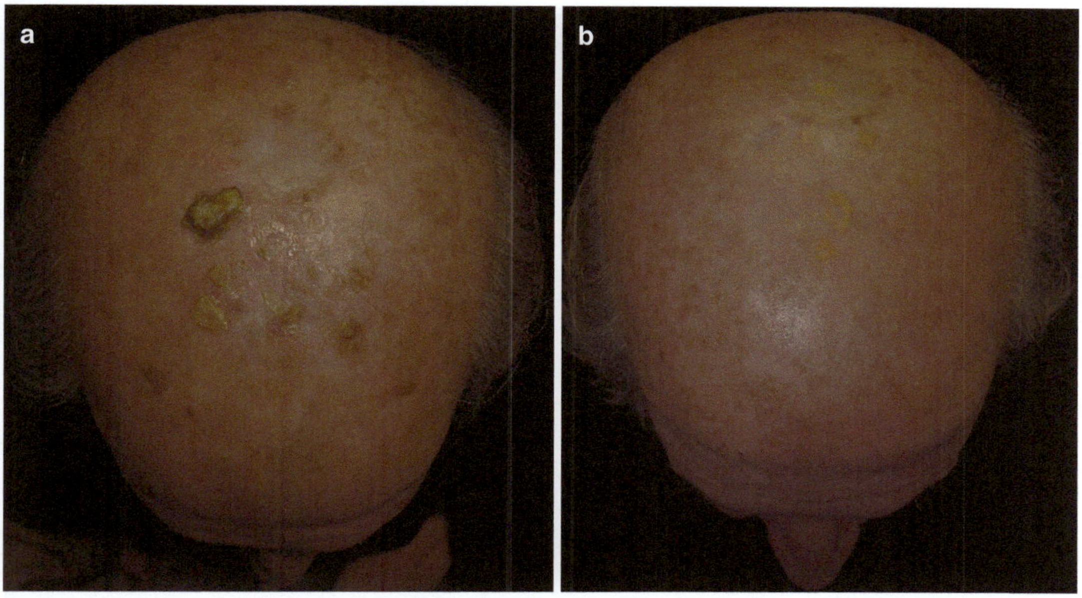

Fig. 16.9 (**a**) Severe sun-damaged scalp. 5 % 5FU was indicated daily for 3 weeks, and then individual residual lesions were treated with one freeze-thaw cycle; (**b**) control image after 13 months

Some combinations with cryosurgery are:

1. *Acitretin/tretinoin*: Oral acitretin has been used in transplant patients with clinical improvement (probably due to peeling off the stratum corneum) although no changes in proliferation were observed. Its potential combination with cryosurgery requires consideration and further studies [27]. The use of topical tretinoin in combination with cryosurgery has no formal support, but it is used in the treatment of AK [28] and for preparation on skin before cryopeelings or treatment of multiple lentigos of face and/or dorsum of hands.
2. *5 Fluorouracil*: Cryosurgery with 5 FU is probably the most used topical treatment but underused in combination despite evidence of its benefit. In fact it is used only on 1.1 % of actinic keratosis treated [29]. Evidence shows that 0.5 % fluorouracil has similar efficacy and is better tolerated than 5 % fluorouracil. It has proven beneficial in 1-week treatments with once-daily use followed by cryosurgery [30]. Extending treatment for up to 4 weeks further improved AK lesion clearance rates [31, 32]. The use of this drug before freezing eliminates some cancerous cells and leaves others in apoptosis; with freezing, there will be increase in cell death when compared to either application alone [33] (Fig. 16.9a, b, 16.10a, b, and 16.11a, b).

   As data of interest, treatment for visceral malignancies used this combination treatment applying cryosurgery followed by 5 FU [34] although new evidence seems to suggest that the sequence used in dermatology (5 FU then cryosurgery) might work better for some internal malignancies [35].
3. *Imiquimod*: Combination of imiquimod with cryosurgery deserves more than one chapter. In Chap. 3, Krunic has reviewed the theoretical aspects of immunocryosurgery while Gaitanis and Bassukas in Chap. 20 have gone through the applications on NMSC. New combinations are using 3.75 % instead of 5 % imiquimod followed by directed (not standardized) cryosurgery [36, 37].
4. *Diclofenac sodium 3 % gel* may work by inhibiting cyclo-oxgenase-2 (COX-2) as an angiogenesis inhibitor and inducing apoptosis; used alone, complete clearance is on the order of 58 % [38]. Some authors have reported clearance of 71 % with diclofenac by the end of the 12-week topical treatment; cryosurgery was

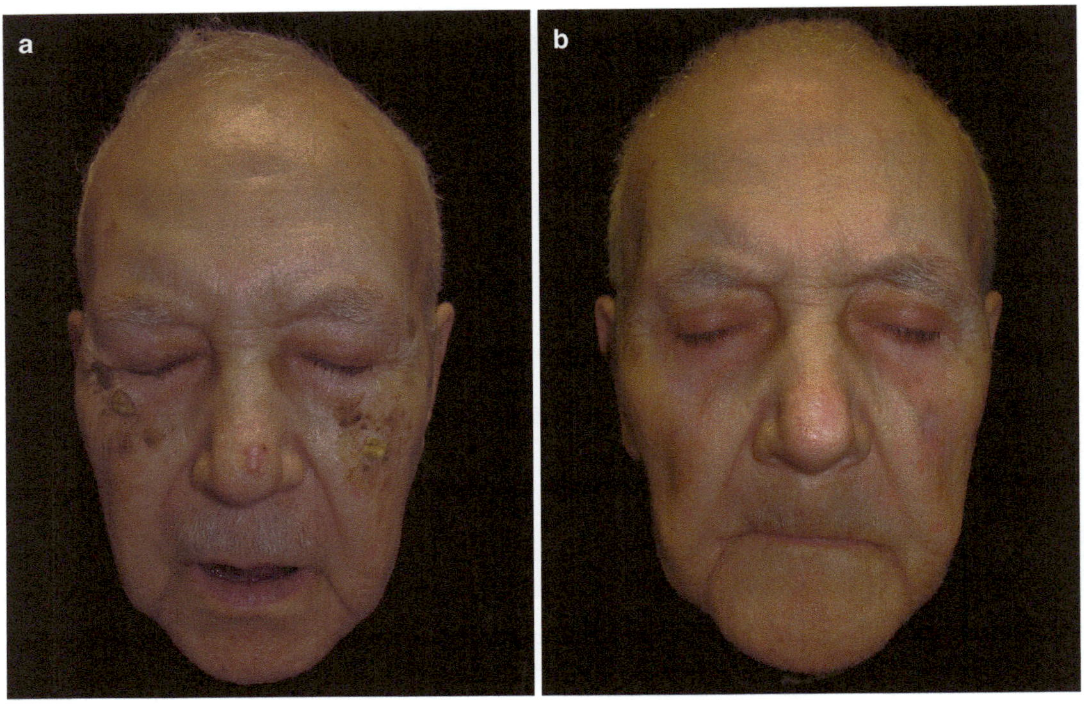

Fig. 16.10 (a) Severe field cancerization on the face. Three weeks of 5 % 5FU in the evenings was followed by cryosurgery (one freeze-thaw cycle on residual lesions). The BCC on the nose was treated with close (probe) technique with a double freeze-thaw cycle. (b) One year later

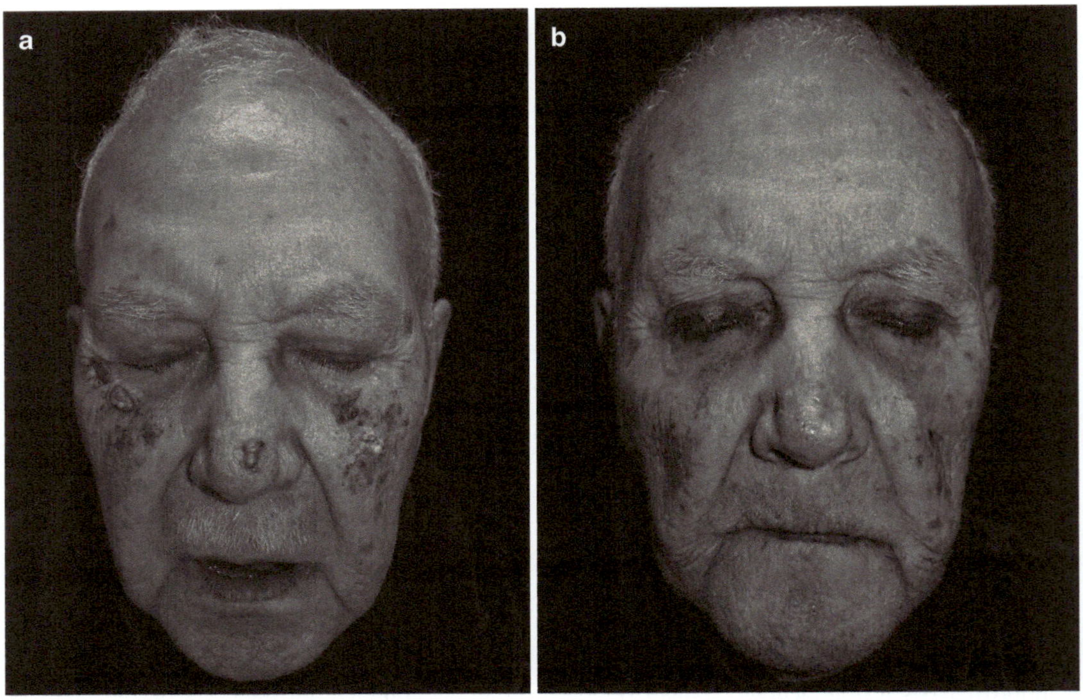

Fig. 16.11 Same patient as in Fig. 16.10a, b. Image processing (infrared) to highlight affected areas before and after treatment

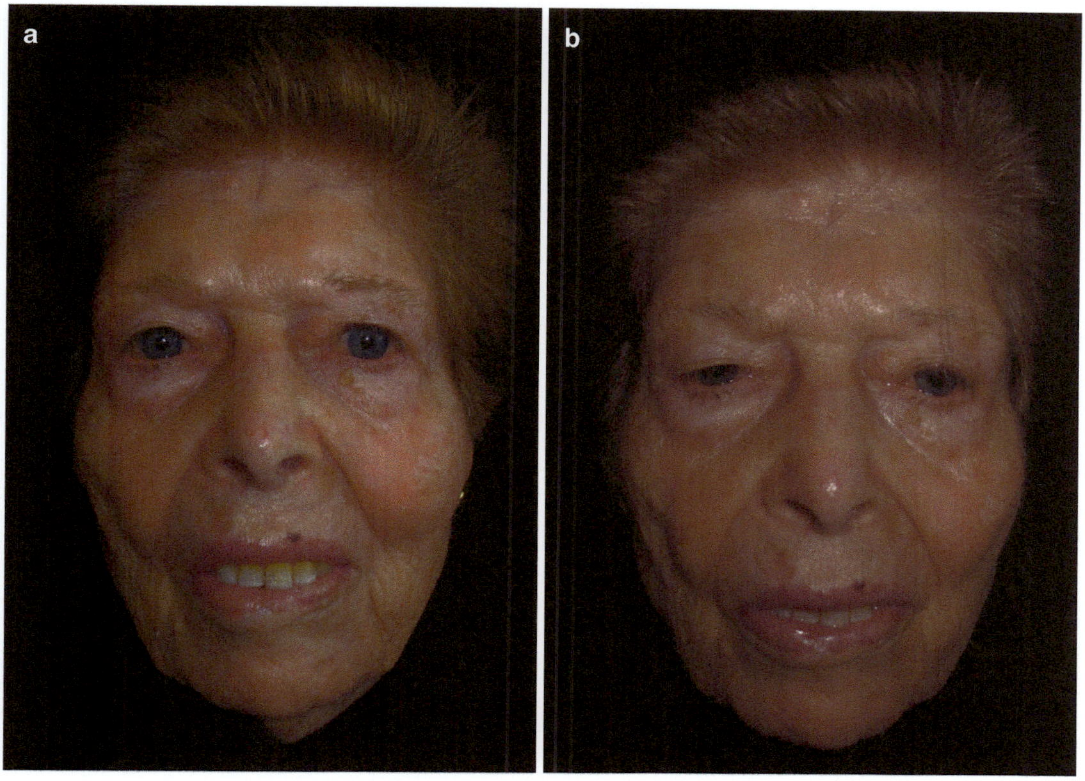

Fig. 16.12 (**a**) Severe skin cancerization of the face treated with Solaraze® (PharmaDerm, Melville, NY) (3 % diclofenac sodium) applied topically twice a day for 3 months; (**b**) 3 months after the end of treatment

done on residual lesions [39]. In another study, cryosurgery on selected lesions followed by 3-months twice-a-day treatment with diclofenac achieved a 100 % clearance [40] (Figs. 16.12a, b, 16.13a, b, 16.14a, b, 16.15a, b, 16.16a, b, and 16.17a, b).

5. *Ingenol mebutate 0.015% gel* has been used either alone or in combination with cryosurgery [41]. Its mechanisms of action include direct cell death followed by recruitment of cytotoxic neutrophils that eliminate residual tumor cells; finally, tumor-reactive antibodies are induced which in turn prevent relapses [42, 43]. Ingenol mebutate has been used in combination with cryosurgery in a double-blind study that evaluated both the short (11-week) and long-term (12-month) efficacy of sequential treatment of open (spray) treatment of individual AK followed by topical ingenol mebutate treatment compared to sole cryosurgery. The clearing rate was superior in the combined treatment [41].

16.3 Actinic Cheilitis

Actinic cheilitis is the premalignant damage present in many patients with skin cancerization. Just as in the skin, precancerous lip lesions need to be recognized and treated on time [44]. Close control is required because the consequences can be highly destructive and surgeries more disfiguring than equivalents in other parts of the face.

Lubritz and Smolewski [45] reported 96 % cure rate in cryosurgical treatment of premalignant leukoplakia of the lips. Cryosurgery has several advantages compared with other treatment modalities: it is inexpensive, very fast to apply, no anesthesia is required, and it does not require the skill level required by vermilionectomy [46]. One single freeze-thaw cycle, with open (spraying) technique, covering the entire surface of the lip is sufficient (Fig. 16.18a–c).

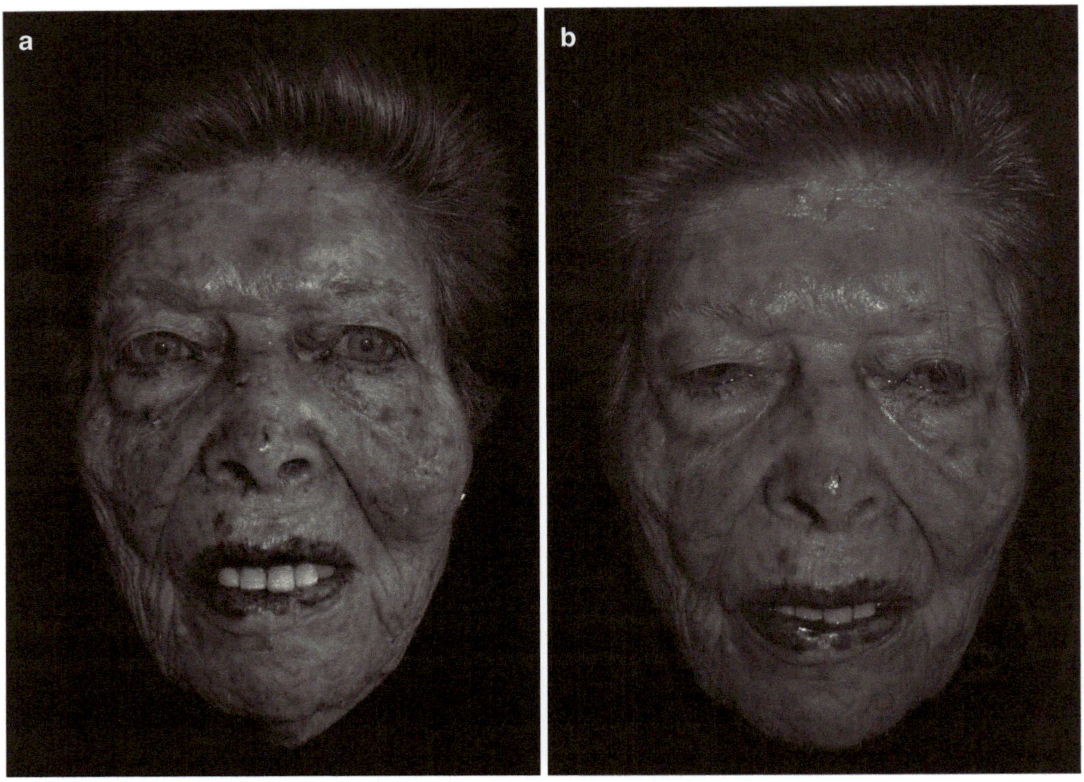

Fig. 16.13 Same patient in Fig. 16.12a, b with image processing (infrared) to highlight sun damage before treatment (**a**) and improvement 3 months after completion of treatment (**b**). Cryosurgery was applied as cryospray over few residual lesions

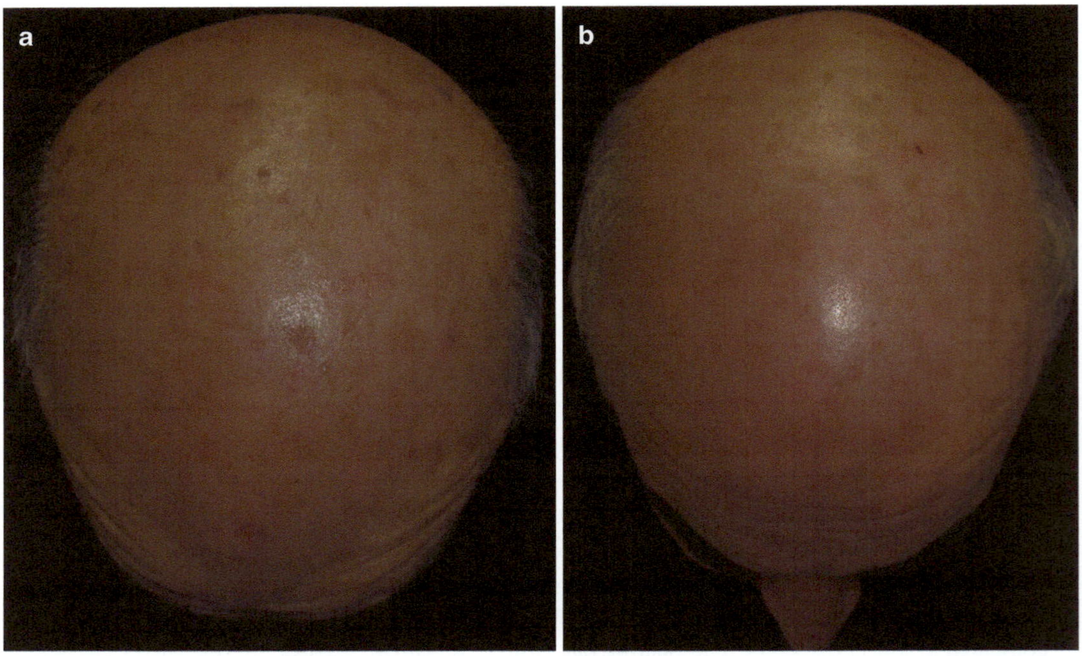

Fig. 16.14 (**a**) Severe field cancerization of the scalp. The patient was asked to apply 3 months of twice daily topical 3 % diclofenac sodium (Solaraze®, PharmaDerm, Melville, NY). Once completed, cryosurgery was done on hypertrophic residual lesions, one freeze-thaw cycle. (**b**) 4 months after completion of treatment

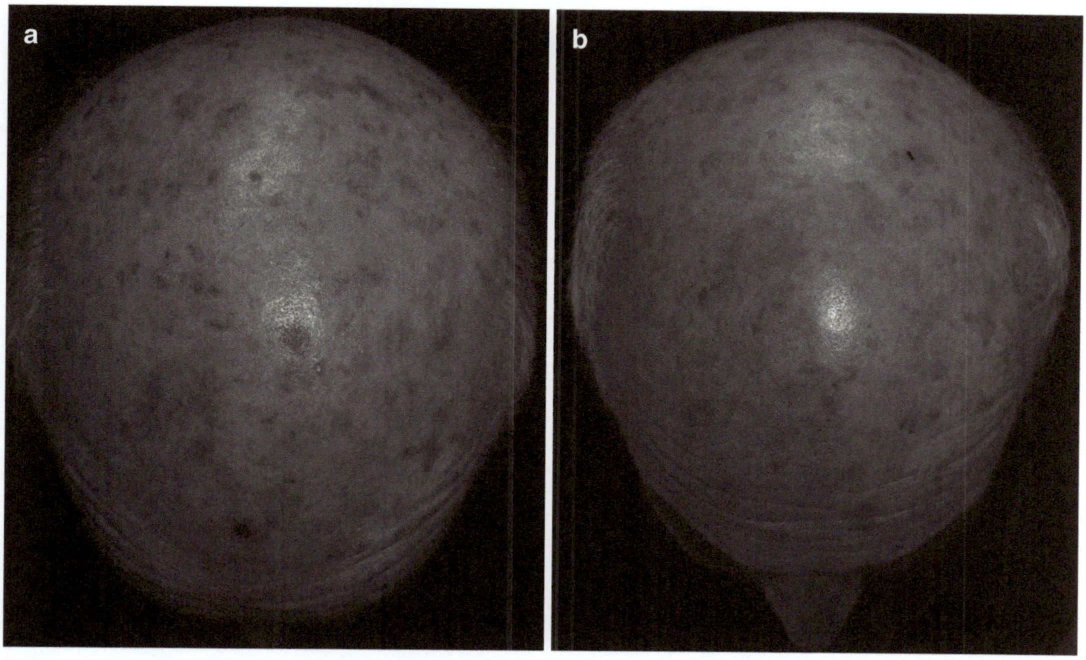

Fig. 16.15 (**a**) Before treatment image of same patient in Fig. 16.14a. The image has been processed (infrared) to make excess keratin more evident (in white). (**b**) After-treatment image of same patient in Fig. 16.14b, 4 months after treatment. The image has been processed (infrared) to make excess keratin more evident (in white)

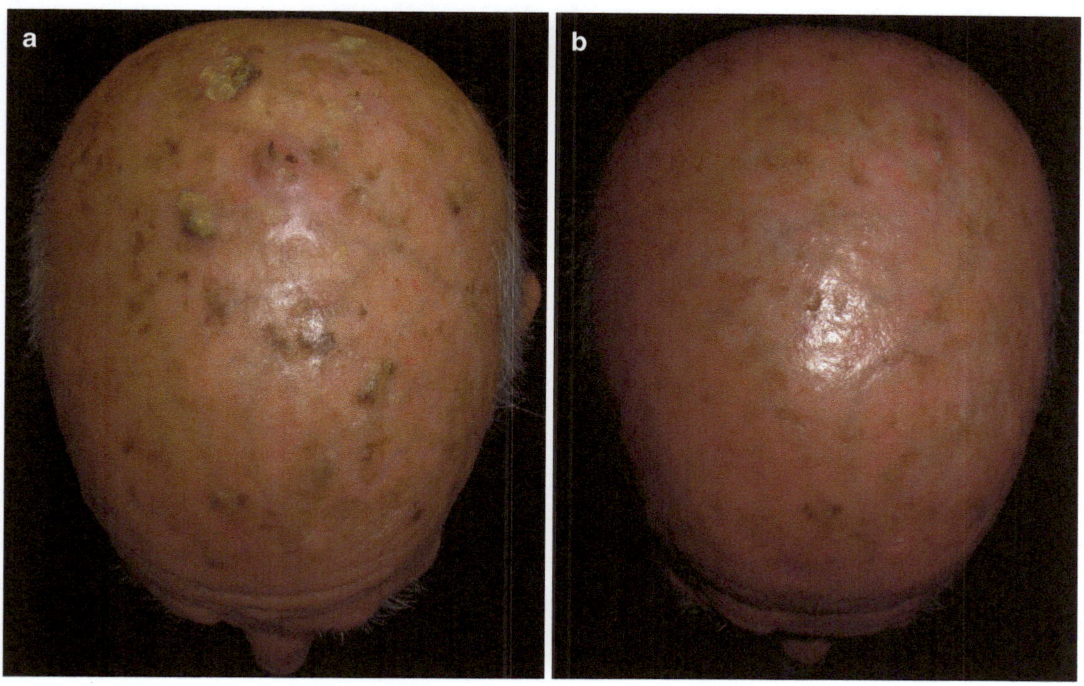

Fig. 16.16 (**a**) Severe field cancerization of scalp treated with twice daily 3 % diclofenac sodium (Solaraze®, PharmaDerm, Melville, NY) for 3 months followed by cryosurgery on residual lesion; (**b**) 1 month after completion of treatment

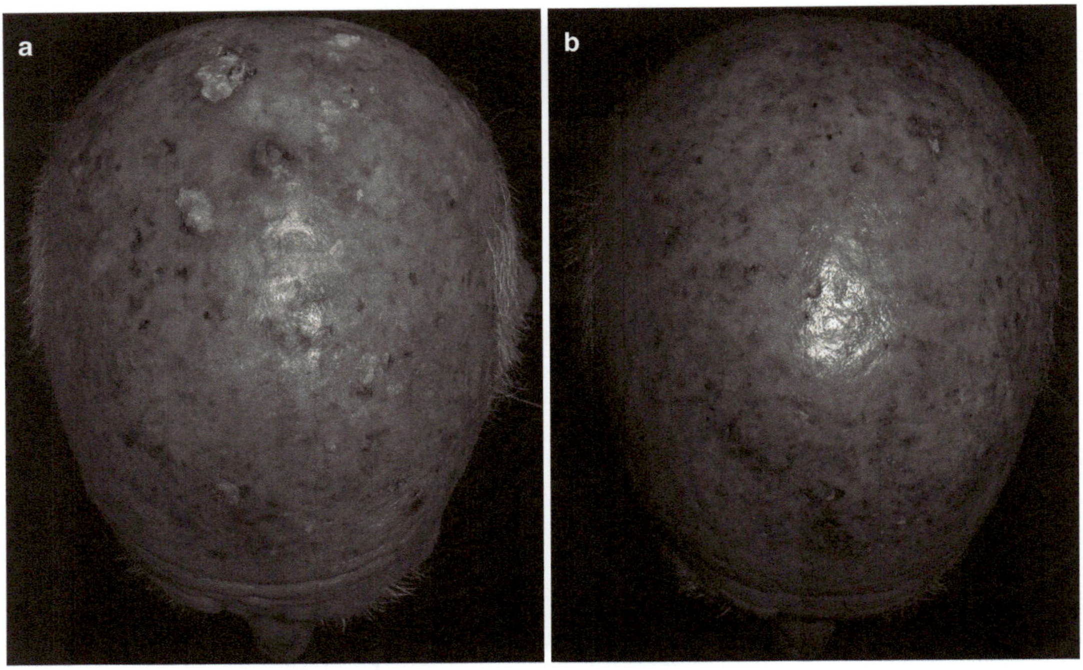

Fig. 16.17 Image processing (infrared) (same on both images) to further highlight white (keratin) vs black (vessel inflammation) and gray (rest of the skin). (**a**) Before; (**b**) after treatment

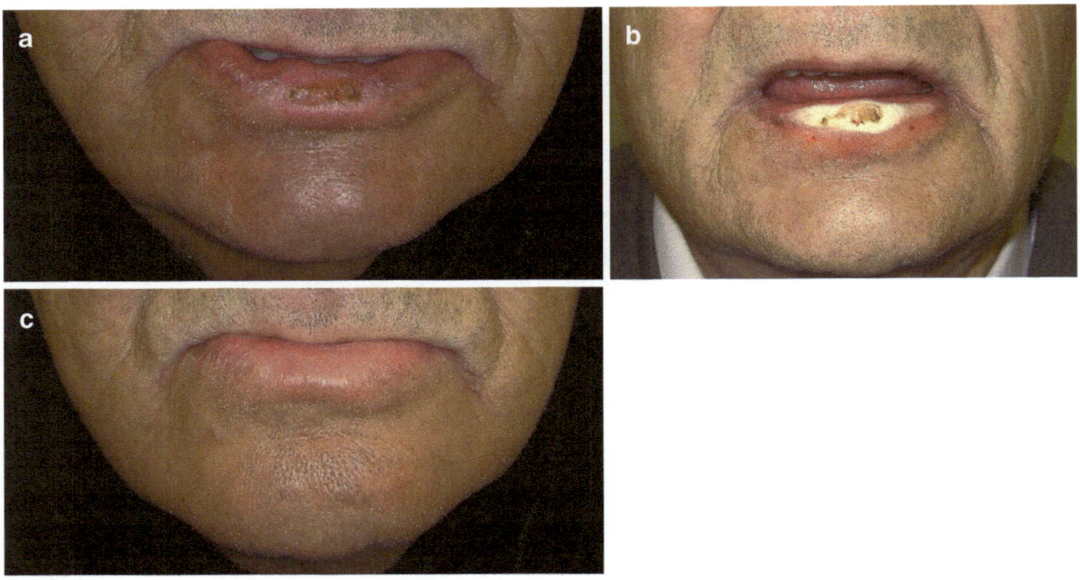

Fig. 16.18 (**a**) Actinic cheilitis on the lower lip treated with cryosurgery; (**b**) one freeze-thaw cycle covering the entire surface of the lip; (**c**) 2 months after treatment

16.4 Oral Leukoplakia

Oral leukoplakia is a potentially malignant disorder [47] that needs close control in order to detect early its malignant transformation into oral squamous cell carcinoma (OSCC), a disease that can have devastating consequences. The annual transformation rate is on the order of 1–2 % per year [48, 49]. Close monitoring of patients with OL is very important in order to diagnose timely any malignant transformation, and it is mandatory to biopsy any suspicious lesion before cryosurgical treatment.

Cryosurgery has been used in the treatment of oral leukoplakia with success [50], with complete remission as high as 89.2 %.

Essential Tidbits

- Pre- and posttreatment photography (with or without image processing) is a prerequisite to assess degree of improvement.
- Combination treatments are multiple, and each has pros and cons. Tailoring treatment to patient's need is fundamental. Degree of damage, anatomical area, extension, availability of medication, and cost are some of the parameters to keep in mind before choosing such a combination.
- Most topical treatment has secondary effects that are not irrelevant: irritation, discomfort, and sometimes systemic symptoms. A patient's appearance can generate concern to the patient and to others. Make sure to properly inform and reassure the patient and any caregivers.

Conclusions

With the large experience accumulated so far, it could be concluded that:

- AK needs to be treated to reduce the possibility of developing NMSC [51]. Criscione et al. (Department of Veteran Affairs Topical Tretinoin Chemoprevention Trial Group) have found that "the risk of progression of AK to primary SCC (invasive or in situ) is 0.60 % at 1 year and 2.57 % at 4 years." 65 % of all primary SCCs and 36 % of all primary BCCs arose in lesions diagnosed as AKs [52].
- AK should be diagnosed not only based on clinical examination. Many noninvasive imaging technologies are available today that aid physicians to reach the correct diagnosis. The most common and practical is dermoscopy. Others like confocal microscopy will be ideal in identifying clinical AK that has progressed to SCC [53], providing information that will allow selection of the best treatment (even before a biopsy is taken). Such a decision will save time and unnecessary costs.
- In case of doubt, a skin biopsy (preferable by shaving) will be necessary to rule out SCC. A cryobiopsy technique (Chap. 7) simplifies this procedure since no local anesthesia is required, and for small AK it can even be curative.
- AK is within an area of sun-damaged skin. The concept of field cancerization imposes a new therapeutic approach for proper management of premalignant skin damage. Treatment of individual (usually thick) lesions needs to be combined with field treatment.
- There are many combination treatment options, most of which have shown good to excellent results. The outcome of these combinations needs to be evaluated for the short and the long term.
- Better standardization of the studies is required. Cryosurgical procedure needs to be standardized in all studies. Temperature measurement at skin surface will probably be the best way to do so. Studies need to compare direct therapy alternatives among themselves or field therapies among themselves to avoid comparing "apples with pears." Similar types of AK and similar severity of field cancerization should be selected.
- Many combination treatments are possible, and each one has advantages and disadvantages [54]. They will need to be tailored to patient's individual needs [55]; in addition, there are differences in availability of products in different countries.
- Noninvasive technology (dermoscopy, eventually confocal microscopy) has become more

indispensable every day in diagnosing and in follow-up of treatments, reducing or avoiding the need of biopsy. As the use of technology becomes more widespread, better management of this condition will be possible.

- Photography and image processing (infrared) is widely available, inexpensive, and still underutilized in treatment management of field cancerization.

Glossary

AK	Actinic Keratosis
BCC	Basal Cell Carcinoma
CM	Confocal Microcopy
OSCC	Oral Squamous Cell Carcinoma
SCC	Squamous Cell Carcinoma

References

1. Salasche SJ. Epidemiology of actinic keratosis and squamous cell carcinoma. J Am Acad Dermatol. 2000;42: 4–7.
2. The Lewin Group Inc. for the Society of Investigative Dermatology and The American Academy of Dermatology Association. The burden of skin diseases. Available at: http://www.lewin.com/~/media/Lewin/Site_Sections/Publications/april2005skindisease.pdf. Accessed 15 Dec 2013.
3. Fenske NA, Spencer J, Adam F. Actinic keratoses: past, present and future. J Drugs Dermatol. 2010;9(5 Suppl ODAC Conf Pt 1):s45–9.
4. Goldberg LH, Mamelak AJ. Review of actinic keratosis. Part I: etiology, epidemiology and clinical presentation. J Drugs Dermatol. 2010;9(9):1125–32.
5. Werner RN, Sammain A, Erdmann R, Hartmann V, Stockfleth E, Nast A. The natural history of actinic keratosis: a systematic review. Br J Dermatol. 2013;169(3):502–18.
6. Gupta AK, Inniss K, Wainwright R, Chow M, Cooper E. Interventions for actinic keratoses (Protocol). Cochrane Database Syst Rev. 2003, Issue 4. Art. No.: CD004415. doi: 10.1002/14651858.CD004415.
7. Stockfleth E. The paradigm shift in treating actinic keratosis: a comprehensive strategy. J Drugs Dermatol. 2012;11(12):1462–7.
8. Terushkin V, Braga JC, Dusza SW, Scope A, Busam K, Marghoob AA, Gill M, Halpern AC. Agreement on the clinical diagnosis and management of cutaneous squamous neoplasms. Dermatol Surg. 2010;36(10):1514–20.
9. Huerta-Brogeras M, Olmos O, Borbujo J, Hernández-Núñez A, Castaño E, Romero-Maté A, Martínez-Sánchez D, Martínez-Morán C. Validation of dermoscopy as a real-time noninvasive diagnostic imaging technique for actinic keratosis. Arch Dermatol. 2012;148(10):1159–64.
10. Zalaudek I, Giacomel J, Argenziano G, Hofmann-Wellenhof R, Micantonio T, Di Stefani A, Oliviero M, Rabinovitz H, Soyer HP, Peris K. Dermoscopy of facial nonpigmented actinic keratosis. Br J Dermatol. 2006;155(5):951–6.
11. Cuellar F, Vilalta A, Puig S, Palou J, Salerni G. New dermoscopic pattern in actinic keratosis and related conditions. Arch Dermatol. 2009;145(6):732.
12. Zalaudek I, Giacomel J, Schmid K, Bondino S, Rosendahl C, Cavicchini S, Tourlaki A, Gasparini S, Bourne P, Keir J, Kittler H, Eibenschutz L, Catricalà C, Argenziano G. Dermatoscopy of facial actinic keratosis, intraepidermal carcinoma, and invasive squamous cell carcinoma: a progression model. J Am Acad Dermatol. 2012;66(4):589–97.
13. Stockfleth E, Zwingers T, Willers C. Recurrence rates and patient assessed outcomes of 0.5 % 5-fluorouracil in combination with salicylic acid treating actinic keratoses. Eur J Dermatol. 2012;22(3):370–4.
14. Ianhez M, Fleury Jr LF, Miot HA, Bagatin E. Retinoids for prevention and treatment of actinic keratosis. An Bras Dermatol. 2013;88(4):585–93.
15. Thai KE, Fergin P, Freeman M, Vinciullo C, Francis D, Spelman L, Murrell D, Anderson C, Weightman W, Reid C, Watson A, Foley P. A prospective study of the use of cryosurgery for the treatment of actinic keratosis. Int J Dermatol. 2004;43(9):687–92.
16. Freeman M, Vinciullo C, Francis D, Spelman L, Nguyen R, Fergin P, Thai KE, Murrell D, Weightman W, Anderson C, Reid C, Watson A, Foley P. A comparison of photodynamic therapy using topical methyl aminolevulinate (Metvix) with single cycle cryotherapy in patients with actinic keratosis: a prospective, randomized study. J Dermatolog Treat. 2003;14(2):99–106.
17. Goldberg LH, Kaplan B, Vergilis-Kalner I, Landau J. Liquid nitrogen: temperature control in the treatment of actinic keratosis. Dermatol Surg. 2010;36 (12):1956–61.
18. Pyne J, Sapkota D, Wong JC. Cutaneous horns: clues to invasive squamous cell carcinoma being present in the horn base. Dermatol Pract Concept. 2013;3(2):3–7.
19. Yu RC, Pryce DW, Macfarlane AW, Stewart TW. A histopathological study of 643 cutaneous horns. Br J Dermatol. 1991;124(5):449–52.
20. Mantese SA, Diogo PM, Rocha A, Berbert AL, Ferreira AK, Ferreira TC. Cutaneous horn: a retrospective histopathological study of 222 cases. An Bras Dermatol. 2010;85(2):157–63.
21. Ceilley RI, Jorizzo JL. Current issues in the management of actinic keratosis. J Am Acad Dermatol. 2013;68(1 Suppl 1):S28–38.
22. Pasquali P. Photography in dermatology. In: Baldi A, Pasquali P, Spugnini EP (eds.) Skin cancer. A practical approach. Springer. Humana Press, New York; 2014: 291–9.
23. Chiarello SE. Cryopeeling (extensive cryosurgery) for treatment of actinic keratoses: an update and comparison. Dermatol Surg. 2000;26(8):728–32.

24. Burkhart CG, Burkhart CN. Can cryosurgery in dermatology be augmented or assisted by pretreatment of skin? Int J Dermatol. 2008;47(10):1082–3.
25. Baust JG, Gage AA, Clarke D, Baust JM, Van Buskirk R. Cryosurgery–a putative approach to molecular-based optimization. Cryobiology. 2004;48(2):190–204.
26. Ondo AL, Padilla RS, Miedler JD, Cockerell CJ, Kerner JD, Steiner RL, Mings SM, Shanler SD. Treatment-refractory actinic keratoses successfully treated using simultaneous combination topical 5-fluorouracil cream and imiquimod cream: a case-control study. Dermatol Surg. 2012;38(9):1469–76.
27. Smit JV, de Sévaux RG, Blokx WA, van de Kerkhof PC, Hoitsma AJ, de Jong EM. Acitretin treatment in (pre)malignant skin disorders of renal transplant recipients: histologic and immunohistochemical effects. J Am Acad Dermatol. 2004;50(2):189–96.
28. Gold MH, Nestor MS. Current treatments of actinic keratosis. J Drugs Dermatol. 2006;5(2 Suppl):17–25.
29. Hagele TJ, Levender MM, Davis SA, Williford PM, Feldman SR. Practice trends in the treatment of actinic keratosis in the United States: 0.5 % fluorouracil and combination cryotherapy plus fluorouracil are underused despite evidence of benefit. J Cutan Med Surg. 2012;16(2):107–14.
30. Jorizzo J, Weiss J, Vamvakias G. One-week treatment with 0.5 % fluorouracil cream prior to cryosurgery in patients with actinic keratoses: a double-blind, vehicle-controlled, long-term study. J Drugs Dermatol. 2006; 5(2):133–9.
31. Menter A, Vamvakias G, Jorizzo J. One-week treatment with once-daily in participants with actinic keratoses. Cutis. 2008;81(6):509–16.
32. Jorizzo J. Topical treatment of actinic keratosis with fluorouracil: is irritation associated with efficacy? J Drugs Dermatol. 2004;3(1):21–6.
33. Clarke DM, Robilotto AT, Rhee E, VanBuskirk RG, Baust JG, Gage AA, Baust JM. Cryoablation of renal cancer: variables involved in freezing-induced cell death. Technol Cancer Res Treat. 2007;6(2):69–79.
34. Le Pivert PJ, Morrison DR, Haddad RS, Renard M, Aller A, Titus K, Doulat J. Percutaneous tumor ablation: microencapsulated echo-guided interstitial chemotherapy combined with cryosurgery increases necrosis in prostate cancer. Technol Cancer Res Treat. 2009;8(3):207–16.
35. Clarke DM, Baust JM, Van Buskirk RG, Baust JG. Addition of anticancer agents enhances freezing-induced prostate cancer cell death: implications of mitochondrial involvement. Cryobiology. 2004;49(1):45–61.
36. Jorizzo JL, Markowitz O, Lebwohl MG, Bourcier M, Kulp J, Meng TC, Levy S. A randomized, double-blinded, placebo-controlled, multicenter, efficacy and safety study of 3.75% imiquimod cream following cryosurgery for the treatment of actinic keratoses. J Drugs Dermatol. 2010;9(9):110.
37. Quist SR, Gollnick HP. Imiquimod 3.75 % cream (Zyclara) for the treatment of actinic keratoses. Expert Opin Pharmacother. 2011;12(3):451–61.
38. Martin GM, Stockfleth E. Diclofenac sodium 3 % gel for the management of actinic keratosis: 10+ years of cumulative evidence of efficacy and safety. J Drugs Dermatol. 2012;11(5):600–8.
39. Mastrolonardo M. Topical diclofenac 3 % gel plus cryotherapy for treatment of multiple and recurrent actinic keratoses. Clin Exp Dermatol. 2009;34(1): 33–5.
40. Berlin JM, Rigel DS. Diclofenac sodium 3 % gel in the treatment of actinic keratoses postcryosurgery. J Drugs Dermatol. 2008;7(7):669–73.
41. Berman B, Goldenberg G, Hanke W, Tyring SK, Werschler WP, Knudsen KM, Goncalves J, Larsson T, Skov T, Swanson N. Efficacy and safety of ingenol mebutate 0.015 % gel 3 weeks after cryosurgery of actinic keratosis: 11-week results. J Drugs Dermatol. 2014;13(2):154–60.
42. Challacombe JM, Suhrbier A, Parsons PG, Jones B, Hampson P, Kavanagh D, Rainger GE, Morris M, Lord JM, Le TT, Hoang-Le D, Ogbourne SM. Neutrophils are a key component of the anti-tumor efficacy of topical chemotherapy with ingenol-3-angelate. J Immunol. 2006;177(11) :8123–32.
43. Hampson P, Kavanagh D, Smith E, Wang K, Lord JM, Ed Rainger G. The anti-tumor agent, ingenol-3-angelate (PEP005), promotes the recruitment of cytotoxic neutrophils by activation of vascular endothelial cells in a PKC-delta dependent manner. Cancer Immunol Immunother. 2008;57(8):1241–51.
44. Zide MF. Actinic keratosis: from the skin to the lip. J Oral Maxillofac Surg. 2008;66(6):1162–76.
45. Lubritz RR, Smolewski SA. Cryosurgery cure rate of premalignant leukoplakia of the lower lip. J Dermatol Surg Oncol. 1983;9(3):235–7.
46. Shah AY, Doherty SD, Rosen T. Actinic cheilitis: a treatment review. Int J Dermatol. 2010;49(11): 1225–34.
47. Boy SC. Leukoplakia and erythroplakia of the oral mucosa–a brief overview. SADJ. 2012;67(10): 558–60.
48. Messadi DV. Diagnostic aids for detection of oral precancerous conditions. Int J Oral Sci. 2013;5(2):59–65.
49. Mehanna HM, Rattay T, Smith J, McConkey CC. Treatment and follow-up of oral dysplasia – a systematic review and meta-analysis. Head Neck. 2009;31(12):1600–9.
50. Yu CH, Lin HP, Cheng SJ, Sun A, Chen HM. Cryotherapy for oral precancers and cancers. J Formos Med Assoc. 2014;113(5):272–7.
51. Rigel DS, Stein LF. The importance of early diagnosis and treatment of actinic keratosis. J Am Acad Dermatol. 2013;68(1 Suppl 1):S20–7.
52. Criscione VD, Weinstock MA, Naylor MF, Luque C, Eide MJ, Bingham SF, Department of Veteran Affairs Topical Tretinoin Chemoprevention Trial Group. Actinic keratoses: Natural history and risk of malignant transformation in the Veterans Affairs Topical Tretinoin in Chemoprevention Trial. Cancer. 2009; 115(11):2523–30.

53. Zalaudek I, Piana S, Moscarella E, Longo C, Zendri E, Castagnetti F, Pellacani G, Lallas A, Argenziano G. Morphologic grading and treatment of facial actinic keratosis. Clin Dermatol. 2014;32(1):80–7.
54. Gupta AK, Paquet M, Villanueva E, Brintnell W. Interventions for actinic keratoses. Cochrane Database Syst Rev. 2012;(12):CD004415.
55. Spencer J. Understanding actinic keratosis: epidemiology, biology, and management of the disease. J Am Acad Dermatol. 2013;68(1 Suppl 1):S1.

Cryosurgery for Malignant Lesions 17

Paola Pasquali

Contents

P. Pasquali, MD
Department of Dermatology, Pius Hospital de Valls, 43800 Tarragona, Spain
e-mail: pasqualipaola@gmail.com

Key Points

- Skin cancer is rising worldwide. No one single treatment option works for the wide range of NMSC.
- Cryosurgery has cure rates of (97–98 %), making it an excellent alternative for the majority of tumors.
- Its excellent cure rates, convenience, low cost, and good cosmetic results (especially in fair-skinned patients) must be balanced with long healing periods, especially in the legs, and unsatisfactory cosmetic results for darker skin types.

17.1 Introduction

Skin cancer, both melanoma and nonmelanoma skin cancer (NMSC), is rising worldwide [1, 2]. NMSC is increasing 3–8 % each year [3], even though it could be said that there are no reliable figures on NMSC since second tumors of the same histology are not registered and many superficial NMSC are not registered at all (especially when they are not biopsied or diagnosed in private practices). Van der Geer et al. [4] have found that nearly half of the patients with NMSC developed multiple tumors and that NMSC should be regarded as a chronic disease. This scenario raises the need for better prevention

P. Pasquali (ed.), *Cryosurgery: A Practical Manual*,
DOI 10.1007/978-3-662-43939-5_17, © Springer-Verlag Berlin Heidelberg 2015

programs and developing cost-effective strategies to manage this huge health problem.

Another obvious conclusion is that such a burden will require a wide range of therapeutic alternatives that range from skin-sparing options to ample excisions that guarantee deep tumor removal. The more alternatives exist, the better for the patient. In addition, common sense says that the best alternative is the one that cures the patient, has the best cosmetic results, imposes less discomfort, and carries the least economic cost.

Having stated all this, cryosurgery is an excellent therapeutic modality and will keep its standing as an excellent therapeutic modality in the future [5], being the first choice of treatment for numerous cases and an alternative in compassionate treatment. It offers a high cure rate (97–98 %) with good to excellent cosmetic results [6–8].

17.2 Principles of Oncologic Cryosurgery

As for any other treatment option, there are several factors that are of utmost importance when considering cryosurgery for the treatment of a skin malignancy.

17.2.1 Tumor Selection

Proper tumor selection is extremely important. There are aspects of the tumor that one should know before attempting to do cryosurgery.

17.2.1.1 Is It Really a Malignant Tumor Amenable to Treatment with Cryosurgery?

There must be certainty on the tumor's nature before attempting to treat a skin lesion with any kind of therapeutic procedure. This seems obvious, but unfortunately bad decisions are not infrequent and can be very costly to both patient and surgeon. Treating a malignant melanoma with open spray technique thinking that it is a pigmented basal cell carcinoma is a deadly mistake that should not occur. Be sure of the diagnosis.

Dermoscopy and confocal microscopy are essential noninvasive imaging tools that will confirm or refute a clinical suspicion of malignancy. If still in doubt, a biopsy is mandatory.

17.2.1.2 What Type of Tumor Is It?

There are criteria universally accepted as to when not to use cryosurgery. They are also the criteria for Mohs micrographic surgery (MMS):

- Recurrent tumors (although not an absolute contraindication [9])
- For BCC: sclerodermiform tumors, morpheaform (Fig. 17.1a, b), fibrosing, sclerosing
- Infiltrating, perineural, perivascular infiltration
- Metatypical/keratotic
- Ill-defined tumors
- Previously irradiated skin
- High-risk tumors
- Micronodular
- For SCC: Poor or undifferentiated, basosquamous
- In prior radiated skin
- Sarcomatoid

  Some criteria are not absolute:
- Tumors larger than 2 cm: treatment can be done by segmental or fractional cryosurgery (see Chap. 21).
- High-risk areas (Fig. 17.2a, b).
- Hair-bearing areas: This is not an absolute contraindication if there is no cosmetic concern as to leaving an alopecic scar.

This leaves an immense field of action for cryosurgeons. With proper tumor selection and correct technique, results will be oncologically and cosmetically excellent.

17.2.1.3 What Volume Does the Tumor Have?

Previous knowledge of the tumor volume and shape will help make the best therapeutic decision. There are tumors that have a subepithelial component larger than the surface lesion (iceberg phenomenon). It is of utmost importance to have this knowledge before treating the tumor otherwise there will be a risk of leaving residual cancerous cells. Previous HFUS (high-frequency ultrasound) imaging of the tumor will help rule out admixture tumors. Biopsy is not necessarily capable of making such a distinction because it

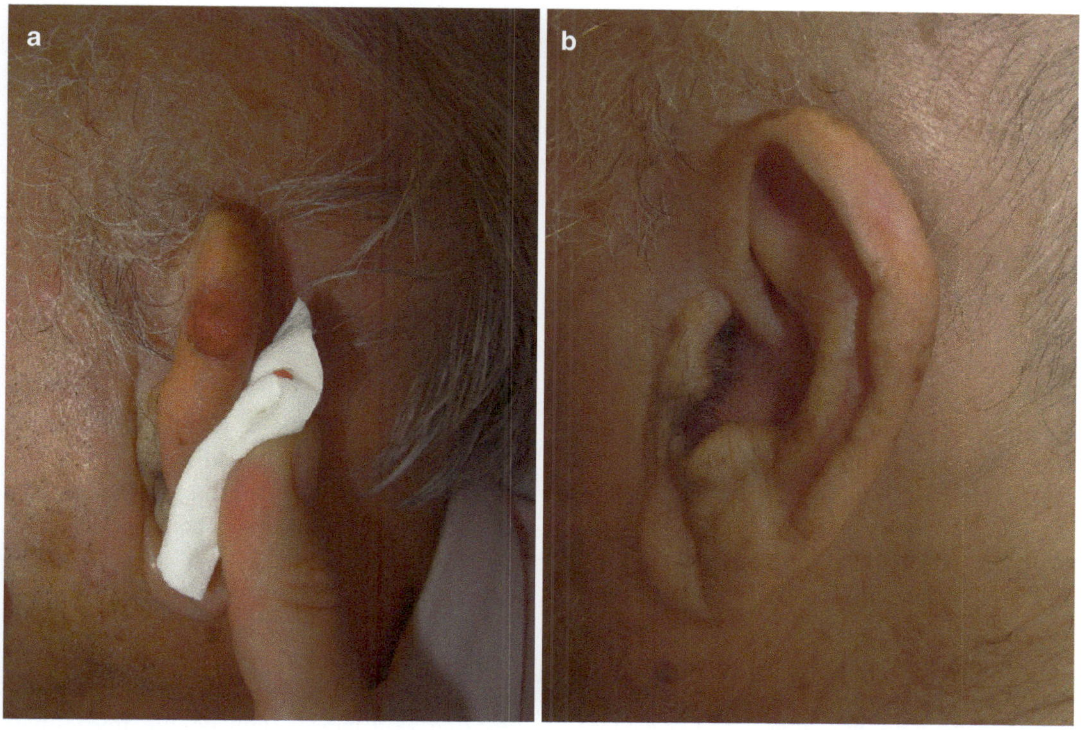

Fig. 17.1 (**a**, **b**) Patient with a morpheaform BCC on the earlobe who did not want surgery. A double freeze-thaw cycle was performed. There has been no recurrence after 3 years

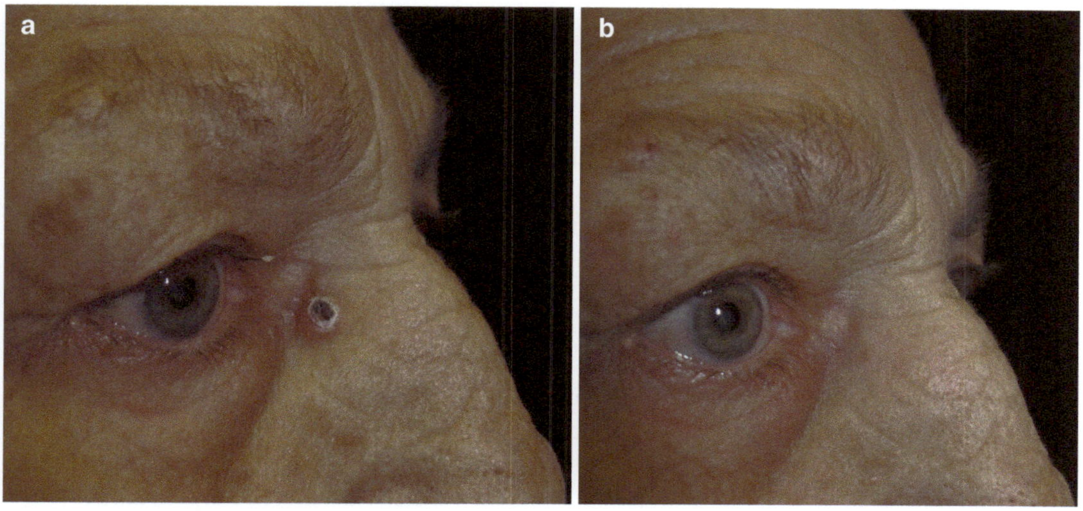

Fig. 17.2 (**a**) Nodular BCC in the medial canthus. The lesion was treated with two freeze-thaw cycles with a 5 mm flat probe. (**b**) One year post treatment

is dependent on the site where the biopsy has been taken. Recognizing an admixture tumor will help choose the proper technique or combination treatment (i.e., a large superficial basal cell carcinoma with a nodular part can be first treated with topical treatment or other tissue-sparing technique and later be treated for the nodular part).

17.2.2 Patient Selection

17.2.2.1 Is the Patient Willing to Be Treated With Cryosurgery?

Patients must understand what the treatment is about. One simple way is by stating that cryosurgery is a fast and low-risk procedure with a long [10] but minimal postoperative care. Patients and/or caretakers need to know in advance and commit themselves to simple instructions of proper wound caring. Time schedule is important: cryosurgery on a low-risk NMSC can be postponed as required. The anatomical area will determine the time of healing: for the same procedure, the face will heal fast and the legs will heal very slowly.

17.2.2.2 Is the Patient's Skin Color Adequate for Treatment?

Cryosurgery can be performed in any type of skin. However, skin cancer treatment can leave hypo- or even achromic scars. Therefore, avoid cryosurgery in darker skin types in visible areas like the face.

17.2.2.3 Does the Patient Have Blood-Borne Infections or Debilitating Conditions? Is the Patient of Advanced Age? Does the Patient Have a Fear of Surgical Procedures?

All of these conditions make patients particularly suitable for skin cancer cryosurgery since it is a low-risk procedure that can be performed even on bedridden or wheelchair-bound patients and in a non invasive manner.

17.2.2.4 Multiple Versus Single Lesions

Multiple-lesion patients will benefit from this procedure because numerous lesions can be treated in one session.

17.2.2.5 Anatomical Area

Some areas heal very nicely: nose, earlobes, and eyelids. Others instead may have unaesthetic scars, for example, the middle of the cheek in a young person. Avoid treating malignancies in the legs because the postoperative healing takes very long and the scar can be cosmetically unacceptable. Use cryosurgery in the lower extremities if patients/caretakers are not concerned about time or cosmesis and other options are not available.

17.2.2.6 Damaged Skin

With healing, the new skin is lighter than the surrounding one. In highly dyschromic skin, the cryosurgical scar will stand out, although with time this improves.

17.2.3 Setting

One of the great advantages of cryosurgery is that it does not require special settings in order to be performed. This is a real advantage when dealing with bedridden or wheelchair-bound patients. No strict asepsis is required.

17.2.4 Anesthesia

Freezing skin cancer with double freeze-thaw cycles requires local anesthesia because freezing will be deeper and last longer. Pain is also related are usually better tolerated than in the nose. For patients allergic to anesthetics, cryosurgery can sometimes be their sole option of curative treatment for a skin malignancy. Some patients tolerate the procedure without any local anesthesia.

17.3 Cryosurgical Techniques

17.3.1 One Versus Two Freeze-Thaw Cycles

In skin cancer amenable to cryosurgery, there are some concepts that must be kept in mind.

Cancerous cells are destroyed at approximately −50 °C. The temperature at the center of the iceball will surely attain values below −50°C which will cause tumor necrosis. The problem might arise if the freezing front is not allowed to extend so that the appropriate margin also achieves this freezing temperature. For most BCC/SCC, a 4–5 mm margin is mandatory.

Recurrences or incomplete treatment are those that leave viable malignant cells behind, and this happens at the periphery, where temperature has not achieved the required −50 °C. Therefore, measure the temperature at the periphery of the tumor and not in the center (see Fig. 13.6). The temperature at the periphery will be the same in depth due to the isotherm within this hemispherical ice ball. The lateral ice spread is approximately equal to the depth of freeze [11]. In a study done by our group, we showed that the mean depth of BCC was 1.73 mm by histology and 2.03 by HFUS (high-frequency ultrasound) and the length was 5.39 mm (histology) and 7.59 mm by HFUS [12]. For example, if one treats a BCC of 6 mm with cryosurgery, freezing 4 mm of margin the ice ball will extend 4 mm in depth. This means that one is freezing a safety margin also in depth. This is true as long as (a) the lateral spreading is from the ice ball (from central freezing) and not an artifact of spiral or paintbrushing on the surface and (b) the −50 °C (killing temperature for cancer cells) is measured at the surface of the lateral spread and not in the center of the lesion.

For small clinical/dermoscopy, superficial BCC in the truncal area can be safely treated with one freeze-thaw cycle [13]. For the rest, BCC should be treated with double freeze-thaw cycles. Histologic cure has been reported for lesions treated with cryosurgery [14].

17.3.2 Technique

Close or probe is the first choice when treating skin cancer. It provides fast freezing that reaches deep into the tissue. Choose a probe that best fits the size of the tumor; when not possible, choose a probe slightly smaller rather than a larger one. This will allow visualization of the lateral extension of the ice ball and avoids overtreating.

Probes need to be placed over surfaces as flat as possible. Irregular surfaces will have "air pockets" separating the tumor from the probe (interphase) that act as insulators. In addition, irregular tumor surfaces many times are caused by excess keratin (mostly seen in squamous cell carcinomas) which is a very bad conductant. Therefore, when probes are to be used, they will require a flat surface to which they can be applied. Finally, some tumors are in areas not easily accessible and a probe cannot be applied to the surface.

As far as the tumor surface is concerned, superficial BCC and some small nodular BCC usually do not pose a problem. For larger lesions, the surface should be flattened down by curettage or simply choose spraying or cryochambers. If curettage has been performed, make sure to leave a blood-free surface before freezing (blood can raise the local temperature) either by using hemostatic solutions or by electrocoagulation (Fig. 17.3a–e). Curetting the tumor down thoroughly and then applying one freeze-thaw cycle has been proposed with excellent results [15]. Remember that if probes have been used on a curette area, it will need to be sterilized (before and after the procedure).

After completing a freeze-thaw cycle, probes occasionally get stuck to the surface even if Teflon covered. Do not attempt a forceful detachment because tissue will tear apart. Just allow thawing and gently detach.

When treating tumors on nasal ala, earlobes, or lips, use your finger beneath the tumor to give further support to the probe and to allow you to feel the advance of the freezing front (Fig. 17.4). Once you feel a cold sensation on your fingertip, stop freezing. In earlobes, it is also possible to see the ice "tattoo" (Fig. 17.5).

After completion of the procedure and before covering the lesion, make sure that there has been total thawing and no bleeding is present. With thawing, there is an immediate vasodilation, and covering the lesion without having made sure that there is no bleeding can result in the patient rushing back in later for a wound dressing change.

If the lesion has been curetted, remind the patient that the bullae can have a bloody content.

Open or spray technique is a good option for large tumors for which correct size probes are not available (Fig. 17.6a–c) and for irregular surface tumors for which no curettage is possible or desired. For very large lesions (superficial BCC), it is best to treat by segments (Chap. 21) to avoid a greater depth destruction. For superficial BCC

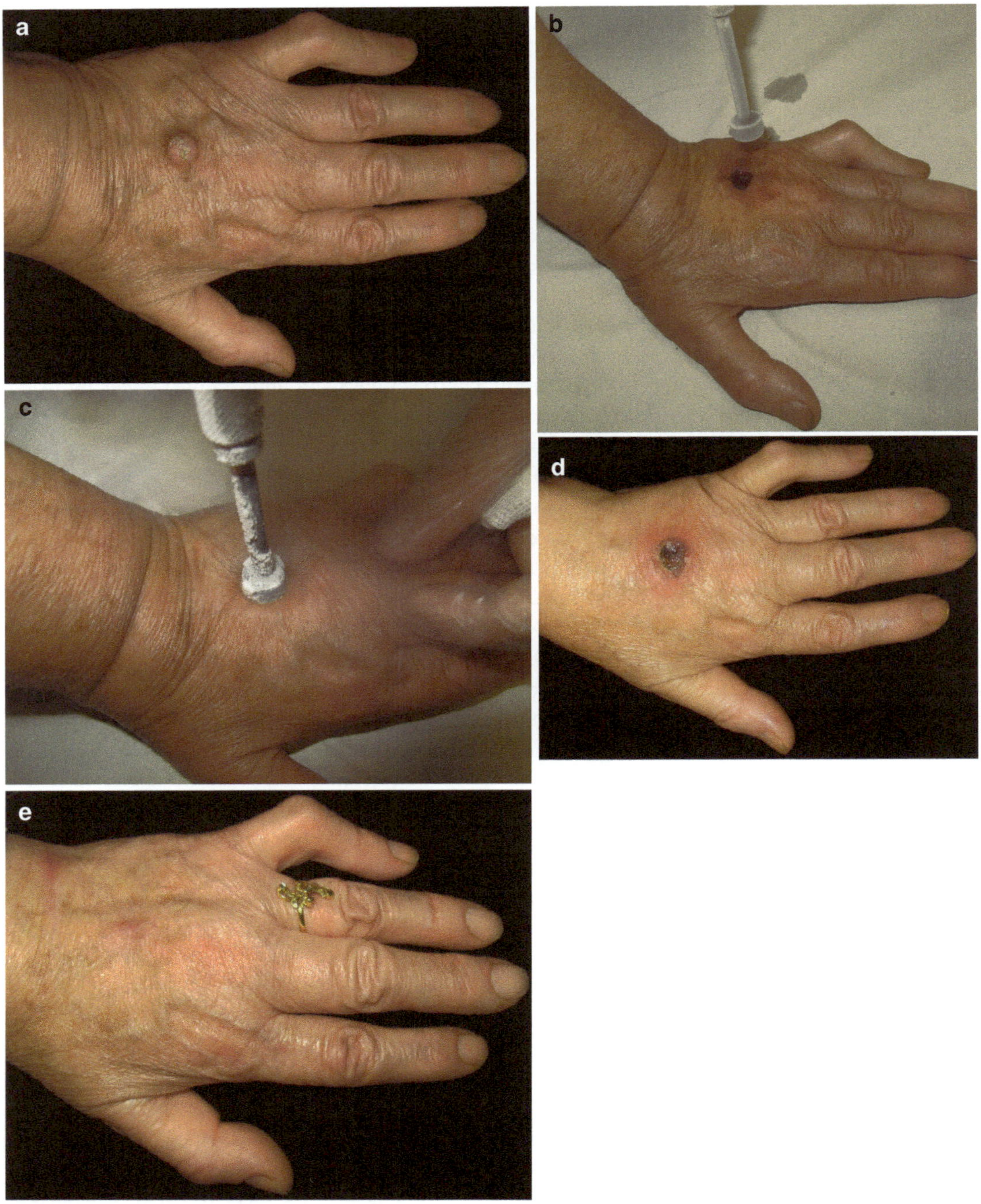

Fig. 17.3 (**a**) Keratoacanthoma of the dorsum of the left hand. After local anesthesia, spray freezing to the surface of the skin, and shaving. Hemostatic solution was applied. (**b**) A double freeze-thaw cycle with flat 1 cm probe (**c**) applied with some pressure until the probe felt fixed to the skin. (**d**) One month after treatment; (**e**) 2 months later

in the truncal area, one freeze-thaw cycle can be sufficient as long as there is certainty that the entire lesion is superficial. Caution should be taken with clinically superficial tumors that in reality are admixture tumors (approximately 30 %) and are the cause of incorrect treatment or technique selection (see Chap. 13 on BCC and high-frequency ultrasound).

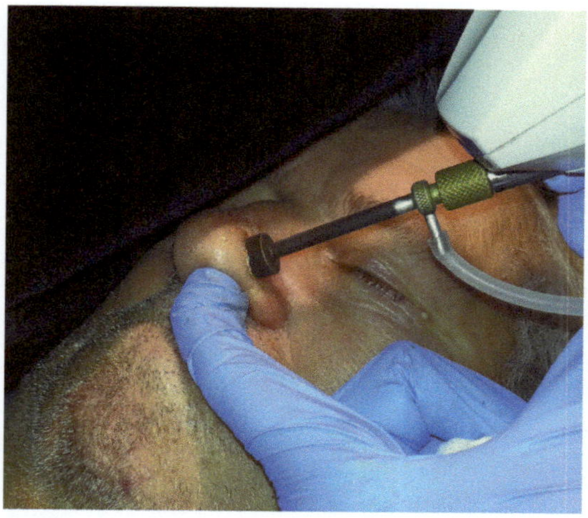

Fig. 17.4 Close (probe) cryosurgery on a nasal ala. Freezing front is palpated at the tip with the left index finger located inside the nostril

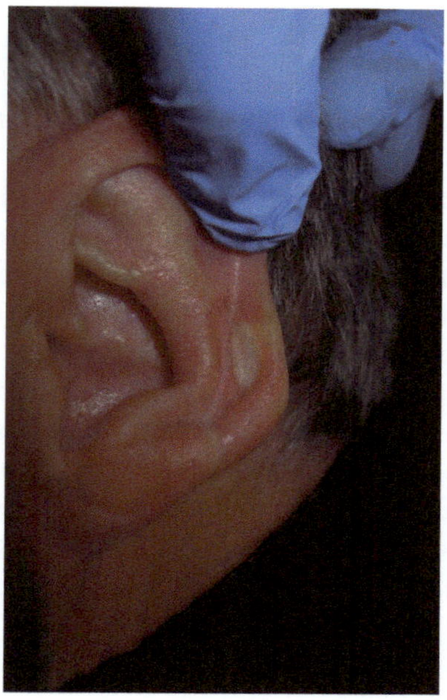

Fig. 17.5 Ice ball tattoo

If the tumor has been curetted down, special care should be taken not to insufflate gas into the skin. To avoid this, one can restrain the LN with a firmly placed cone.

Semi-closed or cryochambers are an excellent option in skin cancer treatment as long as one has the proper-sized chamber so that the whole lesion can be included. It generates a potent and fast freezing. The chamber has to be firmly placed so that it stays stuck during the freezing procedure.

17.3.2.1 Combining Techniques

Large NMSC can be very vascularized, and tumor debulking is avoided for fear of bleeding. One option is to combine cryosurgical treatment modalities: first spray the bulky lesion at the center, allowing the freezing front to advance just to the base of the lesion. At this point, shaving can be performed and the probe can be applied at the base to continue freezing until the desired margin is obtained. Once the freeze-thaw sessions are completed, make sure to do a proper hemostasis.

This combined technique works very well with keratoacanthomas (Figs. 17.7a–c and 17.8).

Table 17.1 shows a summary of the recommendations by type of tumor [16] and patient.

17.4 Combination Treatment for Skin Cancer

Combination treatment in the management of premalignant and NMSC is becoming more frequent. Curiously, very few have pinpointed the concept of neoadjuvant therapy for NMSC [17, 18], although some of these combinations are working as such [19].

NMSC neoadjuvant therapy aims to reduce the size of a large tumor before using a more radical treatment. The result is a smaller tumor that is easier to treat and that will leave a better cosmetic result. These therapies act not only on the tumor but also on the surrounding skin. Although this therapy has been mostly applied on giant inoperable tumors, the concept works also for large superficial BCC, Bowen, or even nodular BCC. The best example of neoadjuvancy is immunocryosurgery [20–22] (see Chap. 20).

Combination treatments, on the other hand, are ideal for those admixture tumors whose deeper parts are not eliminated by superficial therapies like PDT or topical imiquimod.

Several combination treatments are possible. In some, the combination of superficial therapies for the large and shallow components of the tumor and posterior removal of the residual

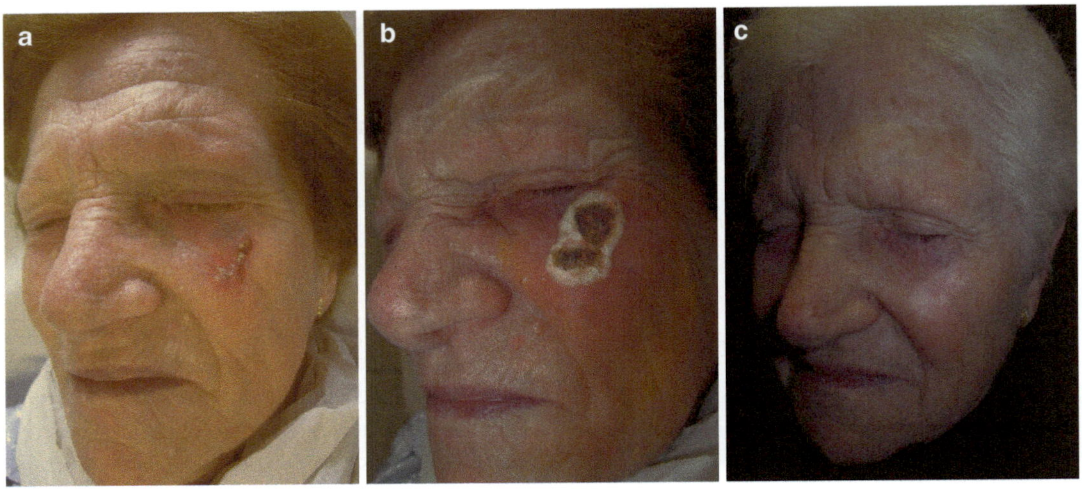

Fig. 17.6 (**a**) Large admixture BCC (superficial and nodular) in the left cheek. (**b**) Two double freeze-thaw cycles with open (spray) technique; (**c**) almost 3 years post cryosurgery

nodular parts by cryosurgery or surgery will result in oncologic cures with excellent cosmetic results. Also reported is a combination with Mohs surgery [23].

17.4.1 Segmental vs Fractional Cryosurgery

Segmental cryosurgery consists of treating a large tumor in multiple overlapping applications. This technique avoids excessive deep destruction (see Chap. 21)

Fractional cryosurgery consists of treating a tumor in the center, letting it heal, and then in the next session treating a smaller tumor. It is a technique designed for large tumoral masses but it can work as well in cases of intermediate-size tumors in difficult to treat areas (Fig. 17.9a, b).

17.5 Other Tumors

17.5.1 Lentigo Maligna

Cryosurgery in lentigo maligna has been proposed and used for several decades [24–28]. Melanocytes are very sensitive to cold; therefore, with the proper technique, results are very good. A double freeze with a wide margin (at least 5 mm) should be done.

It has usually been reserved for elderly people with large lesions where surgery is either disfiguring or not possible because of underlying medical conditions. Nowadays, response of therapy can be monitored using confocal microscopy [29].

Immunocryosurgery has also been proposed as a treatment alternative for lentigo maligna and also for BCC. [30, 31]. It consists of using imiquimod for two weeks, followed by two superficial freeze-thaw cycles, and then 3 more weeks of imiquimod (Figs. 17.10a, b and 17.11a–c) (see Chap. 20).

17.5.2 Kaposi Sarcoma

Cryosurgery has been proposed as treatment option for Kaposi sarcoma [32, 33]. Vascular lesions tend to be very responsive to sub-zero temperature treatments. Cryosurgery should be reserved for those lesions in visible areas that cause psychological discomfort to the patient and that have not responded to retroviral medication.

The treatment is the same as in hemangiomas: precooled probe, applied with pressure, and one freeze-thaw cycle. Take the precaution to

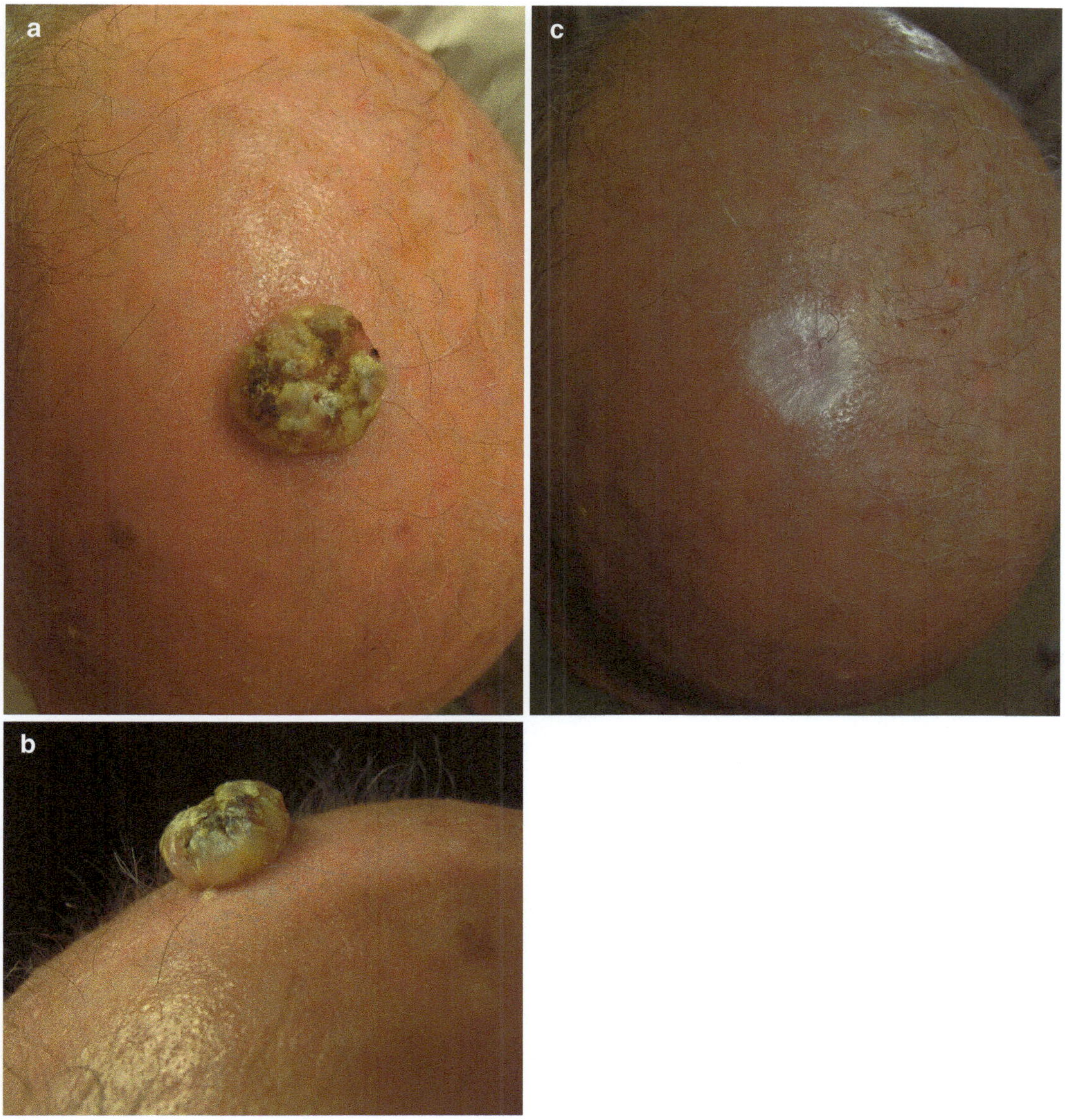

Fig. 17.7 (**a**, **b**) Large keratoacanthoma on the head; one open cycle (spray) from the top just to the skin surface, shaving, hemostasis, and two double freeze-thaw cycles with a 15 mm flat probe. (**c**) One year post cryosurgery

cover the probe with a rubber finger or an ultrasound transducer cover. It does not require local anesthesia.

17.5.3 Squamous Cell Carcinomas and Aggressive Behavior Post Cryosurgery

It has been observed that certain squamous cell carcinomas do not respond adequately to cryosurgery. This fact has been observed as well in certain squamous cell carcinomas treated with PDT [34]. In the case of cryosurgical treatment, this subgroup of tumor has an initial reduction, and a few weeks after treatment they show a very aggressive growth. They become histologically more aggressive. Gonzalez and Juarranz have found that genomic imbalances seem to be involved in the development of resistance to PDT of squamous cell carcinomas. Studies to confirm the same observation on cryosurgery will be required.

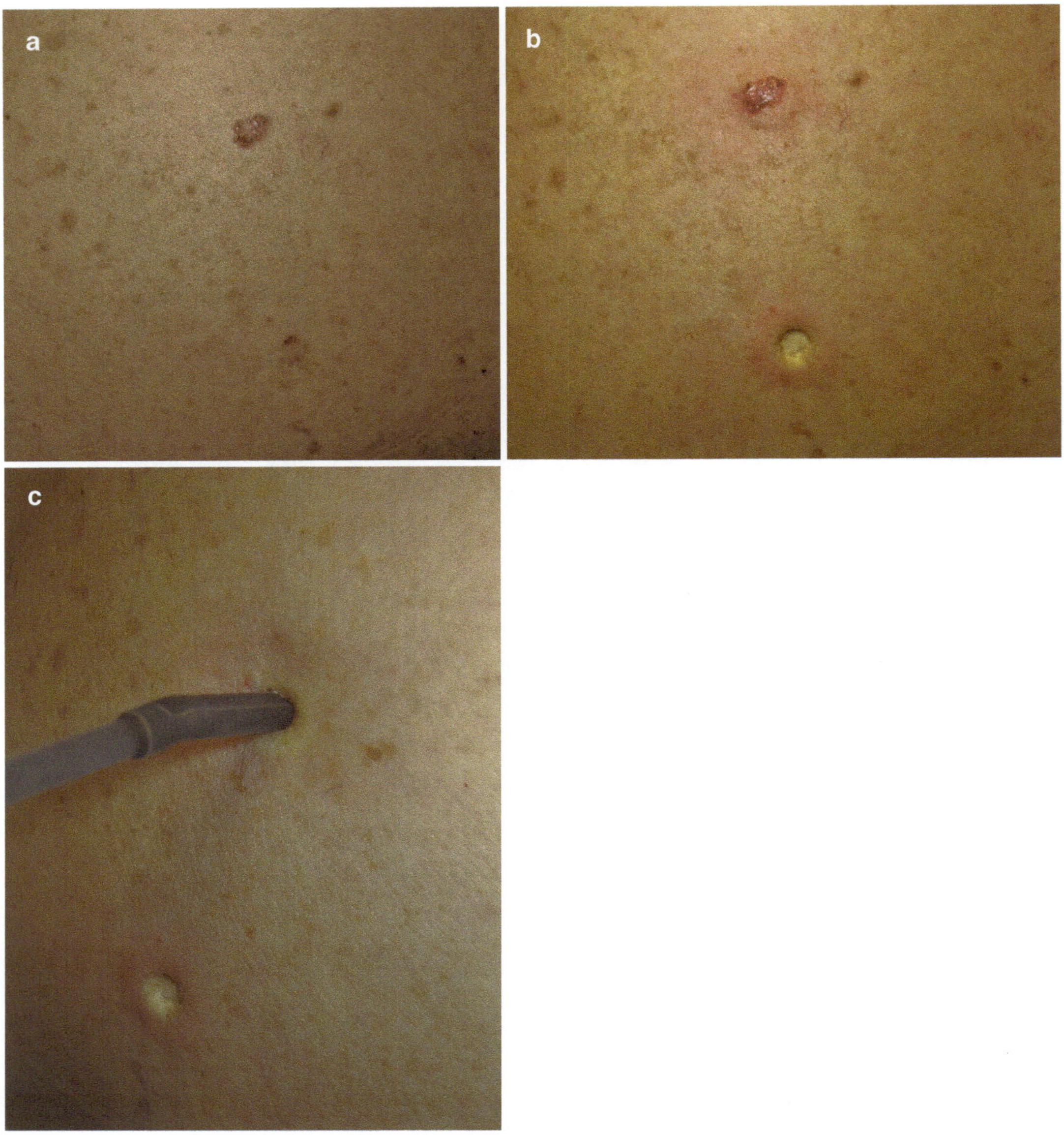

Fig. 17.8 (**a**) Multiple BCC patient. Lesions were measured with HFUS to determine depth. Both were under 1 mm in depth; (**b**) one freeze-thaw cycle on each lesion (**c**) using a "hemorrhoid" probe

Table 17.1 Summary of technique recommendations by type of tumor and patient

Type of tumors
Well-defined superficial or nodular BCC
Well-defined SCC (well-differentiated SCC, small moderately differentiated)
Ideally less than 5 mm in depth
Keratoacanthomas
Lentigo maligna
Kaposi sarcoma
Type of patients
White skin (type I–III)
Multiple BCC patients (Fig. 17.8a–c)
Tumors over bone or cartilage
Especially recommended in elderly patients

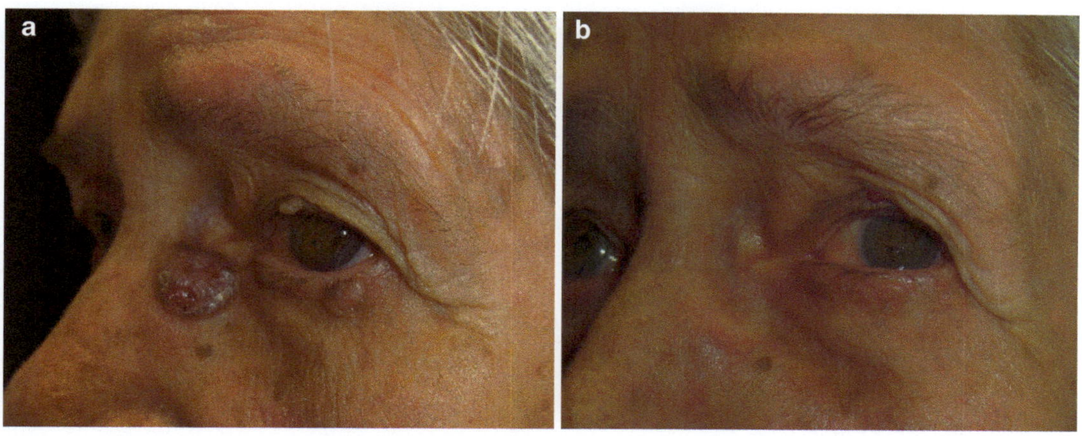

Fig. 17.9 (**a**) Large BCC in the medial canthus. A fractional cryosurgery was performed, freezing the middle of the tumor in one session with a flat 5 mm probe with a double freeze-thaw cycle. One month later, a second freeze-thaw cycle with a 5 mm flat probe was performed. (**b**) One and a half year control

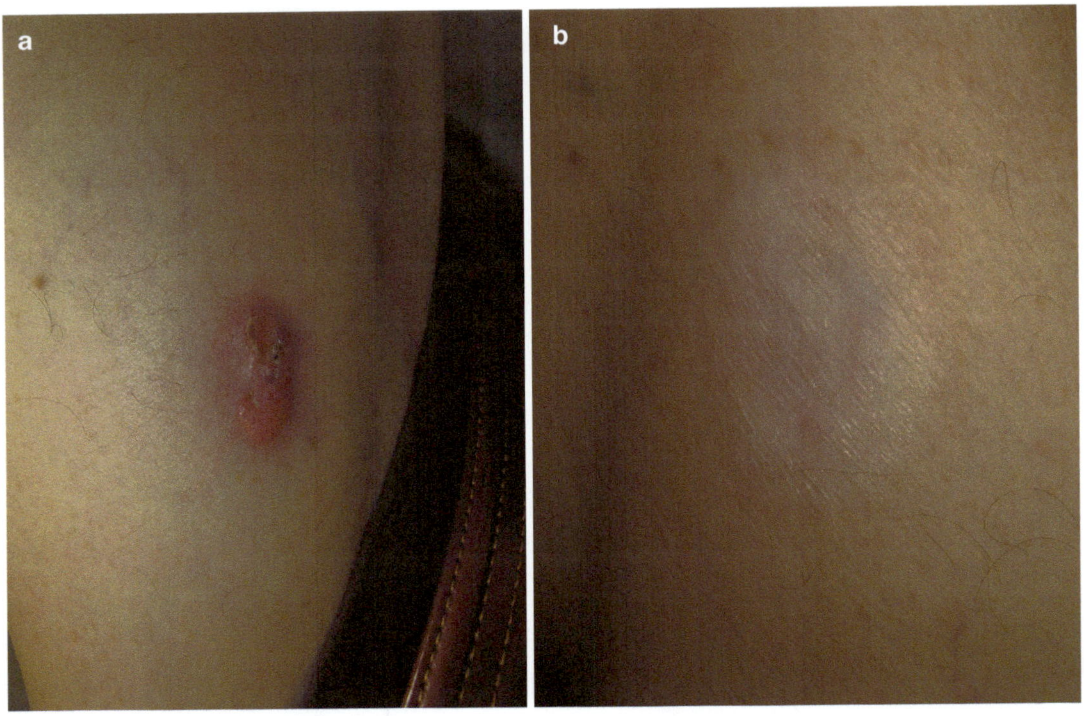

Fig. 17.10 (**a**) A large morpheaform BCC of the thigh treated with Gaitanis and Bassukas's immunocryosurgery protocol. (**b**) Two year control

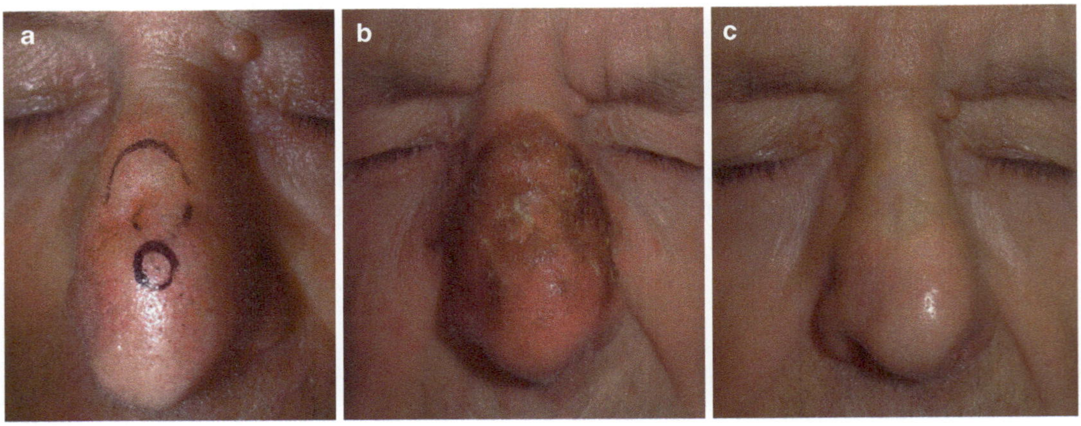

Fig. 17.11 (**a**) Large morpheaform BCC on the dorsum of the nose treated with Gaitanis and Bassukas's immunocryosurgery protocol. (**b**) The day of the cryosurgery session. (**c**) One year control

17.6 Postoperative Care

For details on postoperative care, please see Chap. 22.

Essential Tidbits

- Make sure to know the volume of tumor before treating. This knowledge will allow you to choose the best technique.
- Spraying technique is best for large lesions (superficial BCC, Bowen); probe technique is best for flattened surfaces.
- Previous curettage of a bulky/keratotic lesion improves probe attachment to skin surface.
- Always biopsy before treating if the nature of the lesion is not clear.
- One freeze-thaw cycle is sufficient in small superficial lesions. For the remainder, always use double freeze-thaw cycle.

Conclusions

Cryosurgery is an excellent therapeutic option for most NMSC. Patient, tumor, and technique selection are the key to a successful procedure. This is only possible if one has at hand all possible information on the tumor nature (histologic subtype, volume, depth and length, history of previous interventions) as well as a detailed patient clinical record that includes underlying medical conditions and disposition for treatment. Ideally, all lesions need to be photographed before and after, evaluated with a dermoscope, a HFUS, and confocal microscope/biopsy. As a safe rule, patients with NMSC will benefit from a bi annual check up during the first year of diagnosis and later annually since up to 46% of them may develop second tumors [4].

Glossary

HFUS High-Frequency Ultrasound
NMSC Nonmelanoma Skin Cancer
MMS Mohs Micrographic Surgery

References

1. Etzkorn JR, Parikh RP, Marzban SS, Law K, Davis AH, Rawal B, Schell MJ, Sondak VK, Messina JL, Rendina LE, Zager JS, Lien MH. Identifying risk factors using a skin cancer screening program. Cancer Control. 2013;20(4):248–54.
2. Gordon R. Skin cancer: an overview of epidemiology and risk factors. Semin Oncol Nurs. 2013;29(3):160–9.
3. Skelton LA. The effective treatment of basal cell carcinoma. Br J Nurs. 2009;18(6):346, 348–50.
4. Van der Geer S, Siemerink M, Reijers HA, Verhaegh ME, Ostertag JU, Neumann HA, Krekels GA. The incidence of skin cancer in dermatology. Clin Exp Dermatol. 2013;38(7):724–9.
5. Kokoszka A, Scheinfeld N. Evidence-based review of the use of cryosurgery in treatment of basal cell carcinoma. Dermatol Surg. 2003;29(6):566–71.
6. Kuflik EG. Cryosurgery for skin cancer: 30-year experience and cure rates. Dermatol Surg. 2004;30(2 Pt 2):297–300.
7. Zacarian SA. Cryosurgery of cutaneous carcinomas. An 18-year study of 3,022 patients with 4,228 carcinomas. J Am Acad Dermatol. 1983;9(6):947–56.
8. Graham G, Clark L. Statistical analysis in cryosurgery of skin cancer. In: Breitbart EW, Dachow-Siwiec E, editors. Clinics in dermatology: advances in cryosurgery, vol. 8. New York: Elsevier; 1990. p. 101–7.
9. Kuflik EG, Gage AA. Recurrent basal cell carcinoma treated with cryosurgery. J Am Acad Dermatol. 1997;37(1):82–4.
10. Kuijpers DI, Thissen MR, Berretty PJ, Ideler FH, Nelemans PJ, Neumann MH. Surgical excision versus curettage plus cryosurgery in the treatment of basal cell carcinoma. Dermatol Surg. 2007;33(5):579–87.
11. Jackson A, Colver G, Dawber R. Cutaneous cryosurgery. Principles and clinical practice. 3rd ed. London: Taylor & Francis; 2006.
12. Pasquali P, Camacho E, Fortuño-Mar A. Use of 22 MHz high-frequency ultrasound in the management of skin cancer. In: Baldi A, Pasquali P, Spugnini EP, editors. Skin cancer a practical approach. New York: Humana Press/Springer; 2014. p. 245–56.
13. Mallon E, Dawber R. Cryosurgery in the treatment of basal cell carcinoma. Assessment of one and two freeze-thaw cycle schedules. Dermatol Surg. 1996;22(10):854–8.
14. Giuffrida TJ, Jimenez G, Nouri K. Histologic cure of basal cell carcinoma treated with cryosurgery. J Am Acad Dermatol. 2003;49(3):483–6.
15. Peikert JM. Prospective trial of curettage and cryosurgery in the management of non-facial, superficial, and minimally invasive basal and squamous cell carcinoma. Int J Dermatol. 2011;50(9):1135–8.
16. Graham GF. Cryosurgery in the management of cutaneous malignancies. Clin Dermatol. 2001;19(3):321–7.
17. Wollina U. Update of cetuximab for non-melanoma skin cancer. Expert Opin Biol Ther. 2014;14(2):271–6.

18. Lippman SM, Shimm DS, Meyskens Jr FL. Nonsurgical treatments for skin cancer: retinoids and alpha-interferon. J Dermatol Surg Oncol. 1988;14(8):862–9.
19. Sanmartín V, Aguayo R, Baradad M, Casanova JM. [Oral acitretin and topical imiquimod as neoadjuvant treatment for giant basal cell carcinoma]. Actas Dermosifiliogr. 2012;103(2):149–52. [Article in Spanish].
20. Redondo P, del Olmo J, López-Diaz de Cerio A, Inoges S, Marquina M, Melero I, Bendandi M. Imiquimod enhances the systemic immunity attained by local cryosurgery destruction of melanoma lesions. J Invest Dermatol. 2007;127(7):1673–80.
21. Gaitanis G, Alexopoulos EC, Bassukas ID. Cryosurgery is more effective in the treatment of primary, non-superficial basal cell carcinomas when applied during and not prior to a five week imiquimod course: a randomized, prospective, open-label study. Eur J Dermatol. 2011;21(6):952–8.
22. Moutran R, Maatouk I, Stephan F, Tomb R. Treatment of nodular basal cell carcinoma with cryotherapy and reduced protocol of imiquimod. Cutis. 2012;90(5):256–7.
23. Ruiz Santiago H, Morales-Burgos A. Cryosurgery as adjuvant to Mohs micrographic surgery in the management of subungual squamous cell carcinoma. Dermatol Surg. 2011;37(2):256–8.
24. Graham GF, Stewart R. Cryosurgery for unusual cutaneous neoplasms. J Dermatol Surg Oncol. 1977;3(4):437–42.
25. Dawber RP, Wilkinson JD. Melanotic freckle of Hutchinson: treatment of macular and nodular phases with cryotherapy. Br J Dermatol. 1979;101(1):47–9.
26. Kuflik EG. Cryosurgery for lentigo maligna: a report of four cases. J Dermatol Surg Oncol. 1980;6(6):432–5.
27. McLeod M, Choudhary S, Giannakakis G, Nouri K. Surgical treatments for lentigo maligna: a review. Dermatol Surg. 2011;37(9):1210–28.
28. de Moraes AM, Pavarin LB, Herreros F, de Aguiar Michelman F, Velho PE, de Souza EM. Cryosurgical treatment of lentigo maligna. J Dtsch Dermatol Ges. 2007;5(6):477–80. [Article in English, German].
29. Nadiminti H, Scope A, Marghoob AA, Busam K, Nehal KS. Use of reflectance confocal microscopy to monitor response of lentigo maligna to nonsurgical treatment. Dermatol Surg. 2010;36(2):177–84.
30. Bassukas ID, Gamvroulia C, Zioga A, Nomikos K, Fotika C. Cryosurgery during topical imiquimod: a successful combination modality for lentigo maligna. Int J Dermatol. 2008;47(5):519–21.
31. Messeguer F, Serra-Guillen C, Echeverria B, Requena C, Sanmartin O, Llombart B, Guillen C, Nagore E. A pilot study of clinical efficacy of imiquimod and cryotherapy for the treatment of basal cell carcinoma with incomplete response to imiquimod. J Eur Acad Dermatol Venereol. 2012;26(7):879–81.
32. Tappero JW, Berger TG, Kaplan LD, Volberding PA, Kahn JO. Cryotherapy for cutaneous Kaposi's sarcoma (KS) associated with acquired immune deficiency syndrome (AIDS): a phase II trial. J Acquir Immune Defic Syndr. 1991;4(9):839–46.
33. Kutlubay Z, Küçüktaş M, Yardımcı G, Engin B, Serdaroğlu S. Evaluation of effectiveness of cryotherapy on the treatment of cutaneous Kaposi's sarcoma. Dermatol Surg. 2013;39(10):1502–6.
34. Milla LN, Cogno IS, Rodríguez ME, Sanz-Rodríguez F, Zamarrón A, Gilaberte Y, Carrasco E, Rivarola VA, Juarranz A. Isolation and characterization of squamous carcinoma cells resistant to photodynamic therapy. J Cell Biochem. 2011;112(9):2266–78.

Cryosurgery for Nonmelanoma Skin Carcinomas on the Nose and External Ears

18

Peter Nordin

Contents

P. Nordin, MD
Läkarhuset Hospital, Dermatology Clinic,
S. Vägen 27, Gothenburg 411 35, Sweden
e-mail: peter.nordin2@tele2.se

Key Points

- Nose and ears are areas that can be safely treated with a combination of curettage-cryosurgery.
- It is a tissue-sparing technique that gives optimal oncological and cosmetic result.
- It can be used in most NMSCs of nose and external ear, excluding morpheiform and recurrent BCC.

18.1 Introduction

The nose and external ears are areas where skin cancer often recurs and are areas of obvious functional and cosmetic importance [1, 2]. This highlights the importance of choosing an effective therapy without sacrificing redundant tissue and creating unnecessary deformity. A minimal nonmelanoma skin cancer (NMSC) on the nose or external ear is usually easily treated by any of the standard methods [3–6]. However, in somewhat larger tumors the removal and reconstruction with preserved cosmesis and good healing rates are more laborious. Surgical excisions of such tumors, especially on the ears, tend to be deforming, and the rates of recurrence and morbidity are greater than with skin cancer in general [7, 8]. When available, Mohs micrographic surgery (MMS) is often the preferred treatment and provides the highest cure rates [2, 5, 8–11]. An alternative treatment could, at least in some selected

P. Pasquali (ed.), *Cryosurgery: A Practical Manual*,
DOI 10.1007/978-3-662-43939-5_18, © Springer-Verlag Berlin Heidelberg 2015

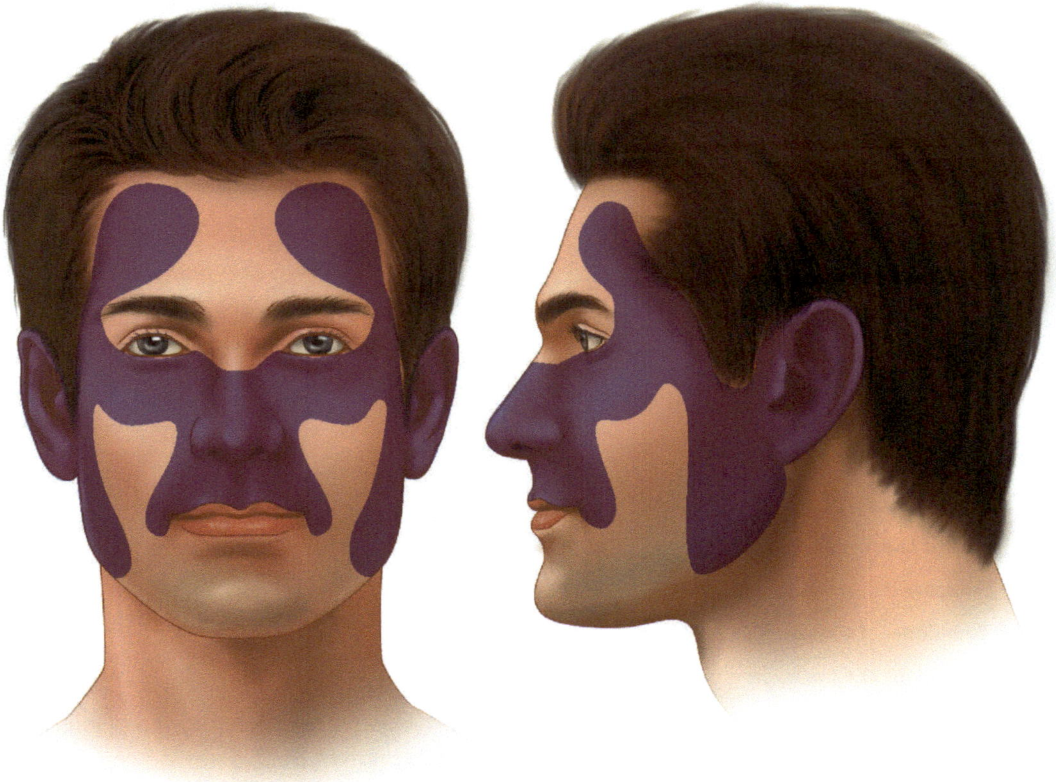

Fig. 18.1 The so-called H-zone of the face is a high-risk area in which the risk for tumor recurrence is about double compared to other regions, irrespective of therapy. The malignancy may grow with silent outgrowths in the dermis, along the perichondrium, the periosteum, and the nerve sheaths

malignancies, be cryosurgery. The NMSCs treated by cryosurgery are by far most often basal cell carcinomas (BCCs), as well as some well-differentiated squamous cell carcinomas (SCCs) and SCCs in situ.

By definition here, the nose also includes its immediate surrounding skin, and the external ear is the pinna, the meatus of the auditory canal, and the immediate periauricular skin, but not the auditory canal.

BCC is the most common cancer in humans. Two-thirds of these tumors occur on the head and neck, and 20–30 % are localized to the nose but only about 3 % to the external ear. SCC is less common [12, 13].

Merely the great number of malignancies on the nose is a therapeutic problem. In addition the nose and ear are located in a high-risk area for tumor recurrence, irrespective of treatment modality, the so-called H-zone (Fig. 18.1). Here the risk of recurrence is about double compared to other regions. An explanation is that many of these cancers, instead of growing exophytically, infiltrate different tissue planes such as the dermis, perichondrium, periosteum, and nerve sheaths and tend to have poorly defined clinical margins, and this is especially true for tumors in the inner canthi, nasolabial furrow, and periauricular area [14–16].

18.2 Patient and Tumor Selection

Before treatment of a malignant tumor, a primary decision must be made concerning the aim of the therapy, namely, cure or palliation. The second decision will be which type of treatment will be the most appropriate in this particular patient. The age and state of health of the patient are important. The histopathological type of tumor, the size of the lesion, and its location are other factors of importance in the choice of therapy.

It is always important to choose the most convenient and safe treatment. Cryosurgery is only one of different therapeutic possibilities.

18.3 Equipment

Liquid nitrogen is the only effective cryogen in the cryosurgical treatment of malignant tumors [17]. In routine clinical practice, liquid nitrogen spray equipment has become the most frequently used device. The most popular units are small handheld, metal or plastic vacuum flasks with four spray tips, with diameters ranging from 0.375 to 1 mm (labeled A, B, C, and D). The author always uses a handheld Cry-Ac (Brymill Corp., New York, USA) with nozzle B.

Additional equipment used in cryosurgery includes cryoprobes, spray-limiting cones of various sizes, protective items, temperature-monitoring devices (not used by the author), stopwatches, ring curettes of different sizes, scissors, punch, scalpel or razor blade, electrosurgical unit, local anesthetic, and hemostatic agents (50 % iron chloride solution) [18]. The equipment used by the author is seen in Fig. 18.2.

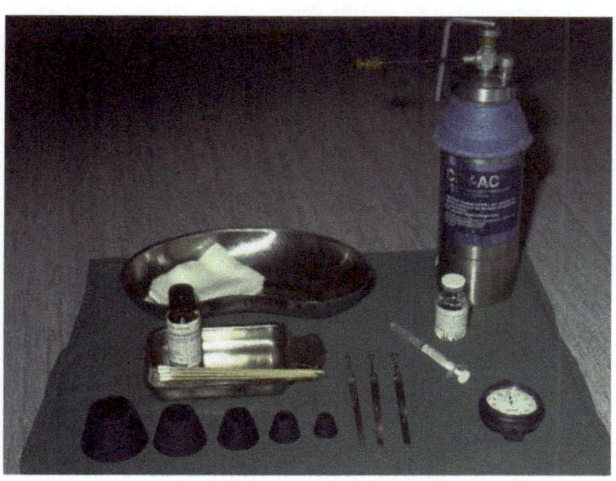

Fig. 18.2 The equipment used in the treatment by curettage-cryosurgery

18.4 Techniques of Cryosurgery

The aim when treating a malignant tumor must be that the first treatment should be the final one. In the treatment with cryosurgery, the tumor has to be frozen sufficiently so that no malignant cells persist.

During the first decades of modern cryosurgery (1960–1970), the goal was a tissue temperature of −20 to −25 °C at the base of the tumor. However, during recent decades, there has been a trend toward a more aggressive treatment with lower temperatures in the range between −40 and −60 °C and a greater use of debulking techniques [19–22]. The freezing time depends on the technique used. With a spray freezing intermittently, about 60 s is needed; with the spot freeze method, about 30 s is needed; and after a thorough curettage, an even shorter freeze time will be adequate for a 1 cm lesion [5, 21–26]. For a larger tumor, the freeze time will increase. In a malignancy larger than 2 cm, the freezing may be divided and applied in sections of the tumor [27]. A double, sometimes even a triple, freeze-thaw cycle should always be performed. This is especially true for tumors in high-risk areas such as the nose and ears.

To register the exact temperature (−50 to −60 °C), some cryosurgeons employ thermocouples at the base of the tumor. Temperature measuring is especially useful for deeper tumors and those in critical locations [28].

Many cryosurgeons do not measure the temperature because an interrelationship exists between the freeze time, the lateral spread of freeze, and tissue temperature, and the adequacy of treatment is based on these [5]. The author uses a special cryosurgery chart with registration of total freeze time, lateral spread of freeze (should be ≥ 5 mm), halo thaw time (should be ≥ 60 s), and total thaw time [21].

Protection in the freezing of tumors close to the external ear canal and the nostrils is needed, and soft cotton is appropriate.

18.5 Indications of Cryosurgery

In general, depending on the cryosurgical technique used, most BCCs – except the morphoeiform types and the recurrent BCCs with

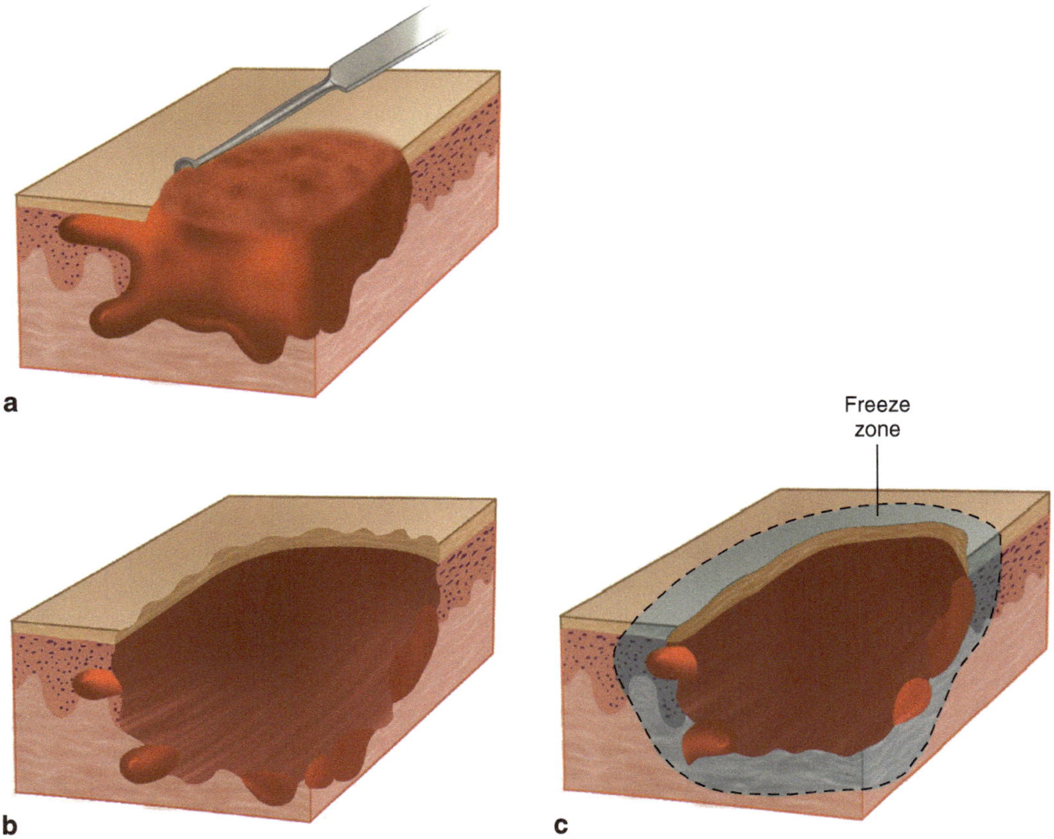

Fig. 18.3 A general outline of curettage-cryosurgery of a nonmelanoma skin cancer. (a) Curettage. (b) After a thorough curettage, there are still tumor extensions left behind not reached by the curettes. (c) Freezing with liquid nitrogen with a lateral spread of freeze of ≥5 mm in a double freeze-thaw cycle will erase any remaining tumor offshoots

secondary sclerosis – are effectively treated by cryosurgery [21–26]. Many SCCs – especially well-differentiated SCCs arising in actinic keratosis and SCCs in situ – are also well suited for cryosurgical treatment [28, 29]. Those tumors overlying cartilage on the nose and ears are often most suitable for cryosurgery, even if they are located in high-risk areas. Cartilage and bone are resistant to freezing injury, and the architecture of the organ is preserved [30, 31].

Unfortunately, the tumors in these areas are often clinically ill defined and thus unsuitable to be treated by cryosurgery alone [29]. However, provided most of the tumor could be removed by curettage and the limits demarcated by a "heavy-handed curettage" [32], cryosurgery would be a suitable therapy, even if any tumor extensions were left behind [20–22]. These remaining outgrowths will then be erased by the freezing with liquid nitrogen in a double freeze-thaw cycle without destroying the stromal framework (Fig. 18.3a–c). A great advantage of cryosurgery on the nose and ears is that stromal tissues such as the cartilage and bone are less cold sensitive than cellular elements [30, 31]. In the healing process, these tissues will serve as a framework [31]. Besides, BCC very rarely invades cartilage or bone [33].

18.6 Contraindications of Cryosurgery

There are no absolute contraindications for cryosurgery except known cold intolerance. Morphoeiform and sclerotic recurrent BCCs are unsuitable for this therapy because the fibrosis does not permit a proper "feeling" of the curettage. Many aggressive tumors in difficult areas, such as the nasolabial fold and the inner canthi and pre- and postauricular fold, are preferably treated with other methods for higher cure rates and better cosmetic results [34].

18.7 Patients

After clinical examination and measuring of the visible size of the tumor, one or more punch biopsies are taken for verification of the diagnosis. Based on the histopathological findings, the morphoeiform tumors are always referred for MMS, and selected tumors of other types are treated by curettage-cryosurgery (CC). According to the present definition, morphoeiform BCC includes fibrosing, sclerosing, and scirrhous types of BCC.

18.8 Author's Method

18.8.1 Curettage-Cryosurgery

A thorough curettage using ring curettes (Thiemann, New York, USA) is performed under local anesthesia (mepivacaine-adrenaline 10 mg/ml+5 μg/ml). At first, a large curette (no.3) is used to remove the bulk of the tumor and then a medium-sized one (no.2), and finally a small curette (no.1) is used to remove any extensions of the malignancy. The curettage material is also sent for histopathological examination, and sometimes the findings are more aggressive than the original one [35]. After meticulous curettage, the tumor is often found to have wider lateral extension and greater depth than expected, and one has to be particularly thorough when treating malignancies in the nasolabial folds, in the inner canthi, and in the pre- and postauricular sulci. The curettage is performed according to the technique described by Strum and Leider [32]. Sometimes undermined edges have to be cut off by a pair of scissors. A cotton stick dipped in 50 % iron chloride solution is used for hemostasis.

Freezing is carried out with a maximal continuous spraying of liquid nitrogen (−196 °C) using a handheld Cry-Ac (Brymill Corp., New York, USA) with the nozzle held as horizontally as possible and, in general, with the patient sitting. By using the vertical position, the problem of liquid nitrogen flowing on the lesion is avoided, and the spraying becomes more standardized. The tumor area is most often, especially on flat surfaces, demarcated by a neoprene cone of appropriate size. The spray tip, size B, is moved in circular motions over the treatment zone, at about 1 cm distance, until the lateral spread of freeze has reached a minimum of 5 mm outside the tumor border or 1–1.5 mm outside the neoprene cone. The skin is always well fixed to the underlying bone by the freezing in spite of the "ballooning" of the local anesthesia. For tumors overlying cartilage on the nasal ala or the pinna of the ear, the freezing continues until the opposing side is frozen.

The goal of the freezing is a fast cooling rate and a slow thawing rate [5]. The procedure is always repeated a second time.

On a special tumor chart registration of the freeze time (10–25 s, depending on the tumor size), the lateral spread of freeze (≥5 mm), the halo thaw time (at least 60 s), and the complete thaw time (2–5 min) are done but no thermocouples are employed. A therapeutic sequence of curettage-cryosurgery of a clinically ill-defined BCC on ala nasi is seen in Fig. 18.4a–e. The same procedure of a BCC on the dorsal aspect of an ear is seen in Fig. 18.5a–e. All treatments are performed at a single outpatient visit.

18.8.2 Complications

It is important to be aware of and inform the patient about the usual and expected postoperative tissue response. Written information about this is handed over to the patient. The incidence of complications is low. They may be classified as temporary or permanent. Pain during and immediately after cryosurgery is common. It may be quite intense but it is usually transient. Edema, especially periorbital, is also very common. However, infection rarely

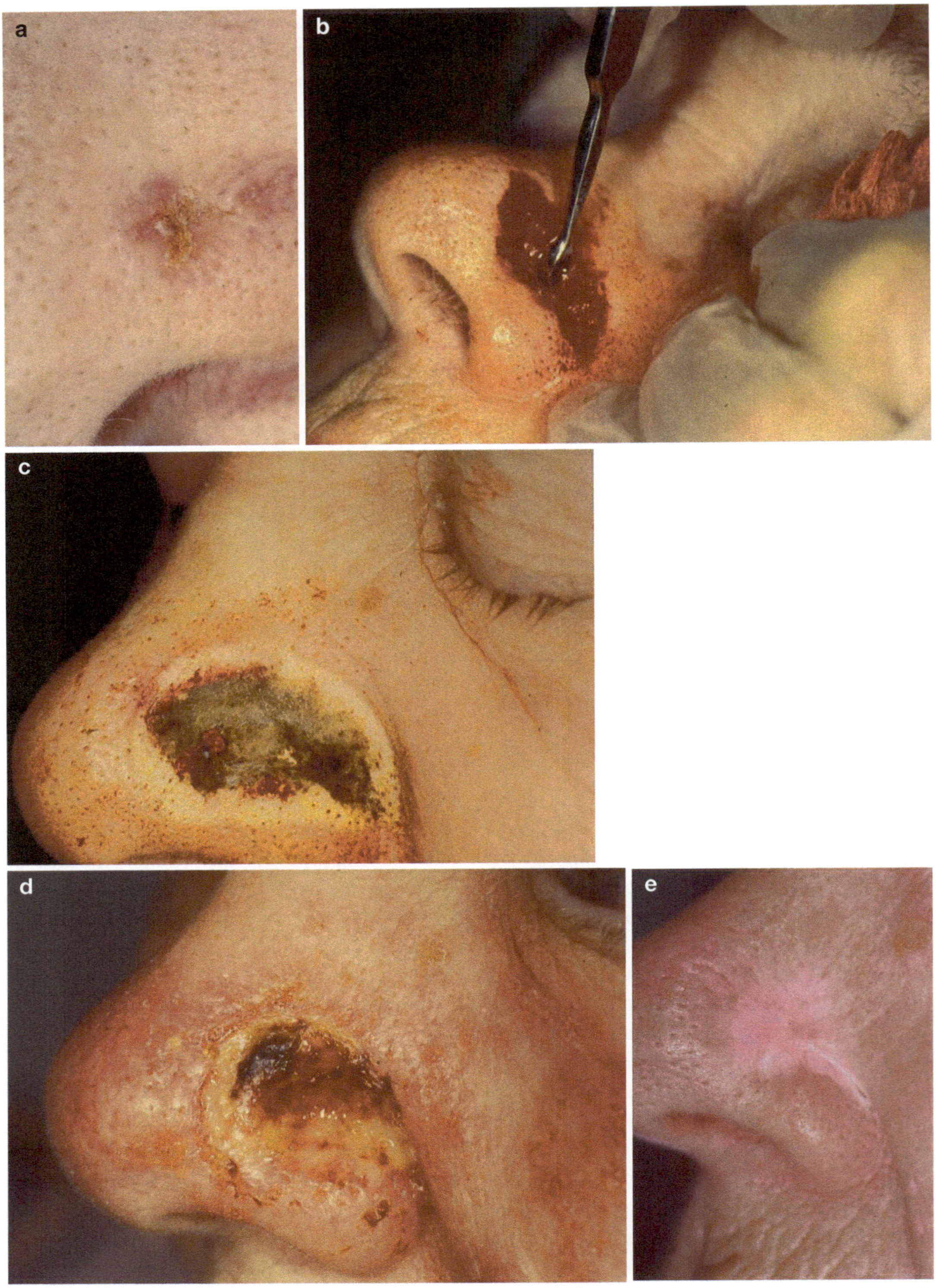

Fig. 18.4 Curettage-cryosurgery of a clinically ill-defined basal cell carcinoma on ala nasi. (**a**) Before treatment. (**b**) After a thorough curettage, the tumor is much larger than expected. (**c**) The tumor area is frozen with liquid nitrogen with a lateral spread of freeze of at least 5 mm. (**d**) The result after 2 weeks. (**e**) The result after 5 years

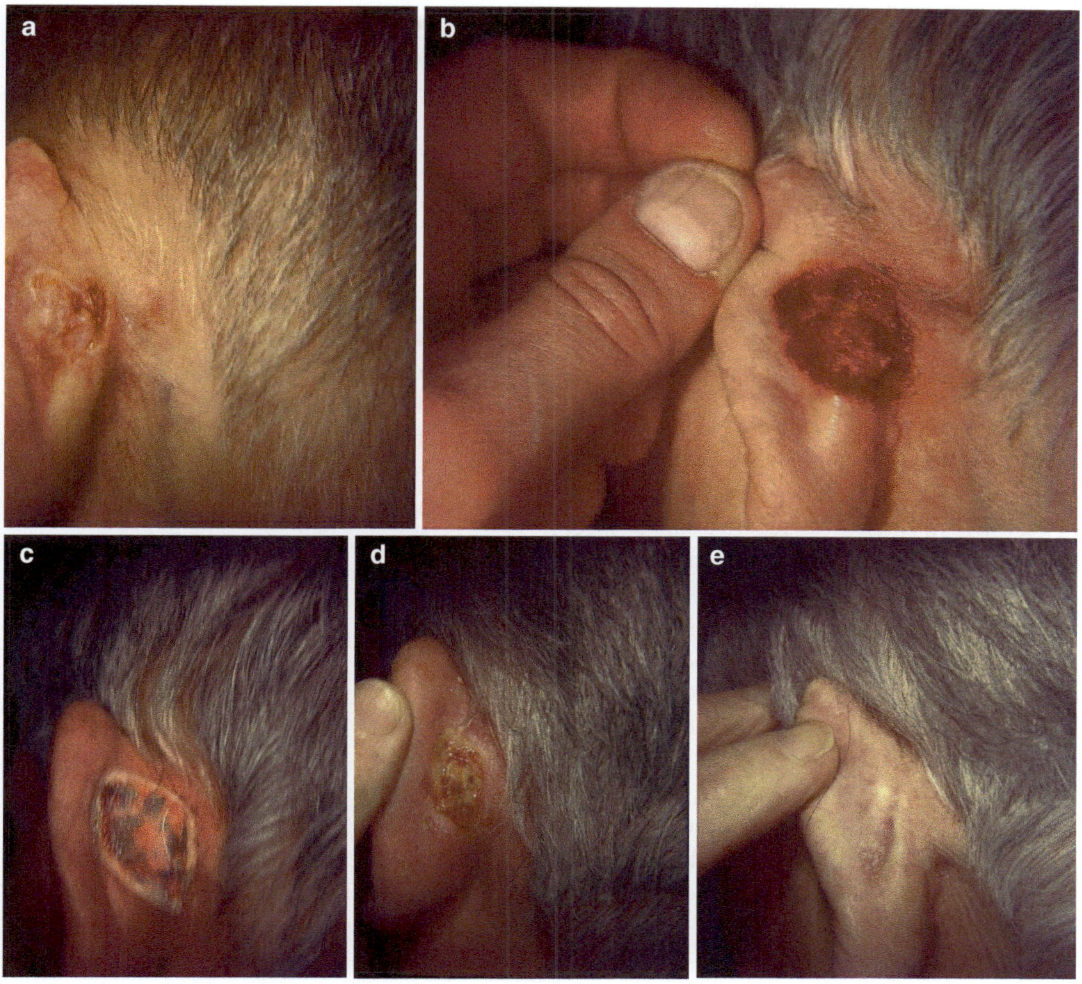

Fig. 18.5 Curettage-cryosurgery of an about 20 mm ulcerated BCC on the dorsal aspect of an ear. (**a**) Before treatment. (**b**) After a "heavy-handed" curettage with different-sized curettes, the diameter is 28 mm and four deeper cavities reaching the cartilage are seen. (**c**) Freezing with liquid nitrogen in a double freeze-thaw cycle. (**d**) Healing by secondary intention after 2 weeks. (**e**) The result obtained after 6 years

occurs. Of the permanent complications, the most common is hypopigmentation. Retraction of tissue and tissue defects as notching of ala nasi may be seen after treatment of tumors overriding the rim of ala. Notching of the ears may occur after treatment of malignancies overreaching the helix. Other complications are rare [34, 36].

18.8.3 Recurrence and Follow-up

The reason for failure to cure a malignancy with cryosurgery may be attributed to poor technique with insufficient treatment. It may also be due to an imperfect assessment of the tumor type and its extension. As mentioned earlier, certain types of skin cancers are unsuitable to be treated by cryosurgery. Recurrences are also more common following treatment of tumors in certain areas such as the inner canthus, the nasolabial fold, and the periauricular area.

Most recurrences following cryosurgery develop during the first 2 years, but they may appear many years later [5, 29, 37].

The patients are usually examined 1–2 weeks after treatment; then after 3, 6, and 12 months;

and, when possible, yearly for 5 years or more. At these visits it is also important to look for new skin tumors as about 40 % of patients treated for a BCC after 5 years have got a new BCC [38].

18.8.4 Results

Cryosurgical treatment – with different techniques – of NMSCs, mainly BCCs, has given excellent 5-year cure rates of 97–98 %.

Zacharian in 1983 reported a cure rate of 97.3 % after treatment of 4,228 epithelial skin cancers in an 18-year study [29]. Kuflik and Gage presented a series of 3,540 new NMSCs with a 5-year cure rate of 98.4 % [26]. Graham has reported similar excellent results [25] as well as Holt [24] and Torre [5]. Most of these tumors in different series were treated with open-spray technique, sometimes preceded by a debulking curettage of the cancer. Many of these malignancies were located on the nose and ears. Nordin et al. used a combination of thorough curettage followed by cryosurgery in the treatment of large primary BCCs on the nose [21] and NMSCs on the external ear [22] with excellent 5-year results. Lindemalm- Lundstam et al. have used the same technique for NMSCs on the scalp and face with similar results [39].

18.8.5 Cosmetic Results

During the first half to 1 year after cryosurgery, the scars are often hyperplastic, but thereafter, they are flat but hypopigmented with good or acceptable cosmesis according to the patients as well as the doctor [21, 22]. A recurrence is easily seen in such a scar. This is in contrast to defects reconstructed by flaps, where recurrences are hard to observe [40]. In general, the cosmetic result is better on concave than on convex surfaces [41].

18.8.6 Advantages and Disadvantages

See Table 18.1 for the advantages and disadvantages of using cryosurgery.

Table 18.1 Advantages and disadvantages of cryosurgery

Advantages	Disadvantages
Tissue sparing	Lack of histopathological tumor margins
Not very resource demanding	Healing by secondary intention
Cheap	Weeping wound for 1–2 weeks
Safe	

Essential Tidbits

- Double freeze-thaw cycles are required.
- A meticulous curettage will help define the tumor.
- For tumors overlying the cartilage on the nasal ala or the pinna of the ear, the freezing continues until the opposing side is frozen: an ice "tattoo" can be seen on the opposite side of the pinna or felt with the fingertip that maintains the nasal ala in place.
- Sprayed LN can be confined by neoprene cones (semiopen technique).

Conclusions

The aim of curettage-cryosurgery is that the first treatment should be the final one. Curettage-cryosurgery is a tissue-sparing, not very resource-demanding, and safe therapy, well suited for outpatient treatment of selected, even large, NMSCs on the nose and external ears. The main disadvantage with curettage-cryosurgery is the lack of histopathological evaluation of the tumor margins. Other drawbacks are the postoperative perilesional edema and the weeping wound which has to heal by secondary intention. However, if a thorough curettage for tumor demarcation is carried out, followed by a deep freeze with liquid nitrogen in a double freeze-thaw cycle, the risk of recurrence should be minimal.

Glossary

NMSCs Nonmelanoma skin carcinomas. These include basal and squamous cell carcinomas.

Mohs micrographic surgery (MMS) Also referred to as chemosurgery. It is a microscopically controlled surgery mostly used in nonmelanoma skin cancer.

Acknowledgment I am very grateful to Bo Stenquist, associate professor and Mohs surgeon, for his valuable comments.

References

1. Levine HL, Bailin PL. Basal cell carcinoma of the head and neck: identification of the high risk patient. Laryngoscope. 1980;90:692–6.
2. Robins P, Reyes BA. Cure rates of skin cancer treated by Mohs micrographic surgery. In: Roenigk RK, Roenigk Jr HH, editors. Dermatologic surgery: principles and practice. New York: Marcel Dekker; 1989. p. 853–8.
3. Albright III SD. Treatment of skin cancer using multiple modalities. J Am Acad Dermatol. 1982;7:143–71.
4. Kopf AW, Bart RS, Schrager D, Lazar M, Popkin GL. Curettage-electrodessication treatment of basal cell carcinomas. Arch Dermatol. 1977;113: 439–43.
5. Torre D. Cryosurgery of basal cell carcinoma. J Am Acad Dermatol. 1986;15:917–29.
6. Smith SP, Grande DJ. Basal cell carcinoma recurring after radiotherapy: a unique difficult treatment subclass of recurrent basal cell carcinoma. J Dermatol Surg Oncol. 1991;17:26–30.
7. Silverman M, Kopf A, Bart R, Grin C, Levenstein M. Recurrence rates of treated basal cell carcinomas. Part 3: surgical excision. J Dermatol Surg Oncol. 1992;18:471–6.
8. Roenigk RK, Ratz JL, Bailin PL, Wheeland RG. Trends in the presentation and treatment of basal cell carcinoma. J Dermatol Surg Oncol. 1986;12:860–5.
9. Mohs F, Larson P, Iriondo M. Micrographic surgery for the microscopically controlled excision of carcinoma of the external ear. J Am Acad Dermatol. 1988;19:729–37.
10. Bumsted RM, Ceilly RI, Panje WR, Cramley RL. Auricular malignant neoplasms. When is chemotherapy (Mohs' technique) necessary? Arch Otolaryngol. 1981;107:721–4.
11. Roenigk R, Roenigk H. Current surgical management of skin cancer in dermatology. J Dermatol Surg Oncol. 1990;16:136–51.
12. Kopf AW. Computer analysis of 3531 basal cell carcinomas of the skin. J Dermatol. 1979;6:267–81.
13. Dahl E, Åberg M, Rausing A, Rausing EL. Basal cell carcinoma. An epidemiologic study in a defined population. Cancer. 1992;70:104–8.
14. Burg G, Hirsch R, Konz B, Braun-Falco O. Histographic surgery: accuracy of visual assessment of the margins of basal-cell epithelioma. J Dermatol Surg Oncol. 1975;1:21–4.
15. Jacobs GH, Rippey JJ, Altini M. Prediction of aggressive behaviour in basal-cell carcinoma. Cancer. 1982;49:533–7.
16. Bailin PL, Levine HL, Wood BG, Tucker HMI. Cutaneous carcinoma of the auricular and periauricular region. Arch Otolaryngol. 1980;106:692–6.
17. Dawber RPR. Cold kills! Clin Exp Dermatol. 1988;13:137–50.
18. Torre D. Cryosurgical instrumentation and depth dose monitoring. Clin Dermatol. 1990;8:48–60.
19. Gage AA. What temperature is lethal for cells? J Dermatol Surg Oncol. 1979;5:459–64.
20. Spiller WF, Spiller RF. Treatment of basal-cell carcinomas by a combination of curettage and cryosurgery. J Dermatol Surg Oncol. 1977;3:443–7.
21. Nordin P, Larkö O, Stenquist B. Five-year results of curettage-cryosurgery of selected large primary basal cell carcinomas on the nose: an alternative treatment in a geographical area underserved by Mohs' surgery. Br J Dermatol. 1997;136:180–3.
22. Nordin P, Stenquist B. Five-year results of curettage-cryosurgery for 100 consecutive auricular nonmelanoma skin cancers. J Laryngol Otol. 2002;116:893–8.
23. Colver GB, Dawber RPR. Cryosurgery-the principles and simple practice. Clin Exp Dermatol. 1989;14:1–6.
24. Holt PJA. Cryotherapy for skin cancer: results over a 5 year period using liquid nitrogen spray cryosurgery. Br J Dermatol. 1988;119:231–40.
25. Graham GF. Cryosurgery. Clin Plast Surg. 1993;20:131–47.
26. Kuflik EG, Gage AA. The five-year cure rate achieved by cryosurgery for skin cancer. J Am Acad Dermatol. 1991;24:1002–4.
27. Kuflik EG. Segmental cryosurgical treatment. J Dermatol Surg Oncol. 1987;13:235–6.
28. Zacharian SA. Cryosurgery in the treatment of skin cancer. In: Friedman RJ, Rigel DS, Kopf AW, editors. Cancer in the skin. Philadelphia: WB Saunders; 1991. p. 451–65.
29. Zacharian SA. Cryosurgery of cutaneous carcinomas: an 18-year study of 3022 patients with 4228 carcinomas. J Am Acad Dermatol. 1983;9:947–56.
30. Shephard JP. The effect of low temperature on dermal connective tissue components. Thesis, University of Oxford, Oxford; 1979.
31. Shephard JP, Dawber RPR. Wound healing and scarring after cryosurgery. Cryobiology. 1984;21: 158–69.
32. Strum HM, Leider M. An editorial on curettage. J Dermatol Surg Oncol. 1979;5:532–3.
33. Robins P. Chemosurgery: my 15 years of experience. J Dermatol Surg Oncol. 1981;9:779–89.
34. Dawber RPR. Cryosurgery: complications and contraindications. Clin Dermatol. 1990;8:108–14.
35. Hendrix Jr JD, Parlette HL. Micronodular basal cell carcinoma. A deceptive subtype with frequent clinically undetected tumor extension. Arch Dermatol. 1996;132:295–8.
36. Scott CM, Graham GF, Hubinette RR. Complications of cryosurgery. In: Nouri K, editor. Complications in dermatologic surgery. Philadelphia: Mosby, Elsevier; 2008. p. 101–35.

37. Rowe DE, Carroll RJ, Day Jr CL. Long-term recurrence rates in previously untreated (primary) basal cell carcinoma: implications for patient follow-up. J Dermatol Surg Oncol. 1989;15: 315–28.
38. Robinson JK, Pollack SV, Robins P. Risk of developing another basal cell carcinoma. Cancer. 1987;60: 118–20.
39. Lindemalm-Lundstam B, Dalenbäck J. Prospective follow-up after curettage-cryosurgery for scalp and face cancers. Br J Dermatol. 2009;161:568–76.
40. Albom MJ. Surgical gems, the management of recurrent basal cell carcinoma. Please no graft or flaps at once. J Dermatol Surg Oncol. 1977;3:382–4.
41. Zitelli JA. Wound healing by secondary intention. A cosmetic appraisal. J Am Acad Dermatol. 1983;9:407–15.

Cryosurgery for Eyelid Basal Cell Carcinomas: A Practical Guide

19

Gun Lindgren and Olle Larkö

Contents

G. Lindgren, MD, PhD (✉)
Department of Ophthalmology,
Sahlgrenska University Hospital,
Göteborgsvägen 31, Mölndal
S-43180, Sweden
e-mail: gun.lindgren@vgregion.se

O. Larkö, MD
Department of Dermatology,
The Sahlgrenska Academy, Sahlgrenska University
Hospital, University of Gothenburg,
Gothenburg SE 413 45, Sweden
e-mail: olle.larko@sahlgrenska.gu.se

Key Points

- Cryosurgery is an excellent alternative treatment for nodular BCC of the eyelids.
- It is fast and tissue sparing and performed under local infiltrative anaesthesia.
- It can be conducted on an outpatient basis.
- Tumours overriding the lacrimal punctum and the medial and lateral canthal areas can be safely treated because the tarsal plate, the lacrimal duct, and the ligaments are exceptionally resistant to cold.

19.1 Introduction

Basal cell carcinomas (BCCs) are the most common of malignant skin tumours and frequently occur on the eyelids [1, 2]. There is an increasing incidence of BCCs in Sweden, and approximately 40,000 cases are now diagnosed every year, nearly one tenth of which appear on the skin of the eyelids or in the canthal area.

Because properly functioning eyelids are vital for protecting the eyes, a treatment modality for BCCs that combines a high cure rate with optimally preserved function is necessary. Cryosurgery of eyelid BCCs, which has also proved to be cost-efficient, is such a modality,

P. Pasquali (ed.), *Cryosurgery: A Practical Manual*,
DOI 10.1007/978-3-662-43939-5_19, © Springer-Verlag Berlin Heidelberg 2015

demonstrated repeatedly over more than 40 years [3–8]. Also, tumours overriding the lacrimal punctum and the medial and lateral canthal areas can be safely treated because the tarsal plate, the lacrimal duct, and the ligaments are exceptionally resistant to cold.

If only well-delineated tumours of low aggressive type are treated, results are excellent, with only minor side effects [9]. Whether cryosurgery should be used to treat tumours exceeding 10 mm is a matter of discussion [10]. However, the size of the tumour per se is no limit to treatment with cryosurgery provided the tumour is well delineated. Treatment of a large tumour, however, creates a large area of necrosis that takes a considerable time to heal; therefore, we limited our treatable tumour size to 25 mm. It has been recommended that tumours in the medial canthal area not be treated with cryosurgery [10]. We, on the other hand, found excellent results treating tumours in the medial canthal area for both high cure rate and cosmetic results. In general, scars resulting from the treatment are less visible in concave areas such as the medial canthal area.

We strongly advise that poorly delineated tumours or BCCs of the morpheic type be treated with Mohs micrographic surgery, even though selected aggressive BCCs can be treated with cryosurgery [11]. Ordinary excisional surgery in these cases is simply not good enough, because only some sections of the specimen are investigated. In Mohs surgery, the entire cut borders are examined and the complete excision can thus be evaluated [12]. The primary treatment of an eyelid BCC should always aim at curing the tumour completely, because the treatment of a recurrence is less likely to be successful [13]. Because a failed treatment can result in the loss of an eye or in an intracerebral extension, it is of utmost importance to select a modality suited to the aggressiveness of the tumour and to extirpate the tumour radically.

19.2 Treatment Technique

Treatment can be conducted on an outpatient basis. Patients should sit comfortably, and those with mobility difficulties may remain seated in their wheelchair with a rest for the head. We advise that tumours be photographed before treatment.

Tumour borders are marked with ink before the tumour area is generously injected with a local anaesthetic with 5 μg/ml adrenalin. The injection is less painful if it starts in the soft tissue away from the tarsal parts of the eyelids; subsequent injections can then move closer to the eyelid margins. The mixture with adrenalin is used to prolong the thaw time. Local anaesthetic drops are applied to the surface of the eye.

If tumours are significantly higher (by approx. >3 mm) than the normal surface, curettage is aimed to reduce the height of the tumour, not to accomplish a thorough curettage. For this purpose, a chalazion forceps can be used to stabilise the tissue (Fig. 19.1). Among the different ways of evaluating the effect of freezing, we have found that

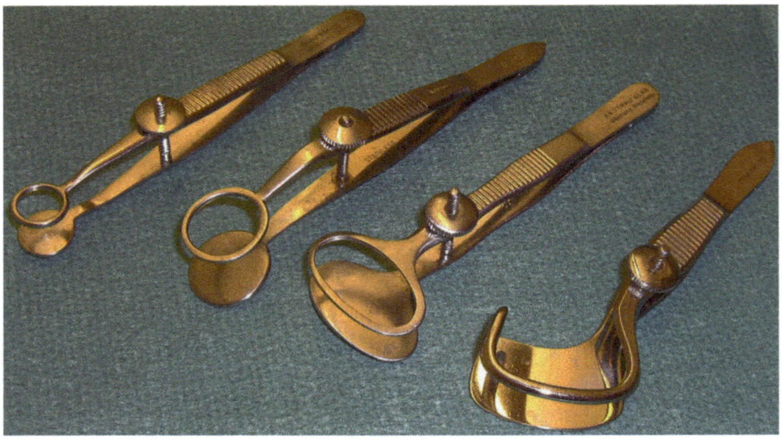

Fig. 19.1 Different-sized chalazion forceps that can be used to stabilise the tissue

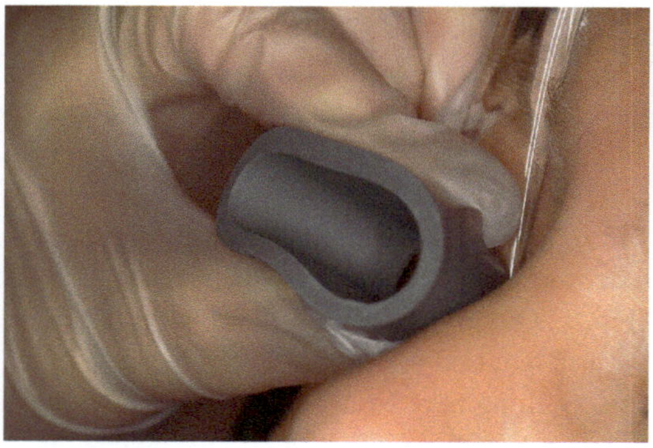

Fig. 19.2 Cone squeezed to an oval to fit the extension of the tumour

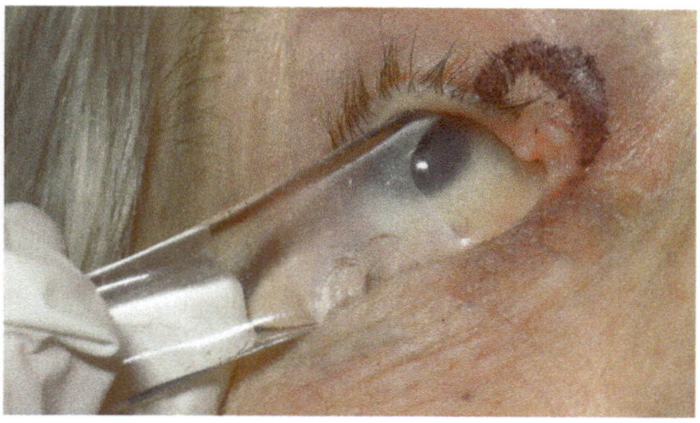

Fig. 19.4 Lid plate positioned horizontally to protect the eye while treating the medial part of both the upper and lower eyelids

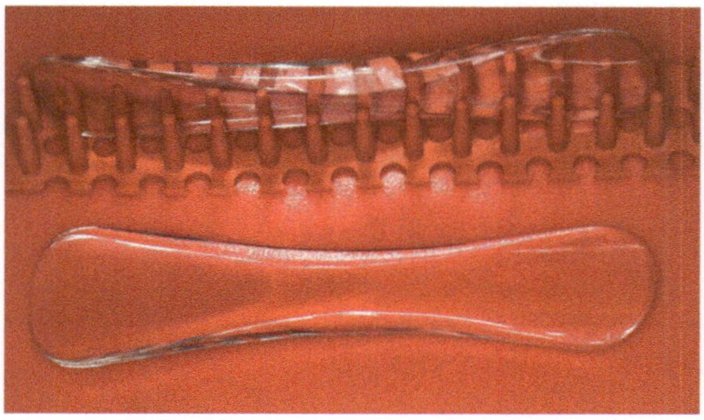

Fig. 19.3 Plastic Jaeger lid plate thick enough to protect the underlying tissue

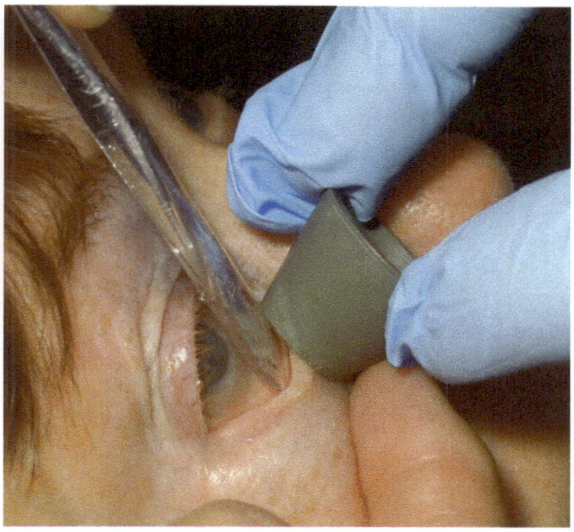

Fig. 19.5 Lid plate lifting the eyelid against the neoprene cone

neoprene cones with a 3 mm thick wall best suit our technique. These cones can easily be squeezed to fit different extensions of tumours and to safely enclose the tumour without damaging healthy tissue. The 3 mm thick wall of the cone also corresponds to the desired lateral extension of the freezing zone (Fig. 19.2). The *inner* diameter of the cone size selected should securely encircle the tumour. Generous administration of local anaesthetic facilitates a tight connection when the cone is applied with some pressure to the surface of the skin, thus avoiding leakage of nitrogen.

A clear plastic Jaeger lid plate is inserted in the eye fornix to protect the eyeball. There are different types of these plates on the market, but it is important that the plate should be thick enough to well isolate the underlying tissues (the eye) during the treatment (Fig. 19.3). Depending on the site of the tumour, the plate is placed vertical in tumours in the central parts of the upper or lower eyelids and horizontal in tumours that are medial or lateral (Fig. 19.4). The plate should be slightly lifted from the globe during the treatment, thus pressing the eyelid towards the cone and further ensuring that no leaked nitrogen can reach the eye (Fig. 19.5). If the tumour is situated far medial (e.g. covering the area above the lacrimal sac), the plate can be placed horizontally on top of the closed eyelid.

The liquid nitrogen coolant, stored in a handheld thermos, is sprayed into the rubber cone. To avoid freezing the fingers that hold the cone, a space with air should be left in the fingertips of the gloves (Fig. 19.6). It is important to freeze without interruption to ensure the freezing is reproducible. The freezing should continue until a small brim of frozen tissue is observed all around the outer border of the neoprene cone. A typical freeze time to achieve the desired extension of iced tissue is 20–30 s of constant freezing. The cone is left until it loosens spontaneously from the skin. The halo, corresponding to the 3 mm mark of the wall of the cone, should be allowed a thaw time exceeding 60 s (Fig. 19.7a, b). The frozen area is left to thaw completely. Two freeze–thaw cycles are carried out. If the halo thaw time is less than 60 s, a third cycle is performed.

After the treatment, an antibiotic ointment is placed in the eye.

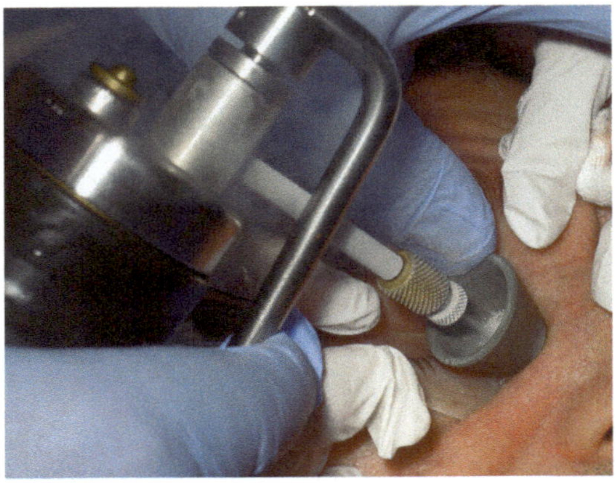

Fig. 19.6 Liquid nitrogen sprayed in the cone; observe the residual air in the fingertips of the glove

19.3 Patient Information

Patients are carefully informed about the procedure. It is particularly important to inform patients about excessive postoperative swelling and oozing of tissue fluid. There are more local reactions in larger tumours than in small ones (Fig. 19.8a, b). Usually, there is little pain. Patients are told that it looks worse than it feels. The swelling may be misinterpreted as infection by those not familiar with its appearance. Antibiotic ointment should be applied in the eye for as long as there is a crust. Patients are encouraged to allow the treated area to get damp during showering, because this facilitates the loosening of the crust, which will then be replaced by a smaller one. The healing period is about 1 month in tumours of 10 mm size. Patients are told about the risk of conjunctival overgrowth and hypo- or hyperpigmentation in the treated area.

19.4 Follow-up

One week following the treatment, the patient is examined by a nurse for signs of infection. The doctor sees the patient 1 month after the cryosurgery. If a crust at that time still covers parts of the treated area, it is removed, or if it is tightly attached to the tissue, the edges are lifted from the wound to facilitate its loosening.

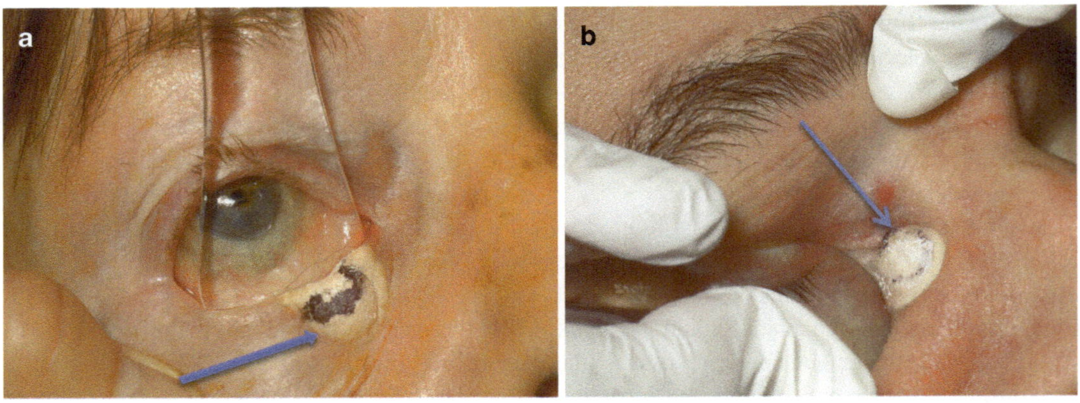

Fig. 19.7 The halo thaw time is the time measured from cessation of freezing to the point at which the thawing has reached any part of the inner aspect of the mark of the cone; in the figures, this is pointed out by the *arrow* (**a**, **b**)

One year after therapy, patients are monitored again and the area palpated for signs of recurrence. The appearance and function of the eyelid are studied and, if possible, photographed. If there is no sign of recurrence and the lid function and appearance are satisfactory, the patients are left to self-assessment. Patients are advised to make contact with the clinic if they suspect the tumour has reoccurred.

19.5 Side Effects

Patients must be informed that correctly performed cryosurgery will permanently destroy the eyelashes. The tumour itself usually destroys lashes in the immediate area, but lashes in the 3 mm treated zone around the tumour also disappear, resulting in a total of at least 6 mm wider loss of lashes than the tumour size. This permanent loss is an inevitable cosmetic side effect of treating tumours on the upper eyelid.

Tumour growths that include and destroy parts of the tarsal plate usually heal with a surprisingly good cosmetic result by secondary intention. Very rarely, defects in the tarsal plate occur. Because tissue healing is dependent on neovascularisation, patients on drugs with a negative impact on this process are at greater risk of having a less favourable outcome [14]. Hence, a word of caution concerning patients on cytostatic or antimetabolites is warranted, since healing by secondary intention may be slower than otherwise in treating these patients with cryosurgery.

The necrosis of the cells after cryosurgery affects the complete thickness of the eyelid, including the conjunctiva on the inside of the eyelid and the skin on the outside. In the healing process, the conjunctiva sometimes is renewed faster and does not stop growing at the margin of the eyelid, but continues to grow on the outside until it meets the skin. Approximately 10 % of patients experience conjunctival overgrowth to some extent (Fig. 19.9). This seldom needs correction, but if the patient finds it bothersome, minor corrective surgery may be carried out. After the treatment, hypopigmentation or hyperpigmentation may occur in the skin (Fig. 19.10a, b). Changes in pigmentation are likely to fade with time [11]. Pronounced scarring is rare, especially in the

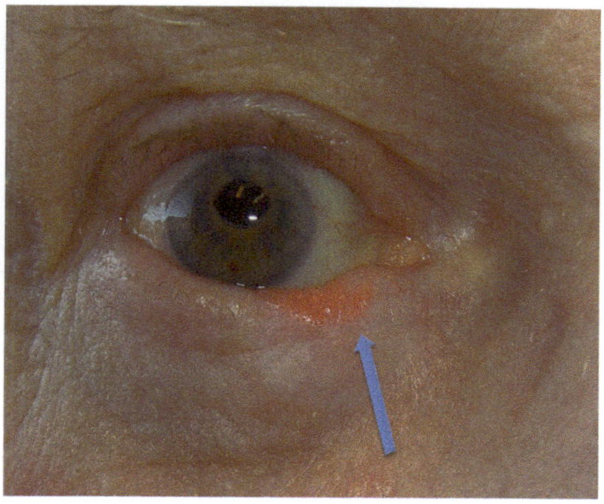

Fig. 19.9 Conjunctival overgrowth to the skin side. The *arrow* indicates the part of the eyelid with conjunctiva on the outside of the eyelid

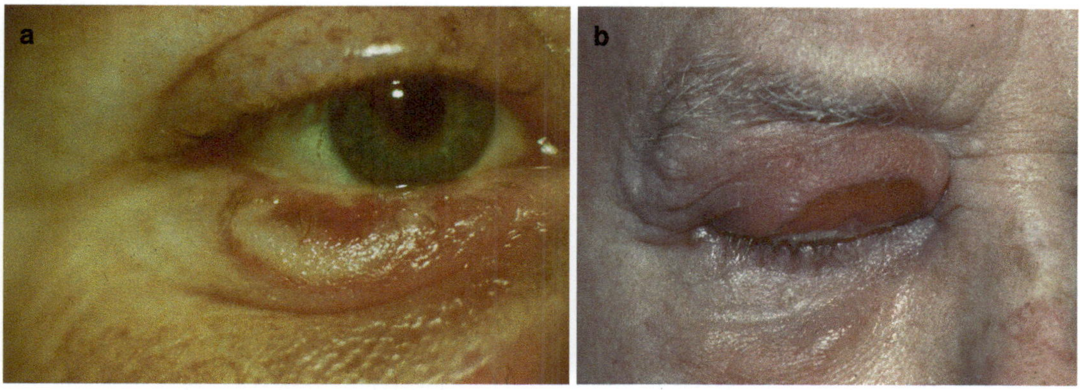

Fig. 19.8 Reaction after 1 week in a small tumour (**a**) and in a large tumour (**b**)

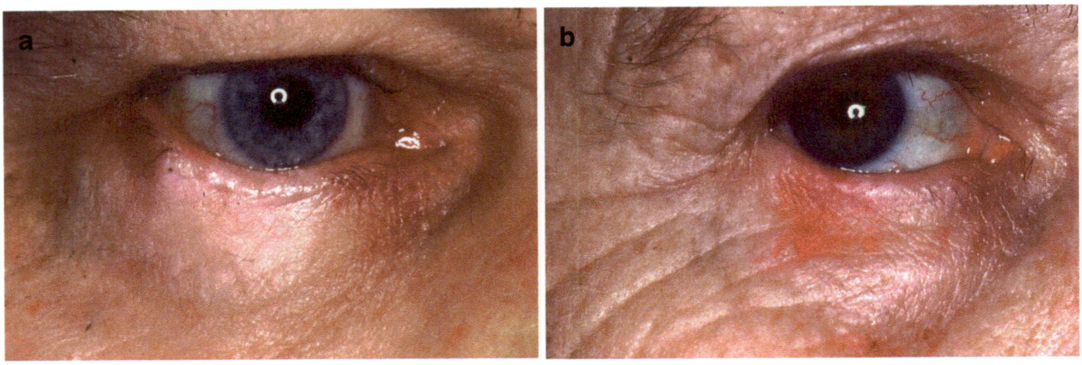

Fig. 19.10 Hypopigmentation in the treated area (**a**) and hyperpigmentation in the treated area (**b**)

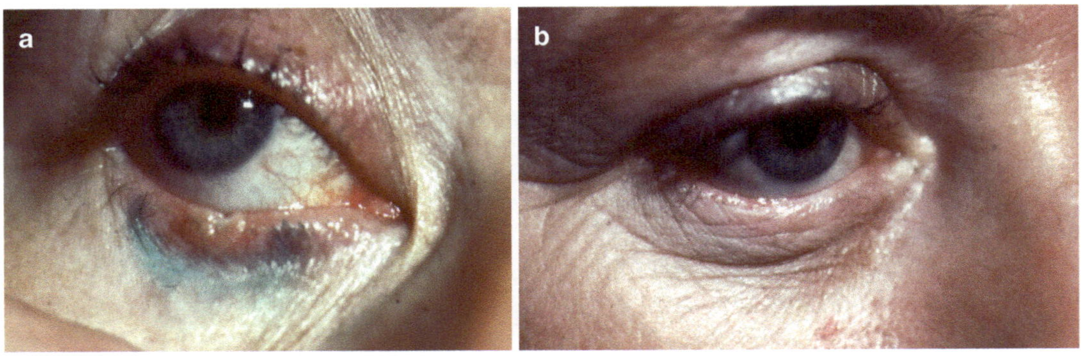

Fig. 19.11 A small basal cell carcinoma in the central part of the lower eyelid before treatment (**a**) and after treatment (**b**)

medial canthal area. In small treated tumours, even the normal skin folds are preserved, giving the area a good cosmetic result (Fig. 19.11a, b).

Essential Tidbits

- Well-defined nodular BCCs are ideal for cryosurgical treatment of the eyelid.
- Protect the eye with nonconductive material shield like plastic.
- Semiopen technique (neoprene cone) will concentrate LN and avoid freezing or splattering LN in surrounding structures.
- Chalazion forceps can be used to stabilise the tissue while performing a biopsy or during curettage.
- Warn patients of the postoperative oedema which is usually short lasting.

Conclusions

Cryosurgery of well-delineated BCCs is effective and has few side effects. A preoperative biopsy should be carried out in order to confirm the nodular type of the tumour. If tumours are poorly delineated, mixed, or morpheiform, we advocate Mohs micrographic surgery. Ordinary excisional surgery is simply not good enough for tumours on the eyelid or in the canthal areas.

Glossary

BCC Basal cell carcinoma

References

1. Loeffler M, Hornblass A. Characteristics and behavior of eyelid carcinoma (basal cell, squamous cell sebaceous gland, and malignant melanoma). Ophthalmic Surg. 1990;21(7):513–8.
2. Saari KM, Paavilainen V, Tuominen J, Collan Y. Epidemiology of basal cell carcinoma of the eyelid

in south-western Finland. Graefe's archive for clinical and experimental ophthalmology. Albrecht Von Graefes Arch Klin Exp Ophthalmol. 2001;239(3):230–3.
3. Biro L, Price E. Basal-cell carcinomas of eyelids: experience with cryosurgery. J Dermatol Surg Oncol. 1979;5(5):397–401.
4. Buschmann W, Linnert D. Stickstoff-Kryotherapie von Lidbasaliomen. [Nitrogen cryotherapy of lid basaliomas (author's transl)]. Klin Monbl Augenheilkd. 1980;177(3):345–53.
5. Fraunfelder FT, Farris Jr HE, Wallace TR. Cryosurgery for ocular and periocular lesions. J Dermatol Surg Oncol. 1977;3(4):422–7.
6. Kuflik EG. Cryosurgery for basal-cell carcinomas on and around eyelids. J Dermatol Surg Oncol. 1978; 4(12):911–3.
7. Zacarian SA. Cancer of the eyelid–a cryosurgical approach. Ann Ophthalmol. 1972;4(6):473–80.
8. Kokoszka A, Scheinfeld N. Evidence-based review of the use of cryosurgery in treatment of basal cell carcinoma. Dermatol Surg. 2003;29(6):566–71.
9. Lindgren G, Larko O. Long-term follow-up of cryosurgery of basal cell carcinoma of the eyelid. J Am Acad Dermatol. 1997;36(5 Pt 1):742–6.
10. Kersten RC, Bartley GB, Nerad JA, Neuhaus RW, Nowinski TS, Popham JK, Beardsley TL. Orbit, eyelid, and lacrimal system. Series: basic and clinical science course, section 7. San Francisco: American Academy of Ophthalmology; 2002.
11. Jaramillo-Ayerbe F. Cryosurgery in difficult to treat basal cell carcinoma. Int J Dermatol. 2000;39(3): 223–9.
12. Mohs FE. Micrographic surgery for the microscopically controlled excision of eyelid cancers. Arch Ophthalmol. 1986;104(6):901–9.
13. Pieh S, Kuchar A, Novak P, Kunstfeld R, Nagel G, Steinkogler FJ. Long-term results after surgical basal cell carcinoma excision in the eyelid region. Br J Ophthalmol. 1999;83(1):85–8.
14. Anderson R. A warning on cryosurgery for eyelid malignancies. Arch Ophthalmol. 1978;96(7): 1289–90.

Immunocryosurgery for Nonmelanoma Skin Cancer: Applications and Practical Tips

20

Georgios Gaitanis and Ioannis D. Bassukas

Contents

G. Gaitanis, MD, PhD (✉) • I.D. Bassukas, MD, PhD
Department of Skin and Venereal Diseases,
School of Health Sciences, University of Ioannina,
S. Niarchou Avenue,
Ioannina 45100, Greece
e-mail: ggaitan@cc.uoi.gr; ibassuka@cc.uoi.gr

Key Points

- Immunocryosurgery is the combination of cryosurgery with immunostimulatory therapy.
- It is a novel approach for the treatment of BCC, also for relatively locally advanced cases.
- It is a recent addition to the therapeutic modalities used for basal cell carcinomas, and current indications include in situ SCC, actinic keratoses, solar cheilosis, Bowen's disease, keratoacanthoma, lentigo maligna, Kaposi sarcoma, and genital warts.

20.1 Introduction

This chapter is a practical guide to the application of immunocryosurgery, a combination modality primarily developed in the authors' institution to treat skin lesions. "Immunocryosurgery" refers to the combination of cryosurgery and immunostimulatory therapy. In the present setting, the immunostimulation therapy is performed with topical imiquimod. Generally, but not universally, rational combination of individual treatment modalities is a reasonable approach to improve efficacy of therapeutic interventions; however, the effectiveness of each proposed combination, even if pathophysiologically predictable, must always be confirmed

P. Pasquali (ed.), *Cryosurgery: A Practical Manual*,
DOI 10.1007/978-3-662-43939-5_20, © Springer-Verlag Berlin Heidelberg 2015

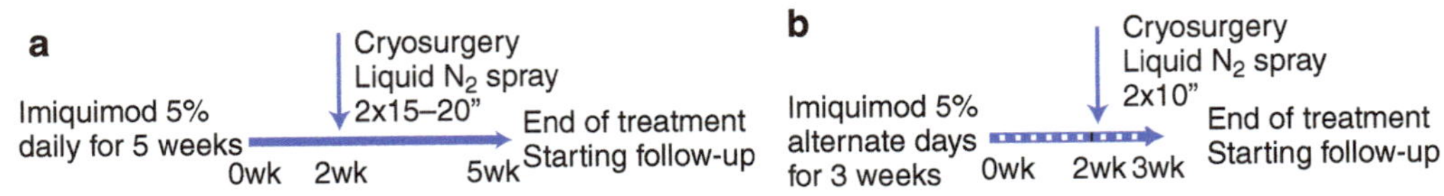

Fig. 20.1 (**a**) The standard immunocryosurgery cycle consists of daily application of imiquimod and a cryosurgery session at the end of the second week. Imiquimod is continued for additional 3 weeks, i.e., 5 weeks in total. (**b**) For benign or premalignant lesions, like genital warts or actinic keratoses, imiquimod is applied every other day, the day prior to cryosurgery and at the same day. Days of imiquimod applications are highlighted with blue color, days off with white

with trial evidence. In the meantime, sufficient evidence has been accumulated to support immunocryosurgery as an alternative therapeutic option for selected patients with certain skin diseases. Clinical data indicate that the efficacy of this combination stems from optimizing the synergistic action of both modalities as determined by the timing of this combination [1, 2]. In this chapter, we have reviewed the therapeutic spectrum of the modality, highlight potential pitfalls of the treatment, and underscore the role of adherence to certain empirical treatment rules that guarantee higher efficacy.

20.2 Standard Immunocryosurgery Protocol

Immunocryosurgery is typically applied in treatment cycles of 5 weeks duration, referred to as the "standard immunocryosurgery protocol" [3–5] (Fig. 20.1a). If required, these cycles can be repeated without restriction. In the standard 5-week immunocryosurgery treatment protocol for malignant skin neoplasms, the patient is instructed to apply imiquimod every night on the target lesion, including an approximately 0.5 cm wide rim of healthy skin around its macroscopic margins. At the end of the second week of daily imiquimod application, the session of cryosurgery is performed on the lesion and a reasonably wide zone of healthy skin around it (usually 0.5–1.0 cm beyond the margins of the lesion). The session of cryosurgery consists of 2 freeze-thaw cycles with the liquid N_2 open-spray method, 10–20 s "effective freezing time" each, depending on the diagnosis and the size of the lesions. With "effective freezing time," the duration of the maintenance of the state of complete freezing of the lesion is defined after maximal freezing condition has been achieved (i.e. tissue ice ball formation). Daily imiquimod applications are continued without interruption for an additional 3 weeks without any interruption, even the same night of the cryosurgery. The local inflammatory response is part of the treatment's mode of action, it is more pronounced after the cryosurgery session, and abates a few days after the end of treatment (Figs. 20.2a–f, 20.3, and 20.4a–f). Patients are encouraged to wash the treated area with soap and tap water in the morning, in order to gently remove some of the scabs that are formed daily. Impressively, by the end of treatment a distinct hard, inelastic relatively firmly adherent scab may cover the treated area (well put recently as "*arbor cutis*") [6]. This can be softened under occlusion with, e.g., fusidic acid cream or petrolatum, for 30–60 min, and then gently removed, revealing the healing skin underneath. As mentioned earlier, in some instances (e.g., incomplete response, large tumors; see discussion later in this chapter), this "basic" treatment cycle can be repeated as required.

There are no specific contraindications for immunocryosurgery; if any, these would be the same as those of cryosurgery and imiquimod. Regarding the known relative contraindications of cryosurgery and imiquimod, we have successfully applied immunocryosurgery to patients under immunosuppressive treatment for either collagen or autoimmune diseases as well as patients with internal, including hematological malignancies and solid organ transplant recipients under immunosuppression without any excess adverse effects attributed to their comorbidities and/or medications. The recommenda-

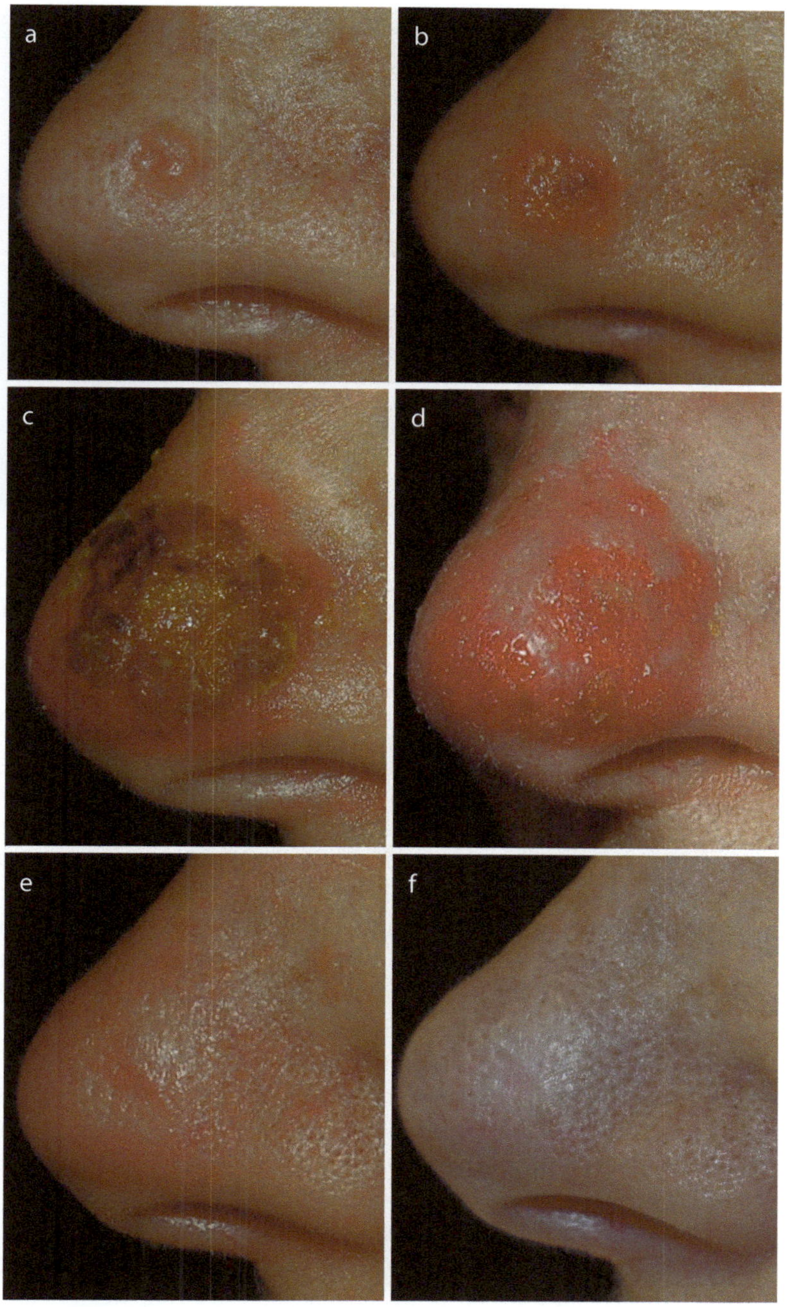

Fig. 20.2 A typical immunocryosurgery cycle treatment in a 75-year-old female patient with a 7 mm basal cell carcinoma on her nose. (**a**) Baseline. (**b**) Day 14, after once daily imiquimod application for 2 weeks and prior to the cryosurgery session (liquid N_2, open spray, 2 freeze-thaw cycles, 15 s each). (**c**) Day 35. End of the 5-week treatment cycle. Extensive scabbing is evident. (**d**) The patient after removal of the scabs. No tumor remnants can be seen and healing is evident ("complete response"). (**e**) The patient at 3 months follow-up. (**f**) The patient at 12 months follow-up. The "tumor ghost," i.e., the skin area that the tumor was infiltrating is evident as a whitish, just perceived scar

tion in the case of a patient with one of the cold precipitated conditions (Chap. 21) should always balance the benefit over the risk of side effects considering the rather mild cryosurgery session which is required for immunocryosurgery.

The side effects of immunocryosurgery present as an aggravation of the side effects of the treatment with either cryosurgery (Chap. 21) or imiquimod [7] and can be divided into acute ones, seen during the treatment, and late ones. From the acute side effects, the major one is the occasional hefty skin inflammation that characteristically peaks the week after cryosurgery. In some cases of exceptionally intense inflammatory responses, flaring up of susceptible skin lesions in rather remote, not directly treated, sites can be observed.

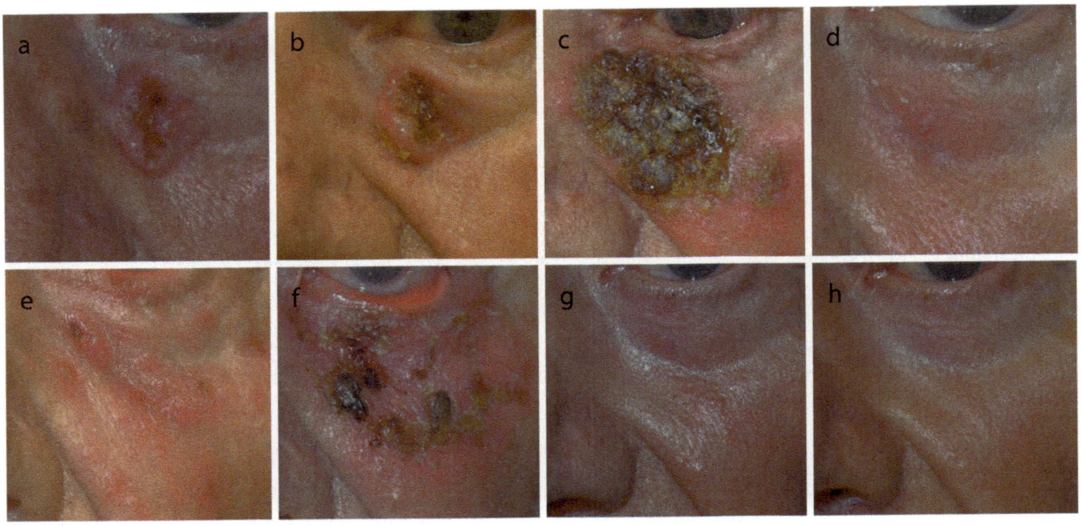

Fig. 20.3 Immunocryosurgery in a large, 17 mm, periocular basal cell carcinoma. (**a**) The tumor at baseline. (**b**) Day 14 of the treatment cycle prior to cryosurgery session (liquid N_2, open spray, 2 freeze-thaw cycles, 15 s each). Please note relatively minimal inflammatory reaction after 2 weeks once daily imiquimod application. (**c**) Day 35. After the cryosurgery session the degree of inflammation was intensified and scabbing is evident. (**d**) 1 month follow-up. Residual tumor is clinically evident and confirmed by biopsy ("partial response"). (**e**) The immunocryosurgery cycle is repeated, and the patient returns after applying imiquimod for 14 days. (**f**) Day 35 of the second cycle: end of treatment. A moderate ectropion is evident; there are no clinical signs of rest tumor ("complete response"); (**g**) 3 months follow-up. The tumor has not relapsed and the ectropion has subsided. (**h**) 12 months follow-up. The tumor has not recurred; no functional sequelae can be observed

Furthermore, in case the tumor is located in the forehead, ears, or around the eyes, the treatment may elicit pain and headache and significant skin and soft-tissue edema. This is more probable to emerge around the middle of the treatment cycle, and in general it progressively subsides towards the end of the treatment cycle, along with the skin inflammation. In a few cases the patient may experience a flu-like syndrome, particularly in the middle of the treatment, i.e., the week after cryosurgery. Almost all patients report tiredness and anorexia that gradually diminishes by the end of treatment.

At the treated sites, hyper- or hypopigmentation may develop, which improves gradually over time. In many cases, a shallow scar is left behind after successful treatment, corresponding to the skin area involved by the growing tumor before treatment ("tumor ghost"). However, the aesthetic outcome is rated as "good" to "excellent" by both patient and physician, for the latter is also compared to that anticipated after surgical treatment. In few patients, a tingling sensation may persist in the treated area for several months after treatment, sometimes with neuropathic character, which however does not interfere with their daily activities [4, 8]. After treatment, the follow-up plan for continuing care is adapted to the initial diagnosis.

The advantages of immunocryosurgery include low cost, easiness of application in the outpatient setting, high efficacy in the indications used, and excellent cosmetic outcome. This is more evident for larger tumors in which the burden of surgery is completely avoided. It can be applied in elderly, multimorbid patients on practically any concurrent medication. Besides optimal cosmesis, a distinctive advantage of immunocryosurgery in contrast to many other nonsurgical therapeutic modalities for skin cancer is that it is not carcinogenic. This side effect is a serious limitation of radiotherapy and potentially also connected to the use of topical antineoplastic agents. Finally, in immunocryosurgery, in contrast to ablative modalities, skin infections are of no concern at the

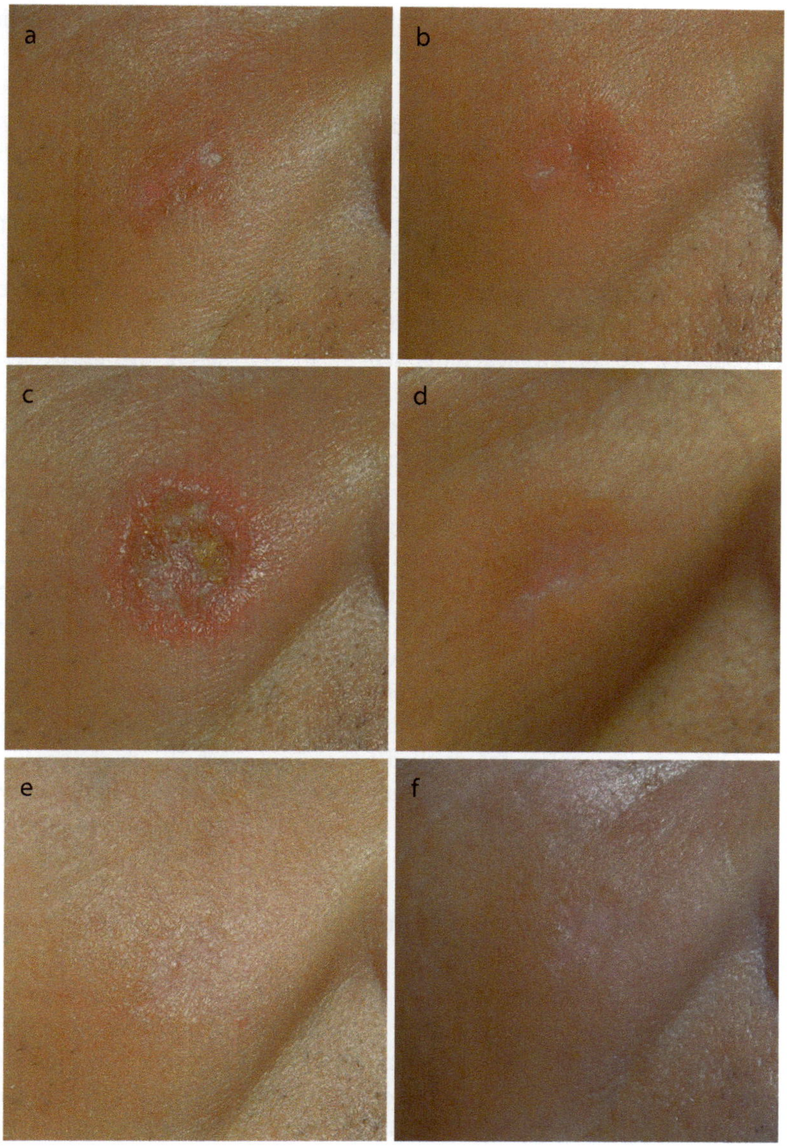

Fig. 20.4 Immunocryosurgery in Bowen's disease of the skin. (**a**) The tumor at baseline; (**b**) Day 14 prior to cryosurgery session (liquid N_2, open spray, 2 freeze-thaw cycles, 15 s each). (**c**) Day 35, end of treatment. (**d**) One month follow-up. A depressed scar is observed. (**e, f**) 12 and 36 months after the end of treatment respectively. The scar has improved and is only slightly obvious

treated sites. Particularly, no case of herpes simplex flare, an important side effect of many other modalities, has been observed.

The main drawback of this modality is the discomfort during treatment and the temporary cosmetic, sometimes also functional embarrassment caused by the inflammation on and around the treated lesion. Patients are encouraged to adhere to treatment by emphasizing the anticipated excellent cosmetic and functional outcome, which are guaranteed by this tissue-sparing modality.

Two special issues that are often encountered during immunocryosurgery and their management are shortly discussed in the following section as a guide to improve the applicability of the treatment in certain cases.

20.2.1 The "Right" Degree of Inflammation

A rather hefty inflammatory reaction of the treated area is generally a hallmark of a successful immunocryosurgery treatment. However, the degree of individual inflammatory reaction to the procedure is unpredictable. Thus, our target is to achieve a sustained inflammatory response that would not be as intense as to deter the patient from therapy. In almost all cases, even in those where the initial 14 days imiquimod course did not provoke a significant degree of local inflammation, this is induced after the cryosurgery session. In the unlikely case of absence of inflammation after cryosurgery, we add a topical retinoid in the treatment schedule (tazarotene or tretinoin once daily in the morning). However, more than absence of inflammation, usually our major concern mostly relates to the occasional immense inflammatory response, especially after the cryosurgery session. In addition, elderly patients are the main target group of this treatment and the treated neoplasm usually lies in photodamaged skin. The free application of imiquimod onto this field will result in areas of extended inflammation. In order to avoid this flair and optimize treatment, detailed instructions of how to control the applied imiquimod quantity per application is mandatory prior and during treatment.

20.2.2 Management of Side Effects

Adherence to instructions is pivotal for the success of immunocryosurgery, as, for example, in the treatment of basal cell carcinoma (BCC), we have observed an increased risk of treatment failure associated with skipping of imiquimod applications for various reasons (misunderstanding, lack of adherence to instructions, etc.), particularly in the last couple of days prior to the cryosurgery sessions. Thus, the key point for the success of the 5-week immunocryosurgery course is the establishment of a caring relationship towards the patient that would strengthen his trust in the physician and support adherence to the treatment. This includes the meticulous discussion of the treatment procedure prior to onset–also with the help of typical case photographs – and the anticipated side effects which constitute part of the treatment's mode of action. Availability of the therapeutic team for extra consultations during the treatment period is essential. All through the treatment period, the patient should be reassured about the temporary nature of the discomfort caused and should be encouraged with the prospect of a favorable outcome with excellent cosmetic results.

In parallel to inflammatory reactions at the site of the treated lesion, usually low-grade systemic symptoms also emerge, which are more intense the week after the cryosurgery and gradually subside during ongoing treatment: low-grade fever in some patients, anorexia, or the feeling of tiredness in most of them, particularly those with larger lesions. As a rule, no antiseptic measures or antiviral medications for infection prophylaxis are required.

20.3 Indications of Immunocryosurgery

Immunocryosurgery is a relatively recent addition to the therapeutic modalities used to treat skin cancer [9], and the spectrum of indications is presently assessed. Immunocryosurgery has been mainly applied to treat skin neoplasms of keratinocytic origin with most experience concentrating in the treatment of BCC. Immunocryosurgery has been used both with primary curative as well as palliative therapeutic intension. Currently, the perspectives of the integration of this modality into treatment protocols for partially responding skin cancer are evaluated (e.g., combination with intralesional bevacizumab [10]). In the following sections, a short review of actual and potential indications of immunocryosurgery is presented (Table 20.1). Special aspects of the use of immunocryosurgery to treat skin lesions at certain anatomical localizations will be separately discussed later in this chapter.

20.3.1 Skin Neoplasms of Epithelial Origin

Histopathological diagnosis, tumor size, and localization are the main neoplasm characteristics that together with the general health status and comorbidities/medications of the patient, frame the optimum treatment plan of an individual

Table 20.1 Indications of immunocryosurgery

1. Skin neoplasms of epithelial origin
(a) Keratinocyte precancer and in situ SCC
(i) Actinic keratoses
(ii) Solar cheilosis (actinic cheilitis)
(iii) Bowen's disease of the skin
(iv) Paget's disease
(v) Keratoacanthoma
(b) Basal cell carcinoma
2. Non-epithelial skin neoplasms
(a) Lentigo maligna and MM
(b) Kaposi sarcoma
(c) Merkel cell carcinoma
3. Benign skin growths and conditions
(a) Genital warts
(b) Pyogenic granuloma
4. Potential applications
(a) Skin metastases
(b) Skin infections
(c) Skin lymphoma
(d) Hypertrophic scars and kelloids

tumor in a certain patient. Especially the value of the precise histopathological diagnosis emerges as a core parameter for the newer modalities, including immunocryosurgery, in the expanding area of nonsurgical therapeutic interventions for malignant skin diseases.

20.3.1.1 Keratinocytic Precancer and In Situ SCC

Treatment outcome of these neoplasms with immunocryosurgery strongly depends on the stage of tumor progression. Overall high cure rates have been achieved with in situ neoplasms; however, the effectiveness against invasive squamous cell carcinomas (SCC) is highly unpredictable. This uncertainty underscores the need for accurate diagnosis.

Actinic Keratoses (AK)

Actinic keratoses can appear as single lesions or involve extensive skin areas (field cancerization) and are amenable to treatment with both cryosurgery and imiquimod [11]. Many authors regard cryosurgery as a first line modality for the treatment of most AK. Immunocryosurgery is highly effective in AK. Due to its vast efficiency and the involvement of large skin areas, we adapted the standard treatment protocol in order to minimize side effects and improve feasibility without reducing efficacy. Imiquimod is applied every other night for 2 weeks, with the patient applying it also the day prior to the cryosurgery session (Fig. 20.1b). Subsequently, mild cryosurgery is applied (open spray, liquid N_2, 2 freeze-thaw cycles of 10 s each effective freezing time), and imiquimod is continued for another week on alternate days on the treated area, starting at the day of cryosurgery, i.e., for additional four times (a total of 11 imiquimod applications). In practice, this is guaranteed by providing the patients with a detailed calendar plan of imiquimod application. The patient is followed up, and treatment is repeated on persisting lesions. As in the case of BCC (see discussion later in this chapter), in the absence of inflammation, a local retinoid can be added as an adjuvant, once daily in the morning for the duration of the treatment.

Solar Cheilosis (Actinic Cheilitis)

A standard immunocryosurgery protocol has been used to treat cases of solar cheilosis (Spyridonos et al. 2014). Data with sufficient follow-up periods ≥1 year are available in 8 patients and demonstrate both feasibility and efficacy of the method. However, lip treatment with immunocryosurgery imparts a significant burden on the patient's quality of life for the duration of treatment as local inflammation can prevent the patient from the consumption of solid food for the remaining period after the cryosurgery session. Based on our current experience, this approach is suggested exclusively for highly motivated patients and only after explicit explanation of the transient, yet significant, burden of the side effects of therapy.

Bowen's Disease of the Skin (BD)

Both cryosurgery and imiquimod are moderately effective modalities for Bowen's disease [12]. However, immunocryosurgery achieves excellent treatment outcomes in this condition (Fig. 20.2a–f) [13]. BD can sometimes be quite extensive or involve difficult-to-treat localizations, like the fingers [14], and immunocryosurgery can offer sufficient field therapy with excellent outcomes in these cases. Relatively small BD lesions are treated with the standard 5-week immunocryosurgery protocol. When larger areas are involved, especially on the head, the diseased area can be treated in subsections of 4–5 cm^2. Monomodal cryosurgery can be employed for small sites of residual disease or recurrences within the treated area (up to 0.5 cm in diameter); for more extensive lesions immunocryosurgery can be repeated. In the literature, there is some concern about the possibility of BD progression to invasive SCC during imiquimod treatment [15]; however, to date such cases have not been observed with immunocryosurgery.

Keratoacanthoma

Immunocryosurgery might offer an efficacious alternative in the treatment of keratoacanthoma. Treatment with add-ins is suggested. Intralesional injection of 5-fluorouracil (50 mg in 1 ml solution) on day 0 followed by subsequent treatment with immunocryosurgery has been quite efficacious in inducing disease involution (unpublished data).

20.3.1.2 Squamous Cell Carcinoma (SCC)

The results of the treatment of squamous cell carcinoma (SCC) with immunocryosurgery are generally disappointing despite protracted and intensive treatment schedules used as palliative therapy in certain cases (unpublished data). In some of these patients, the tumor could be restricted in size; however, early relapses or even relapses under continuing treatment were observed, and thus this modality cannot be recommended for the treatment of SCC. Similar experience with progression of SCC during monomodal imiquimod treatment has been repeatedly reported in the literature [16–19], an additional argument against the use of this modality for SCC. This contrasts initial optimism regarding the use of imiquimod to treat SCC [20–23] and theoretical predictions about targeted imiquimod and cryosurgery actions on SCC [24] and also obviates the central value of clinical trials for the establishment of therapeutic indications. Moreover, the divergence in the susceptibility of basal cell carcinoma (BCC) and SCC to this therapeutic approach underscores the vast differences in biological nature and clinical behavior of these two families of keratinocytic neoplasms, a difference to date largely concealed because of the predominance of the pathophysiologically "indifferent" surgical-ablative approaches for the treatment of these lesions.

20.3.1.3 Basal Cell Carcinoma (BCC)

Locally Confined BCC

To date, most experience with the use of immunocryosurgery is in the treatment of locally confined BCC (Fig. 20.3a–h) [3–5, 8]. With one standard immunocryosurgery cycle, initial tumor clearance can be achieved in up to 97.5 % of unselected BCC with macroscopic diameter ≤2 cm, i.e., for the vast majority (80–90 %) of all BCC at the time of reference for treatment [25, 26]. Treatment is performed as detailed earlier in this chapter, with 15–20 s effective freezing time, and follow-up visits are scheduled at 1, 3, and 6 months after the end of treatment (end of imiquimod application), every 6 months for the rest first 2 years, and yearly thereafter. For comparing effectiveness with other treatment modalities, this single immunocryosurgery cycle can be considered as the equivalent of a conventional surgical excision with at least comparable therapeutic efficiency. In the few cases of incomplete (partial) responses with the repetition of this treatment cycle, tumor clearance is essentially achieved in all cases (>99 %) of primary and relapsed BCC ≤2 cm (Fig. 20.4a–f) [4]. This high clearance rate is coupled by the equally high cure rates with relapse free >97 % of the treated tumors 3 years after treatment. This effectiveness is significantly higher than (a) that reported for either monomodal imiquimod (<65 %; [27]) or cryosurgery (based on common experience probably <50 % for the herein applied treatment parameters; [compare: [28, 29]) and also (b) anticipated for the simple additive action of the two modalities [2]. It is worth noting that the core reasons for the reference of a BCC for Mohs' surgery, i.e., recurrent tumor with poorly defined margins and located in a so-called high risk area [25], are no limitations for the application of immunocryosurgery [4]. Moreover, relapse rate profile compares successfully with corresponding outcomes after conventional surgery, after which relapse rates of 5–10 % are expected during follow-up [30].

Immunocryosurgery for Locally Advanced Tumors

For locally advanced BCC (usually >2 cm in diameter), the effectiveness of a single standard 5-week immunocryosurgery treatment cycle declines with increasing tumor size, and cure rates of about 75 % are achieved for tumors with maximal diameter of 3–5 cm after the first treatment cycle (unpublished data). The only scheme modification for the treatment of larger tumors is the slightly longer cryosurgery freezing cycles (2×20 s). Moreover, cryosurgery is performed in slightly overlapping tumor surface sections of about 2×2 cm that are treated sequentially in a session. One month after the end of treatment, the treated area is examined for BCC remnants, also with the help of explorative biopsies if necessary, and therapy cycles are repeated, if required. Presently, efforts to optimize immunocryosurgery treatment protocols for larger, locally advanced BCC (>2 cm diameter) are under evaluation in our department. The role of extended imiquimod treatment periods, repeated cryosurgery sessions, and the integration of further modalities into the treatment schedule (e.g., the anti-VEGF monoclonal antibody bevacizumab [10]) are in focus.

Multiple BCC

BCC can appear as multiple tumors in elderly patients that have a history of extensive exposure to carcinogenic and/or immunosuppressive agents (i.e., ultraviolet radiation, arsenic, ionizing radiation, solid organ transplant recipients, etc). These patients sometimes present with almost confluent tumors that cover large areas of the skin of the face and build up surgery fields of many centimeters in diameter that involve functionally important structures. Not only concurrent but also relapse tumors present a real challenge for surgery and also for radiotherapy in many of these cases. Immunocryosurgery, as an extremely tissue-sparing modality, is often an ideal choice for patients with numerous synchronous and metachronous tumors that protects them from multiple, sometimes inevitably disfiguring surgical excisions or radiotherapy with important functional sequels [31]. At this point, a special mention of patients with the Gorlin-Golz syndrome is essential. Although we have had no opportunity to treat a patient with the latter condition, we are convinced that this combination will also be effective in patients with this syndrome.

Palliative Therapy for Locally Advanced BCC

There are some BCC patients where a palliative approach is a more realistic treatment target than tumor clearance. Although most cases of BCC, if referred in a timely manner, can be successfully treated, if neglected, severely destructive-invasive advanced BCC may develop. Radical therapeutic methods are not always a realistic goal in these patients. In addition in some other cases despite intense therapeutic efforts, cure of BCC cannot be achieved. All these patients with devastating locally advanced BCC are candidates for palliative interventions, especially for protection of important structures from unrestrained tumor expansion. Conventional modalities are usually less effective in these patients. As most of these tumors are observed in elderly, multimorbid patients, treatment decisions have to be tailored to each patient and the burden of therapy to his overall condition. The advent of the newer targeted pharmacologic modalities may offer a therapeutic option for these patients, especially after multiple surgeries with local flaps or recurrences after radiotherapy. Immunocryosurgery offers a further effective alternative for these patients that, although not generally curative, in most cases can contain the tumor tissue and protect important anatomical structures from destruction. Our main focus in these cases is to concentrate treatment efforts to control the expanded tumor front towards the aforementioned threatened anatomical structures, preserve their functional integrity, and minimize overall tumor load. The use of immunocryosurgery as a potential adjuvant of emerging pharmacologic modalities, like vismodegib, for advanced BCC needs further evaluation.

20.3.2 Non-epithelial Skin Neoplasms

20.3.2.1 Lentigo Maligna and Malignant Melanoma

Lentigo maligna is a melanoma in situ with a 5 % risk of becoming invasive during lifetime, amenable to treatment with imiquimod and cryosurgery [32, 33]. Interestingly, the first published case on immunocryosurgery involved a patient with lentigo maligna [34]. Subsequent use in additional cases has been as rewarding as the first one. After treatment, close follow-up with elective biopsies is recommended until we are certain that we have eradicated the malignant melanocyte nests.

Primary malignant melanomas are not an indication for immunocryosurgery. However, there are two settings in which immunocryosurgery could be an adequate therapeutic alternative in strictly selected cases: (a) after diagnostic excisional tumor biopsy for tumor margins sterilization instead of wide re-excision and (b) as palliative therapy for melanoma skin metastases. In the latter lesions should be treated with extended imiquimod application schemes and repeat cryosurgery sessions every 2 weeks, until the tumors treated have regressed. The induction of an inflammatory response locally in the treatment field seems to be essential for the successful therapy of this condition and should be always provoked, if necessary also with the advent of adequate adjuvant modalities, like topical retinoids ([35, 36]; own unpublished observations). Meticulous follow-up is mandatory and appearance of new lesions or relapses should be promptly treated in order to prevent the development of invasive malignant melanoma.

20.3.2.2 Kaposi Sarcoma

Skin lesions of Kaposi sarcoma respond swiftly to immunocryosurgery sessions. Our experience to date is restricted to cases of classical Kaposi in elderly patients, with most of them under parallel systemic interferon-alpha treatment as well. As the disease can be extensive, we prefer to treat the tumors in skin sections that can be covered by a sachet of 5 % imiquimod, the maximum approved daily dose. In this cohort of patients, not much inflammatory response is observed, yet the outcome is rewarding. Prompt clearing of the treated lesions as opposed to persistence of those awaiting the onset of topical therapy underlines the local impact of immunocryosurgery to the observed treatment outcome.

20.3.2.3 Merkel Cell Carcinoma

Merkel cell carcinoma is a rare skin tumor of elderly individuals characterized by high rates of locoregional recurrences that usually constitute a therapeutic challenge. Recently, we reported the successful treatment of a multinodular *in transit* locoregional Merkel cell carcinoma recurrence in a patient 6 months after surgical excision of the primary tumor [37]. More than 15 cutaneous-subcutaneous metastases responded to the standard 5-week immunocryosurgery courses. Interestingly, a concurrent paraneoplastic arthritis resolved in this patient after treatment of the metastases too.

20.3.2.4 Benign Skin Growths and Conditions

Certain skin conditions are amenable to treatment with a modified immunocryosurgery protocol. Hefty inflammatory responses as those intended in the treatment of BCC are not always observed during the treatment of these lesions.

Genital warts respond swiftly to immunocryosurgery. However, care should be given to contain the inflammatory response which can cause extreme discomfort due to the localization of the lesions. The alternate day scheme described in the AK section (Fig. 20.1b) is also followed in this case. However, for larger, exophytic lesions that do not respond to treatment promptly, we do not interrupt imiquimod application and repeat cryosurgery sessions every 2 weeks, until clinical cure. In this way, we ascertain efficacy and feasibility of treatment. With this method, not only treated warts clear but in many cases involution of remote, not directly treated lesions (e.g., intraanal) has been observed in parallel (unpublished data).

20.3.2.5 Pyogenic Granuloma

The combination of the antiangiogenic effects of imiquimod and cryosurgery is effective in the treatment of pyogenic granuloma. However, the need for repeated sessions of cryosurgery (2 cycles, 10 s each) has been observed. Imiquimod is applied daily and cryosurgery is performed every 2 weeks as needed. Use of imiquimod under occlusion [38] could be an alternative approach to intensify therapy instead of repeat cryosurgery sessions. Outcome is rewarding as no scaring has been recorded; however, we have to be certain of the diagnosis in order to avoid the erroneous treatment of an amelanotic malignant melanoma [39].

20.4 Adaptations for the Treatment in Certain Anatomic Localizations

Successful immunocryosurgery depends on understanding and acceptance of the instructions and adherence of the patient to some simple treatment rules that help her/him understand and manage any, sometimes though temporary, quite hefty side effects. Currently, there is not much experience on the use of imiquimod in relatively "sensitive" areas like the orbit, ear, and the perioral area. Much more this applies to immunocryosurgery. Side effects are expected to be more prominent during treatment cycles that involve these anatomical localizations (periorbital and eyelids, nose, ears, perioral and lips, shins). Localization of a skin lesion in these areas is by no means a contraindication for the treatment with immunocryosurgery [4, 40]. In the following sections, details on the difficulties anticipated in the treatment of tumors in these areas are described, and certain practical rules are discussed to ensure high feasibility of the method in these localizations.

20.4.1 Periorbital Region and Eyelids

The relatively intense conjunctivae congestion that follows imiquimod application and cryosurgery is transient and will abate shortly after stopping therapy. Measures to protect conjunctivae during treatment, like the application of a viscous ophthalmic topical, lessens eye surface irritation and improves acceptability of treatment. Prior to the cryosurgery session, the conjunctivae are anesthetized with local prilocaine (or equivalent) ophthalmic drops and are further protected with the use of an antibiotic ophthalmic ointment. Cryosurgery is performed with protection of the eye surface as required. Treatment of BCC on the eyelids and around them is really rewarding both for the patient and the physician as the functional and aesthetic outcomes is excellent (Fig. 20.4a–f) [40, 41].

20.4.2 Ears

Treatment of lesions on the ear is as rewarding as that of the orbit [31]. For BCC, a standard 5-week immunocryosurgery cycle is usually sufficient to achieve tumor clearance, and in more complicated cases, like extended tumor relapses, treatment can be repeated as required. Standard care measures are taken to protect the acoustic meatus (e.g., with a cotton pledge) as for conventional cryosurgery in this localization.

20.4.3 Nose

This is an area in which immunocryosurgery has a superb outcome, both in curative and cosmetic terms [3, 4, 8, 10, 31]. Actually, a susceptible tumor is removed with the immunocryosurgery in a fashion that we term "scalpel-free Mohs" as what is actually left behind after a successful treatment cycle is merely the "shining ghost" of the previous tumor, i.e., a shallow scar that projects on the skin surface the contours of the area of the dermis that the growing tumor had destroyed. Healing is usually excellent and even large, multiple-confluent and recurrent tumors on the bridge of the nose heal with minimal scaring. In the alae, sometimes a more prominent depressed scar might be visible [4], which however improves significantly through time.

20.4.4 Perioral

As in the case of solar cheilosis, the difficulty in the treatment of lesions close or proximal to the oral cavity stems from the unavoidable implication of the lips during the inflammatory response to immunocryosurgery. This happens as almost all patients have concurrent photodamage and/or solar cheilosis that will flare during treatment leading to extended inflammatory skin fields. Possibly for reasons related to lymph drainage, this is more prominent in tumors involving the upper lip [3]. However, the temporary burden of immunocryosurgery treatment should be weighed against the permanent functional outcomes of an extensive surgical procedure in this area.

20.5 Potential Immunocryosurgery Applications

Based on pathophysiologic considerations (pathophysiology of the lesion, known effectiveness of imiquimod and cryosurgery), immunocryosurgery could be proposed for a series of further indications (Table 20.1). Because of the possibility for considerable burden of local side effects connected to the use of immunocryosurgery, feasibility should be always reviewed before starting any therapeutic attempt. Thus, for example, in the case of infantile hemangiomas, although immunocryosurgery may be a potentially efficacious modality, the feasibility of the treatment in a young patient can be anticipated as quite low. Although we have in much experience in our department with the treatment of infantile hemangiomas with cryosurgery, based on these considerations, we do not recommend immunocryosurgery for this indication.

On the other hand, immunocryosurgery can be proposed for the treatment of skin metastases. Besides skin neoplasms (malignant melanoma, Merkel cell carcinoma) based on their known susceptibility against imiquimod and cryosurgery, metastases from certain other cancer types, particularly renal cell carcinoma and breast cancer, can be evaluated for treatment with immunocryosurgery. Similarly favorable outcomes can be anticipated for specific skin infiltrations from hematologic malignancies. Also in the setting of palliation of huge neoplasms or metastases, e.g., thoracic wall or axilla infiltrations from underlying neoplasms or lymph node metastases, immunocryosurgery (with increased freezing times) has been helpful in certain cases (unpublished data).

Primary skin lymphomas, including infiltrations of mycosis fungoides, certain chronic skin infections (e.g., cutaneous leishmaniasis), and hypertrophic scars and keloids, are further potential indications of immunocryosurgery to be explored in future studies.

Essential Tidbits

- Immunocryosurgery combines the best of both immunomodulation and cryosurgery. This combination enhances the final result compared to either option applied individually.
- The standard 5-week treatment protocol consists of daily topical imiquimod with a session of cryosurgery at the end of the second week (2 freeze-thaw cycle, spraying technique).
- Patients have to be warned beforehand of topical and possible systemic effects of immunocryosurgery.

Conclusions

With meticulous selection of the indications and the adequate guidance of the patient, immunocryosurgery is a powerful and versatile, though simple, method for the stationary and office-based treatment of a series of skin lesions. Proper histopathological diagnosis of the target skin lesion will guide the appropriate application of the method and determine the successful treatment outcome in keratinocytic carcinoma and precancerous lesions, as well as the other indications covered in this chapter. The required training for the physician is minimal and mostly requires overcoming the restrain of the application of cryosurgery on an inflamed by imiquimod skin lesion and subsequently just treating a few patients. The combination can be appraised in the future in lesions that have been shown or are expected to respond either to imiquimod or cryosurgery. Likewise, the combination of immunocryosurgical interventions with the newer hedgehog targeting treatment modalities for BCC will probably be a further fascinating approach.

Glossary

Immunocryosurgery Is a term used to refer to the combination of cryosurgery with topical imiquimod application.

Imiquimod Is a prescription medication, patient applied, that acts as an immune response modifier.

Tazarotene Is a third generation topical retinoid cream.

Bevacizumab Is a monoclonal antibody that inhibits angiogenesis mediated by VEGF-A (vascular endothelial growth factor A).

Synchronous tumors Refer to tumors arising at the same time.

Metachronous tumor Refers to those tumors that appear at different time from the tumor of interest. Multiple, separate, or consecutive tumors.

Gorlin-Golz syndrome Also called nevoid basal cell carcinoma syndrome. It is an autosomal dominant condition involving several body systems. In the skin, patients are prone to develop multiple basal cell carcinomas.

Abbreviations

AK Actinic keratoses
BCC Basal cell carcinoma
BD Bowen's disease
SCC Squamous cell carcinoma

References

1. Bassukas ID, Gaitanis G. Combination of cryosurgery and topical imiquimod: does timing matter for successful immunocryosurgery? Cryobiology. 2009;59: 116–7.
2. Gaitanis G, Bassukas ID. Immunocryosurgery for basal cell carcinoma: an audit for combination, minimally invasive approaches [Internet]. Treatment strategies – dermatology, volume 2, issue 2. c2012. [Cited 2013 Oct 27]. Available from: http://viewer.zmags.com/publication/cd22c9f9#/cd22c9f9/56.
3. Gaitanis G, Nomikos K, Vava E, Alexopoulos EC, Bassukas ID. Immunocryosurgery for basal cell carcinoma: results of a pilot, prospective, open-label study of cryosurgery during continued imiquimod application. J Eur Acad Dermatol Venereol. 2009;23: 1427–31.
4. Gaitanis G, Bassukas ID. Immunocryosurgery for Non-superficial Basal Cell Carcinoma: A Prospective, Open-label Phase III Study for Tumours ≤2 cm in Diameter. Acta Derm Venereol. 2014;94(1):38–44.
5. Gaitanis G, Alexopoulos EC, Bassukas ID. Cryosurgery is more effective in the treatment of primary, non-superficial basal cell carcinomas when applied during and not prior to a five week imiquimod course: a randomized, prospective, open-label study. Eur J Dermatol. 2011;21:952.
6. Knabel P, Cleaver L. Arbor cutis: hyperkeratotic plaque secondary to the use of imiquimod for the treatment of squamous cell carcinoma in situ. Dermatol Surg. 2013;39:655–7.
7. Gollnick H, Barona CG, Frank RG, Ruzicka T, Megahed M, Maus J, Munzel U. Recurrence rate of superficial basal cell carcinoma following treatment with imiquimod 5 % cream: conclusion of a 5-year long-term follow-up study in Europe. Eur J Dermatol. 2008;18:677–82.
8. Nakuçi M, Bassukas ID. Office-based treatment of basal cell carcinoma with immunocryosurgery: feasibility and efficacy. Acta Dermatovenerol Alp Panonica Adriat. 2013;22:35–8.
9. Bader RS, Santacroce L, Diomede L, Kennedy AS. Surgical treatment of basal cell carcinoma [last actualized: 22. Oct 2013]. Available from: http://emedicine.medscape.com/article/27778-overview Accessed 30 Oct 2013.
10. Gaitanis G, Bassukas ID. Intralesional bevacizumab as in-add adjuvant to immunocryosurgery for locally advanced basal cell carcinoma. J Eur Acad Dermatol Venereol. 2013. doi:10.1111/jdv.12327. Published online Nov 29.
11. Nashan D, Meiss F. MüllerM. Therapeutic strategies for actinic keratoses – a systematic review. Eur J Dermatol. 2013;23:14–32.
12. Shimizu I, Cruz A, Chang KH, Dufresne RG. Treatment of squamous cell carcinoma in situ: a review. Dermatol Surg. 2011;37:1394–411.
13. Gaitanis G, Mitsou G, Tsiouri G, Alexis I, Bassukas ID. Cryosurgery during imiquimod cream treatment ("immunocryosurgery") for Bowen's disease of the skin: a case series. Acta Derm Venereol. 2010;90:533–4.
14. Benmously-Mlika R, Hammami-Ghorbel H, Koubaa W, Debbiche A, Mokhtar I. Bowen's disease of the digit successfully treated with immunocryosurgery. Int J Dermatol. 2013;52:514–6.
15. Gong HS, Cho JH, Roh YH, Chung MS, Baek GH. Bone invasion by squamous cell carcinoma in situ (Bowen's disease) of the finger during treatment with imiquimod 5 % cream: case report. J Hand Surg Am. 2010;35:999–1002.
16. Singh S, Bunker CB. Squamous cell carcinoma on the scalp following treatment with 5 % imiquimod cream. Clin Exp Dermatol. 2007;32:594–5.

17. Goh MS. Invasive squamous cell carcinoma after treatment of carcinoma in situ with 5 % imiquimod cream. Australas J Dermatol. 2006;47:186–8.
18. Fernández-Vozmediano J, Armario-Hita J. Infiltrative squamous cell carcinoma on the scalp after treatment with 5 % imiquimod cream. J Am Acad Dermatol. 2005;52:716–7.
19. Matin RN, Gibbon K, Rizvi H, Harwood CA, Cerio R. Cutaneous mucinous carcinoma arising in extramammary Paget disease of the perineum. Am J Dermatopathol. 2011;33:656–7.
20. Hengge UR, Schaller J. Successful treatment of invasive squamous cell carcinoma using topical imiquimod. Arch Dermatol. 2004;140:404–6.
21. Martin-Garcia RF. Imiquimod: an effective alternative for the treatment of invasive cutaneous squamous cell carcinoma. Dermatol Surg. 2005;31:371–4.
22. Flórez A, Feal C, de la Torre C, Cruces M. Invasive squamous cell carcinoma treated with imiquimod 5 % cream. Acta Derm Venereol. 2004;84:227–8.
23. Oster-Schmidt C. Two cases of squamous cell carcinoma treated with topical imiquimod 5 %. J Eur Acad Dermatol Venereol. 2004;18:93–5.
24. Clark RA, Huang SJ, Murphy GF, et al. Human squamous cell carcinomas evade the immune response by down-regulation of vascular E-selectin and recruitment of regulatory T cells. J Exp Med. 2008;205:2221–34.
25. Leibovitch I, Huilgol SC, Selva D, Richards S, Paver R. Basal cell carcinoma treated with Mohs surgery in Australia. I. Experience over 10 years. J Am Acad Dermatol. 2005;53:445–51.
26. Gulleth Y, Goldberg N, Silverman RP, Gastman BR. What is the best surgical margin for a basal cell carcinoma: a meta-analysis of the literature. Plast Reconstr Surg. 2010;126:1222–31.
27. Chitwood K, Etzkorn J, Cohen G. Topical and intralesional treatment of nonmelanoma skin cancer: Efficacy and cost comparisons. Dermatol Surg. 2013;39:1306–16.
28. Kuflik EG. Cryosurgery for skin cancer: 30-year experience and cure rates. Dermatol Surg. 2004;30:297–300.
29. Ng J, Chong A, Foley P. Destructive management of skin cancers in organ transplant recipients. Cancer Treat Res. 2009;146:447–60.
30. Kuijpers DI, Thissen MR, Berretty PJ, Ideler FH, Nelemans PJ, Neumann MH. Surgical excision versus curettage plus cryosurgery in the treatment of basal cell carcinoma. Dermatol Surg. 2007;33:579–87.
31. Gaitanis G, Nomikos K, Vlachos C, Bassukas ID. Immunocryosurgery for patients with therapeutically challenging basal cell carcinomas: report of two representative cases. J Dermatolog Treat. 2012;23: 70–1.
32. McLeod M, Choudhary S, Giannakakis G, Nouri K. Surgical treatments for lentigo maligna: a review. Dermatol Surg. 2011;37:1210–28.
33. Ellis LZ, Cohen JL, High W, Stewart L. Melanoma in situ treated successfully with imiquimod after non-clearance with surgery: review of the literature. Dermatol Surg. 2012;38:937–46.
34. Bassukas ID, Gamvroulia C, Zioga A, Nomikos K, Fotika C. Cryosurgery during topical imiquimod: a successful combination modality for lentigo maligna. Int J Dermatol. 2008;47:519–21.
35. Cotter MA, McKenna JK, Bowen GM. Treatment of lentigo maligna with imiquimod before staged excision. Dermatol Surg. 2008;34:147–51.
36. Hyde MA, Hadley ML, Tristani-Firouzi P, Goldgar D, Bowen GM. A randomized trial of the off-label use of imiquimod 5 % cream with vs without tazaroten, 0.1 %, gel for the treatment of lentigo maligna followed by conservative staged excisions. Arch Dermatol. 2012;148:592–6.
37. Voulgari PV, Gaitanis G, Markatseli TE, Kempf W, Bassukas ID. In transit recurrence of Merkel cell carcinoma associated with polyarthritis, effectively treated with immunocryosurgery. Acta Derm Venereol. 2014. doi:10.2340/00015555-1812. [Epub ahead of print].
38. Georgiou S, Monastirli A, Pasmatzi E, Tsambaos D. Pyogenic granuloma: complete remission under occlusive imiquimod 5 % cream. Clin Exp Dermatol. 2008;33:454–6.
39. Bassukas ID, Kuhnert A, Diepgen TL, Hornstein OP. Clinically relevant differences between amelanotic malignant melanoma and granuloma pyogenicum. Dermatologica. 1991;182(2):81–4.
40. Gaitanis G, Kalogeropoulos C, Bassukas ID. Imiquimod can be combined with cryosurgery (immunocryosurgery) for locally advanced periocular basal cell carcinomas. Br J Ophthalmol. 2011;95: 890–2.
41. Apalla Z, Karteridou A, Lallas A, Tzellos T, Lefaki I, Sotiriou E, et al. Letter: immunocryotherapy for difficult-to-treat basal cell carcinoma of the eyelid. Dermatol Surg. 2013;39:146–7.

Palliative Treatment with Cryosurgery

21

Paola Pasquali

Contents

P. Pasquali, MD
Department of Dermatology, Pius Hospital de Valls, 43800 Tarragona, Spain
e-mail: pasqualipaola@gmail.com

Key Points

- Cryosurgery for palliation is an excellent alternative for the treatment of selected inoperable tumors.
- It is safe and easily performed even in patients who are bedridden or in wheelchairs.
- It can be used in primary skin malignancies or in metastatic tumors.

21.1 Introduction

The goal of cryosurgical palliative treatment is to improve the quality of life of patients who suffer from advanced skin cancer disease. In palliation, to cure is not the ultimate goal although this is sometimes achieved (Fig. 21.1a, b). The aim is to alleviate symptoms and in doing so improve the quality of life. Inoperable tumors can be primary skin malignancies or metastasis from a skin cancer or from an internal malignancy. The objective of palliative care is to prevent or to treat, as early as possible, the symptoms and side effects of the disease and its treatment (painful scars, radiodermatitis, etc.). Not less important are the related psychological, social, and spiritual problems. Palliative care is also called comfort care, supportive care, and symptom management [1].

Since most large inoperable tumor masses are in older patients, it is not infrequent to have other

P. Pasquali (ed.), *Cryosurgery: A Practical Manual*,
DOI 10.1007/978-3-662-43939-5_21, © Springer-Verlag Berlin Heidelberg 2015

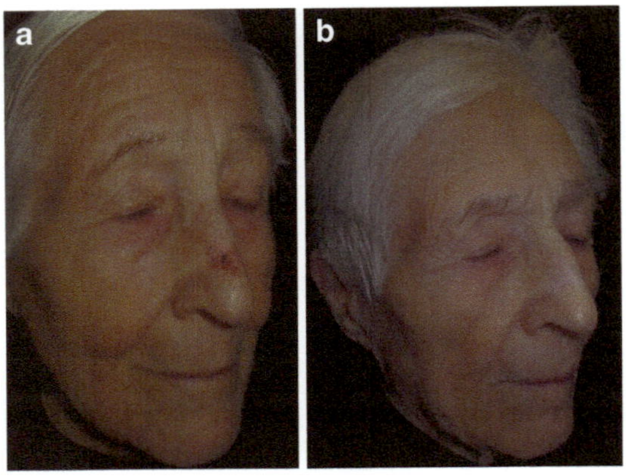

Fig. 21.1 (**a**) A 92-year-old patient with a morpheiform basal cell carcinoma on the nose. The patient did not want Mohs surgery. A double freeze-thaw cycle with open technique (spraying). (**b**) Almost two years later, no recurrence

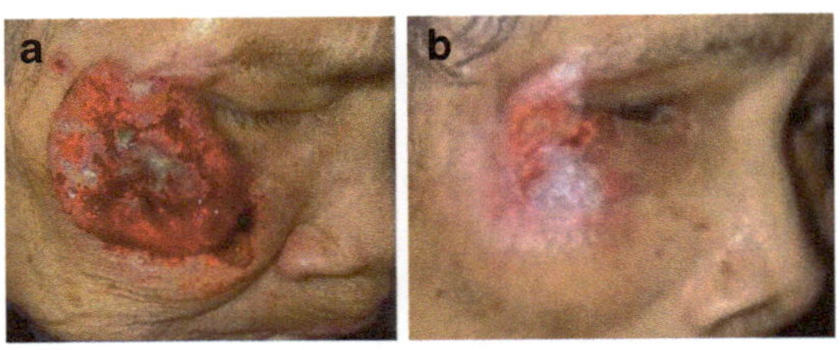

Fig. 21.2 (**a**) Patient with dementia who lived in a nursing home. She presented a poorly differentiated squamous cell carcinoma that bled easily. Double freeze-thaw cycle with semi-open technique (cone) in one session. (**b**) After 2 months, there was tumor left but no bleeding. Cryosurgery was repeated

underlying medical conditions which make alternative forms of therapy difficult or prevent them altogether. Some patients have lost the capacity to make decisions on their own; therefore, treatments have to be discussed with family or other caretakers.

Some tumors are life threatening per se or may be the cause of bothersome symptoms which include oozing, bleeding (Fig. 21.2a, b), pain, foul smell, and functional problems (like tumors located in anatomical areas that prevent the wearing of glasses, the use of hearing aid, the wearing of shoes, etc.). Sometimes tumors may give off unpleasant odors due to superinfection, causing social isolation from family, caretakers, and even pets [2].

More than any other type of surgery, palliative treatment needs to focus on the patient's or the caretaker's expectations. Since suffering is the origin of consultation, reducing it becomes the final goal. False expectations can be a terrible blow even after a successful surgical treatment. Treatment needs to be tailored to the needs and expectations of the patient. Inoperable tumors require multidisciplinary approaches, and the team must include nurses and psychologists/psychiatrists, without losing sight at any moment the cultural aspects of the individual.

Most patients have gone through numerous surgeries, radiotherapy, and chemotherapy. Some are tired of treatments that have left them weaker, and others are just not willing to go through them for any number of reasons.

Cryosurgery stands as an excellent alternative [3, 4] that can be used alone or in combination with other treatment modalities [5]. It is safe and easily performed on bedridden patients or patients constrained to a wheelchair. One session is usually sufficient. This aspect is one of the strong points in favor of cryosurgery: the reduction of the need to move the patient from one place to another for numerous sessions (as required in radiotherapy).

21.2 When

Palliative treatment with cryosurgery is proposed when [6] (Table 21.1):

- The patient's underlying medical conditions are too risky for alternative therapies: this includes serious illnesses such as heart disease, chronic obstructive pulmonary disease, emphysema, kidney disease, or diabetes. Surgery of a large tumor in a patient with an underlying heart condition or coagulopathy can be a threat to his/her life.
- Patients with underlying mental conditions that make surgical management or radiotherapy difficult (Fig. 21.3a, b).
- The proposed alternative treatments are disfiguring and not accepted by the patient and/or family/caretakers (Fig. 21.4a, b).
- The tumor(s) has/have not responded to other treatments, such as chemotherapy, radiotherapy, surgical treatment.

Table 21.1 Summary of the most frequent conditions under which palliation can be considered in order to alleviate symptoms

Related to the tumor
An actively growing tumor that could reach vital structures around the tumor
Pressure of the tumor on nearby structures producing discomfort and the need to assume antalgic positions
Pain caused by local destruction and disfigurement
Episodes of bleeding/oozing/secretions which tend to weaken the patient, stain clothing, require constant change of gauze, and risk bacterial infection
Infection of an exposed tumoral mass. Foul smell caused by local infection which can be severe and affect patient and caretakers. The impact on caretakers can in turn impact the patient's well-being
Related to the patient
The patient's underlying medical conditions are too risky for alternative therapies
Patients with underlying mental conditions make other therapeutic treatments difficult
The proposed alternative treatments are disfiguring and not accepted by the patient
Lack of response to other treatment modalities
The secondary effects of other treatments are not accepted by the patient
Patients refuse other treatment alternatives out of fear or due to advanced age
Related to the social environment
Not feasible to transfer the patient one or more times to obtain treatment in other centers

- The secondary effects of other treatments are not accepted by the patient and/or caretakers.
- Patients refuse other treatment alternatives out of fear, due to advanced age, or because of the impossibility or difficulty of transferring the patient from one center to another.

21.3 How

21.3.1 Spray or Open Technique

Spraying or open technique is probably the most utilized mode used to treat a large tumoral mass. Most palliative treatments are performed on protruding masses of irregular surface. Curetting down (debulking) is recommended [7] but is not always possible because it increases the risk of bleeding since most of these tumors are per se vascularized.

Spraying with large opening tips (0.8–1.0 mm) should be done from the center of the mass, allowing the freezing front to advance gradually toward the base of the tumor and expanding 0.5 cm or more toward the periphery. Depending on the size of the tumor, thawing can take a long time (over 30 min). Freezing should be repeated at least two times.

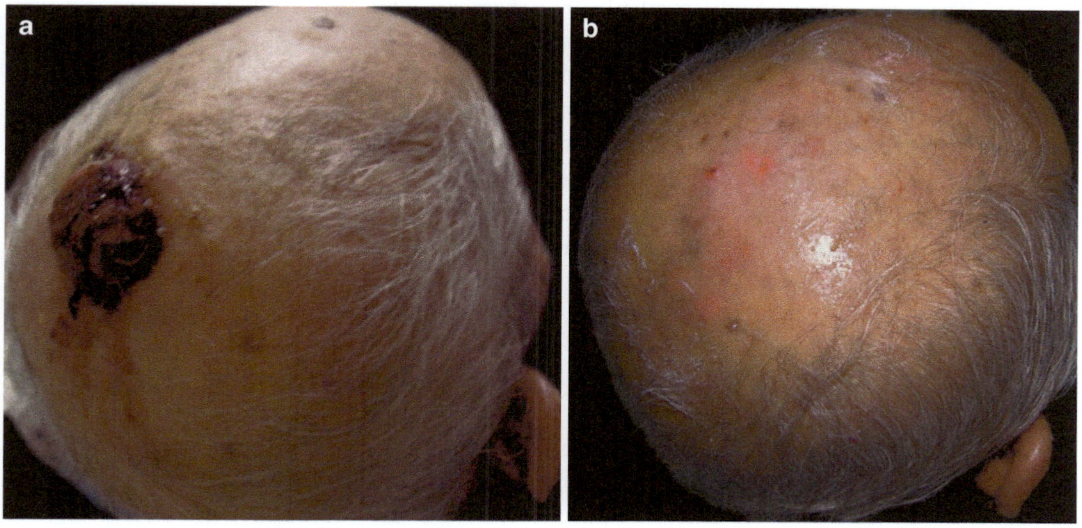

Fig. 21.3 Patient in a nursing home with Alzheimer and confined to a wheelchair. (**a**) Large bleeding squamous cell carcinoma on the head which was treated in one session with a double freeze-thaw cycle semi-open technique (rubber cone) while sitting in a wheelchair. (**b**) One month after treatment. No recurrence 6 months later

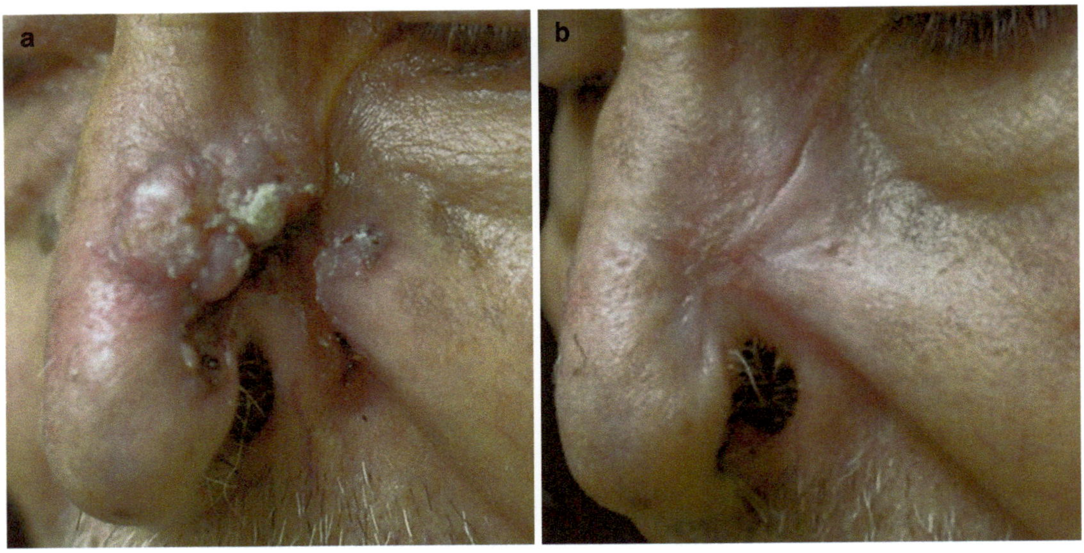

Fig. 21.4 (a) Patient with a destructive basal cell carcinoma on the nose. He refused any other treatment modality. One session treatment with a double freeze-thaw cycle with open technique (spraying). (b) Five weeks later

Allow for the complete postoperative process to occur and then repeat treatment over areas with residual tumor [8].

21.3.2 Semi-open or Cone Technique

Rubber cones are very useful to circumscribe freezing. They are commercially available in different sizes, up to 38 mm. The idea is to include the tumor and up to a 1 cm margin and spray the tumor until the whole area is frozen. The cone has to adhere to the skin surface in order to avoid liquid nitrogen (LN) leakage from the sides. Temperature at the margin should be on the order of −50 °C. A double freeze-thaw cycle is required.

21.3.3 Probe or Close Technique

The use of probe in palliative treatment is reserved for those large tumors that do not have an irregular surface or can be safely scraped down to the base. The size of the probe has to fit the size of the tumor. The use of probes in palliative cryosurgery is usually reserved for segmental cryosurgery (see discussion later in this chapter) or in relative small and multiple skin metastases.

21.3.4 Cryochamber or Semi-close Technique

In small to medium metastatic tumors, cryochambers work very well. They generate a very potent freezing in a short time. Their only limitation is size: one needs to have the chamber that corresponds to the size of the tumor. It has to fit completely in the chamber, and the base must rest firmly on the skin surface, without leaving spaces in order to avoid LN leakage.

21.3.5 Intralesional Technique

Large masses can be treated using the intralesional technique. This has the advantage that the freezing front expands from the center toward the periphery reducing the total time and guarantying freezing of the whole tumor. The needle needs to be located in place with ultrasound guidance, and it is better if placed slightly off-center in order to freeze the desired margin (Figs. 21.5a–c and 21.6a–d).

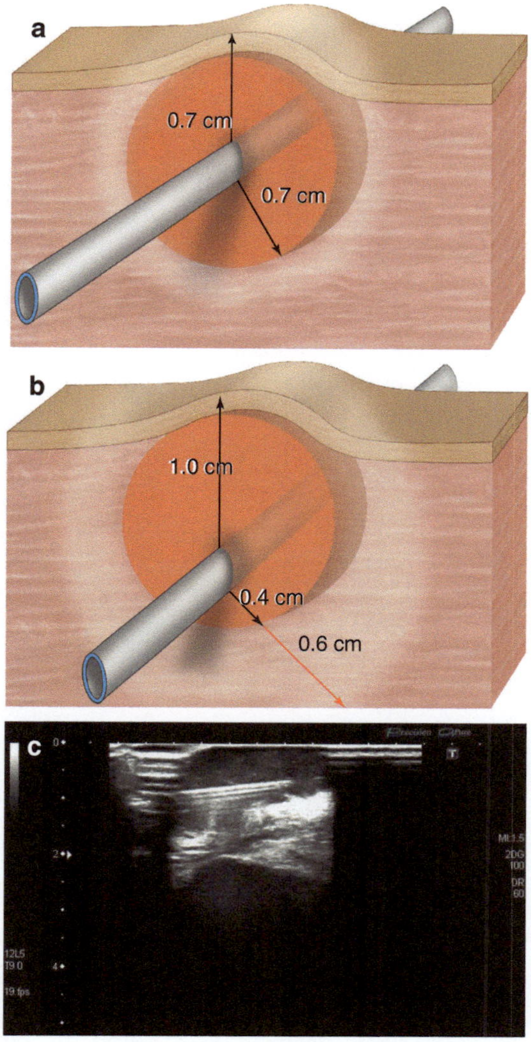

Fig. 21.5 (**a**) By placing the needle in the center, the freezing front will expand symmetrically. Once the surface of the tumor is frozen, the surgeon knows the whole tumor is frozen but has no way of knowing how much of the depth margin has reached the desired temperature. (**b**) By placing the needle via ultrasound guidance off-center, when the freezing front has reached the surface and the desired temperature is reached, the desired temperature is also achieved in the safety margin depth. (**c**) Off centered needle placement shown by ultrasound for tumor on patient on Fig. 21.6

21.4 Techniques

For large tumoral masses (over 3–4 cm), freezing from the center outward will cause an excess freezing of the center while still not reaching the periphery of the tumor. For a tumor of 7 cm of length, freezing the entire tumoral mass plus a 1 cm safety margin will cause destruction of underlying structures.

There are two possible techniques that can be used: segmental and fractional technique (Fig. 21.7a, b).

21.4.1 Segmental Technique (Fig. 21.7a)

Originally described by Zacarian, it consists of dividing a large tumor by imaginary lines and freeze each sector separately, allowing the freezing fronts to overlap at the periphery until the whole tumor is covered [9] (Fig. 21.8a–f).

It is a technique that can also be used in large benign superficial tumors (such as large lentigines or seborrheic keratosis) in which case freezing is done by segments but superficially.

In large and shallow tumors, it is necessary to measure by HFUS (high-frequency ultrasound) the depth over the entire surface of the tumor. HFUS will give information regarding depth for tumors of less than 0.8 cm. In large and deep tumors, US with Doppler will give information on depth, presence of large vessels, and proximity to high-risk structures. Once established that the whole tumor has approximately the same depth, draw, with a presurgical marker pen, dividing lines and create as many sectors as needed. Larger tumors will need to be divided into a larger number of sectors. Start freezing each sector just as it would be done for an individual tumor [10]. Overlapping of margins will occur, and no sector should be left untreated.

It is a technique ideal for large and relatively shallow tumors.

21.4.2 Fractional Technique (Fig. 21.7b)

First described by Gonçalves [11, 12], it is a technique developed for large and deep tumoral masses. It is performed in stages (Fig. 21.9a–d). First, the center of the lesion is frozen (by spraying technique; these large tumoral masses seldom have flat surfaces to which a probe can be applied). Once the center of the tumor is destroyed and healing takes place, there will be a central retraction of

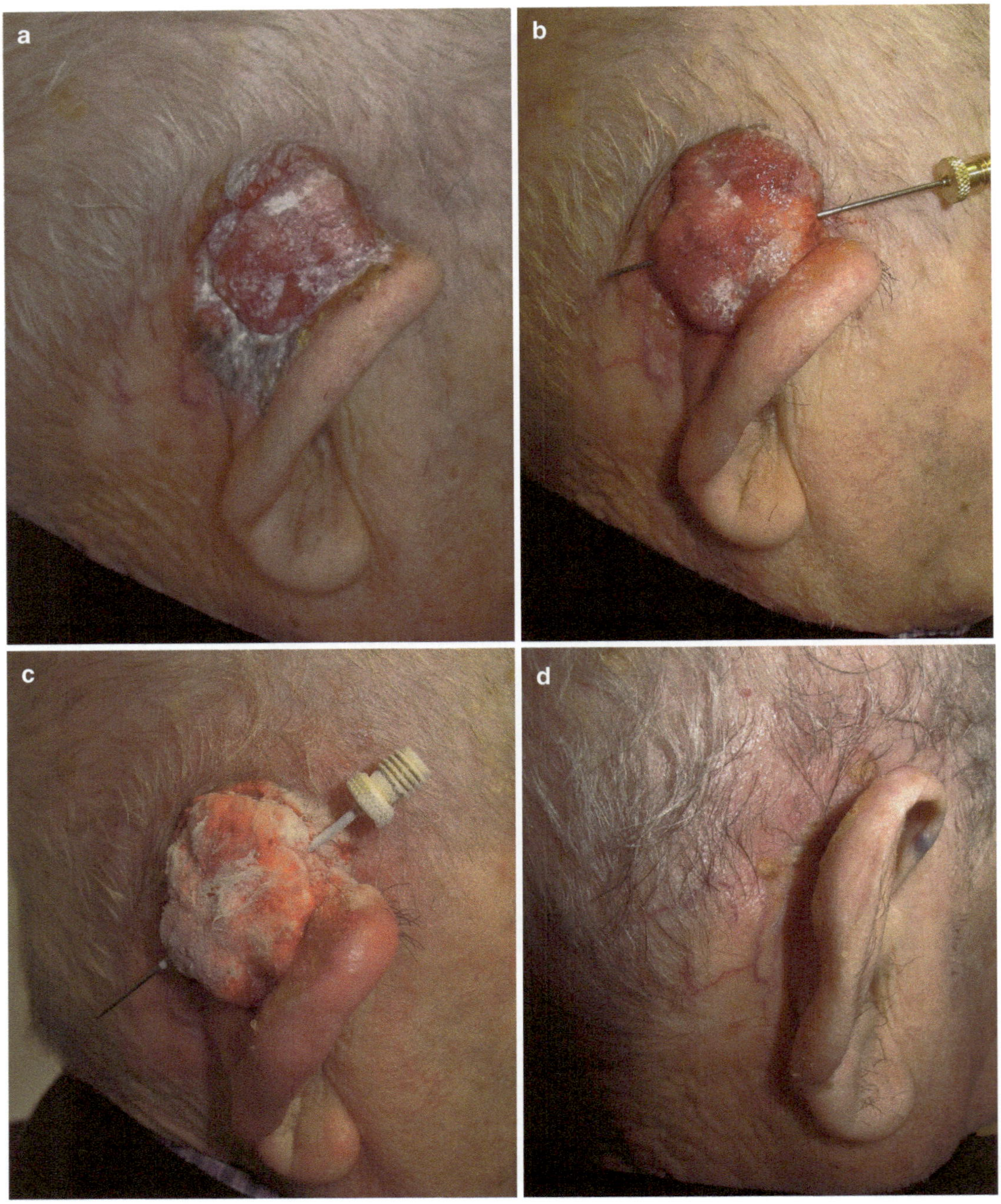

Fig. 21.6 (**a**) Patient with a severe heart condition connected to a portable oxygen device with a rapidly growing squamous cell carcinoma that caused pain and difficulty in the use of the oxygen mask and glasses. (**b**) The needle had been placed off-center with ultrasound guidance as shown in Fig. 21.5. (**c**) The tumor was treated with double freeze-thaw cycles of intralesional cryosurgery under local anesthesia, with the patient sitting in his wheelchair. (**d**) 2 months postoperative

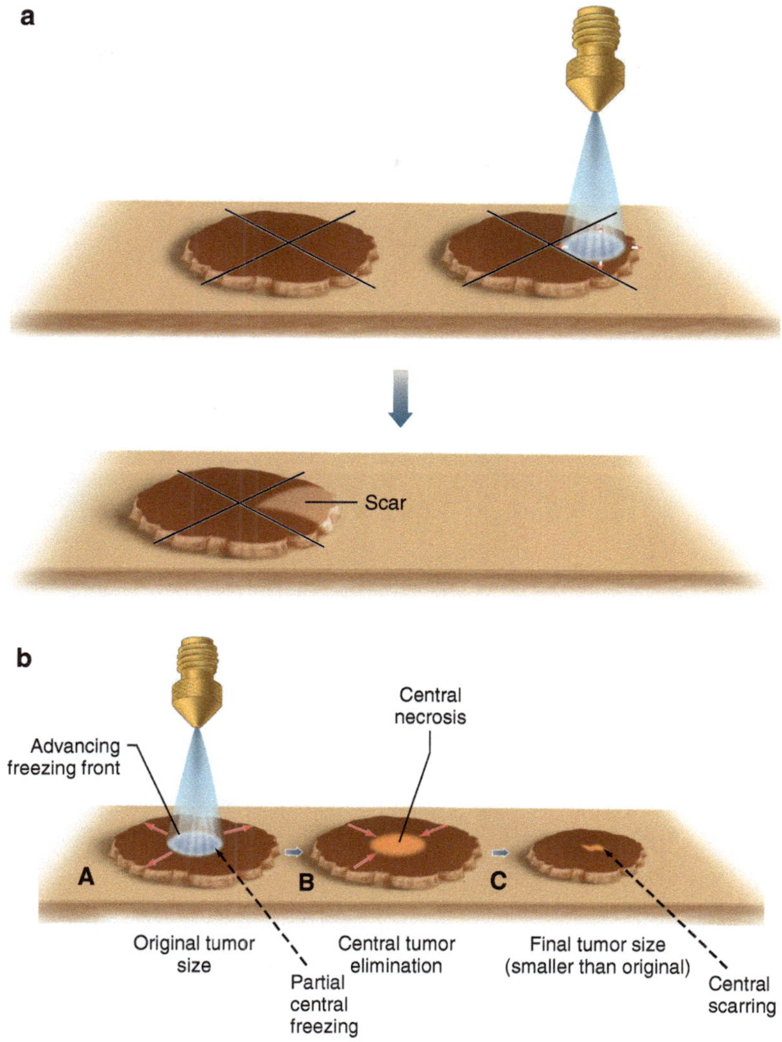

Fig. 21.7 (**a**) Segmental technique: the tumor is divided with imaginary lines and each segment is frozen separately overlapping the margins. (**b**) Fractional cryosurgery. The tumor is first treated in the centre, allowed to heal. The remaining tumor will be smaller than the original. If it is still too large, the fractional procedure can be repeated

the tumor and consequently a reduction in the diameter of the whole tumor. The procedure can be repeated as necessary until the tumor diameter is small enough to be treated entirely in one session with a standard cryosurgical procedure. For large and deep tumors, the final scar will correspond to the size of the lesion preceding the last cryosurgical procedure (Fig. 21.10a, b).

21.4.3 Postoperative Care

Palliative cryosurgery tends to be on large tumoral masses or on small metastatic lesions; the expected secondary effect will be proportional to the time, depth, and volume treated.

The expected time of final healing will be different from one anatomical area to another with the face healing faster and the legs healing slower. Oozing takes longer for deep freezing procedures than for superficial ones. Warn both patient and caretaker of the need to change dressings two to three times a day during the period of severe oozing. A weekly evaluation to check on the healing is recommended. Weekly necrectomy (eschar debridement) helps speed healing and reduces the chances of bacterial infection.

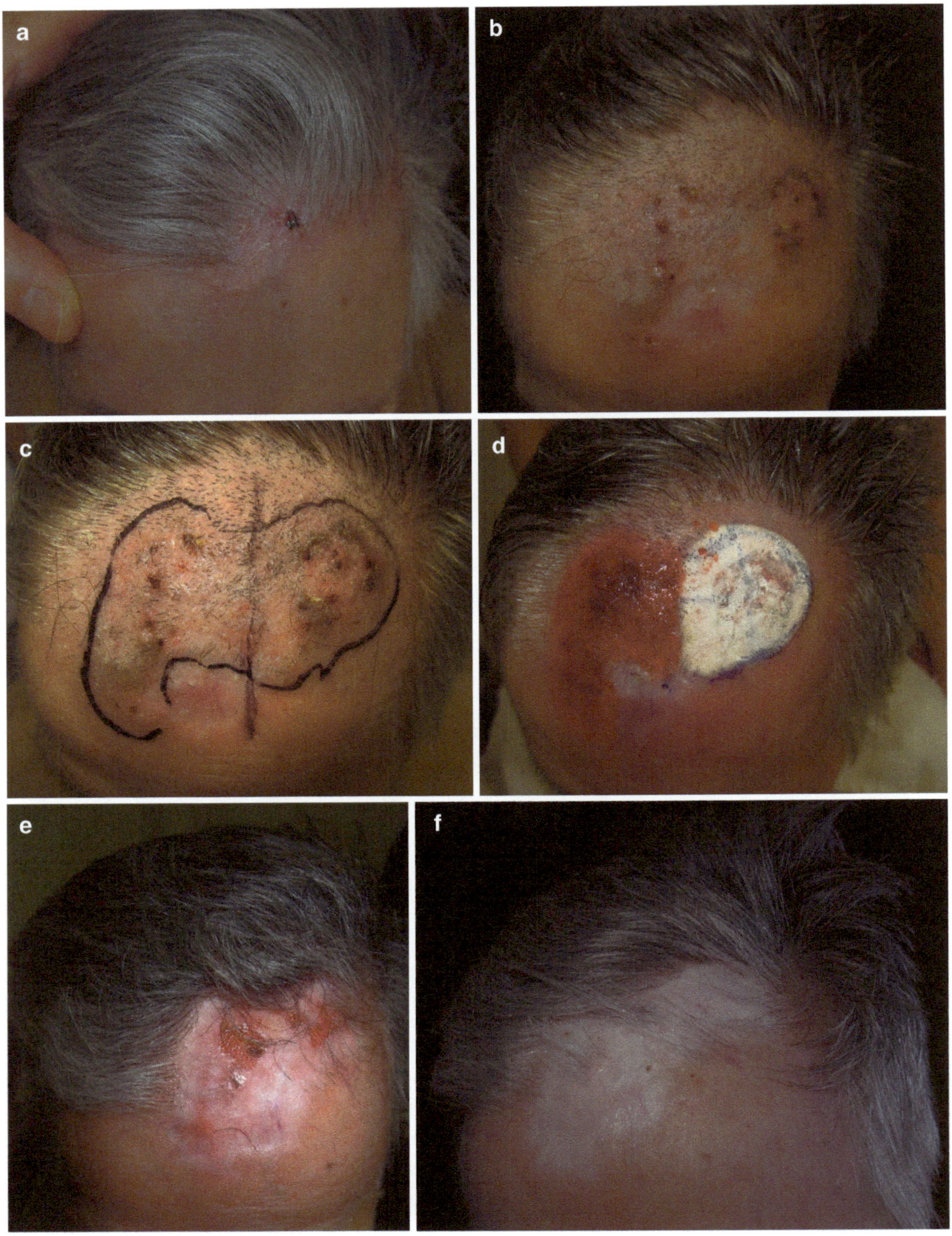

Fig. 21.8 (**a**) Superficial basal cell carcinoma. The first treatment included exclusively the visible area not covered by hair. (**b**) After shaving the head, a tumor of over 10 cm is shown. (**c**) The tumor was divided into sectors for segmental cryosurgery. (**d**) Double freeze-thaw cycle with open or spraying technique was performed on the entire tumor in one session. (**e**) Follow-up 3 months later. (**f**) Control at 2 years. No recurrence

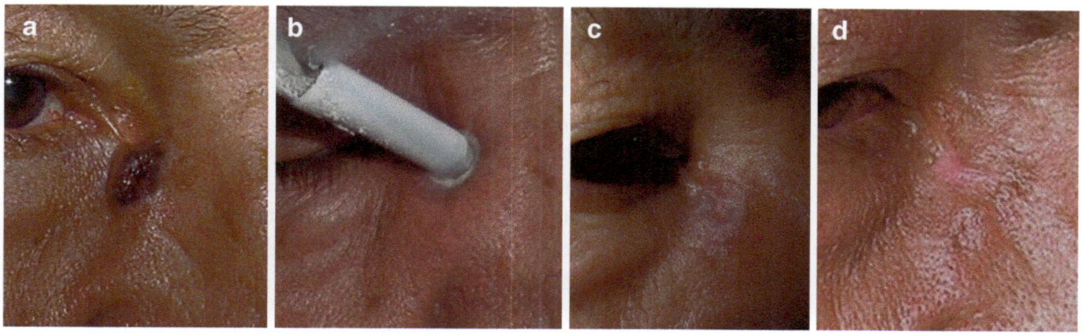

Fig. 21.9 (**a**) Curative fractional cryosurgery was performed on a 1 cm pigmented BCC in a patient with type IV skin. (**b**) Freezing was done with contact (5 mm probe) cryosurgery (double cycle) in the center of the lesion. (**c**) After complete healing from the first cryosurgery, a second cryosurgery of the remaining tumor was performed with a round 4 mm probe. (**d**) End result a year later

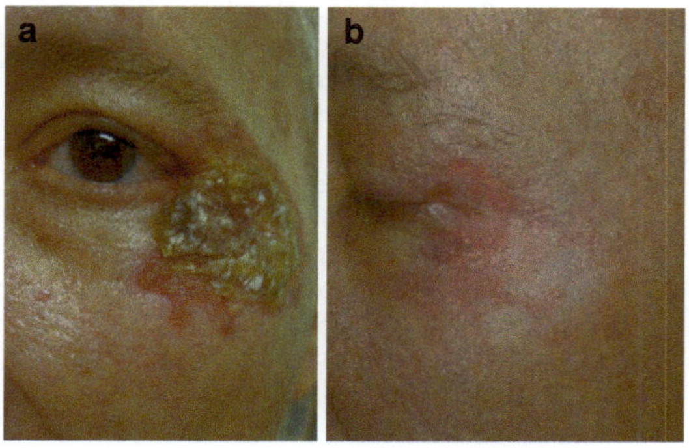

Fig. 21.10 (**a**) A large basosquamous tumor at the outer angle of the left eye in a patient who refused surgery. A fractional cryosurgery was performed: first stage, double cycle, on the center of the lesion; second stage, remainder of the tumor. (**b**) Result after 9 months

Essential Tidbits

- The purpose of the treatment should be made clear to the patient and/or to the family in order to avoid false expectations.
- Make sure the patient can count on someone for local care (a family member, a nurse).
- Close follow-up is important for necretomies: suggest the most appropriate dressing for each stage of healing and help the patient/caregiver decide when to repeat treatment if necessary.

Conclusions

Cryosurgical palliative treatment stands as an excellent treatment modality [13]. It is easy to perform and can be performed even on bedridden patients or on those constrained to wheelchairs. There are no special contraindications besides the ones already known for any cryosurgical procedure. These treatments can be performed under local anesthesia.

They can be repeated as many times as needed and have the advantage that for certain tumors one session can be sufficient to obtain the desired results. This latter point is important considering that many older patients have difficulties being transferred from their home/nursing home to the hospital.

The postoperative healing is the sole drawback because it takes time, but it is not painful. It will require daily cleaning and a nurse or a relative must be available to perform it. A regular visit is convenient for eschar debridement.

Glossary

Palliative surgery Is a treatment when cure is not the ultimate goal. It is performed to assuage pain or discomfort in an effort to improve the quality of life in patients who suffer from advanced cancer disease.

Segmental cryosurgery Is a procedure by which large tumors are divided by sectors and cryosurgery is applied on each sector separately. It is used for large tumors.

Fractional cryosurgery Is a staged procedure where a large tumor is treated in the center and allowed to heal. During follow-up procedures, the tumor will be smaller thanks to the retraction caused by the central scar. It is used for large tumors.

Eschar Slough or a piece of dead tissue that is cast off from the surface of the skin after a burn injury or cryosurgical procedure

References

1. Palliative care in cancer. National Cancer Institute from National Institutes of Helath. Weblog. [Online] Available from: http://www.cancer.gov/cancertopics/factsheet/Support/palliative-care [Accessed 1 Dec 2013].
2. Figueroa G. Bioethics of Sigmund Freud's death: euthanasia or appropriation? Rev Med Chil. 2011;139(4):529–34. [Article in Spanish].
3. Jaramillo-Ayerbe F. Cryosurgery in difficult to treat basal cell carcinoma. Int J Dermatol. 2000;39(3): 223–9.
4. Gage AA. Cryosurgery of advanced tumors. Clin Dermatol. 1990;8(1):86–95.
5. Ruiz Santiago H, Morales-Burgos A. Cryosurgery as adjuvant to Mohs micrographic surgery in the management of subungual squamous cell carcinoma. Dermatol Surg. 2011;37(2):256–8.
6. Pasquali P. Cryosurgical palliation for advanced malignancies. In: Dyall-Smith D, Marks R, editors. Dermatology at the millennium. New York: Parthenon Publishing Group; 1999. p. 564–5.
7. Goncalves JC, Martins C. Debulking skin cancers with radio frequency before cryosurgery. Dermatol Surg. 1997;23:253–6; discussion 256–7.
8. Scala M, Gipponi M, Queirolo P, Mereu P, Solari N, Monteghirfo S, Cafiero F. Cryosurgery for advanced malignant melanoma of the facial skin. A case report. In Vivo. 2006;20(1):153–6.
9. Zacarian SA. Cryosurgery in the treatment of skin cancer. In: Friedman RJ, Rigel DS, Kopf AW, editors. Cancer in the skin. Philadelphia: WB Saunders; 1991. p. 451–65.
10. Graham GF. Cryosurgery in the management of cutaneous malignancies. Clin Dermatol. 2001;19(3):321–7.
11. Goncalves JC. Fractional cryosurgery. A new technique for basal cell carcinomas of the eyelids and periorbital area. Dermatol Surg. 1997;23:475–81.
12. Gonçalves JC. Fractional cryosurgery for skin cancer. Dermatol Surg. 2009;35(11):1788–96.
13. Kuflik EG. Cryosurgery for palliation. J Dermatol Surg Oncol. 1985;11(9):867–9.

Part V

Post-operative Care/Management and Future Considerations

Post-operative Care for Cryosurgery

22

Paola Pasquali

Contents

P. Pasquali, MD
Department of Dermatology, Pius Hospital de Valls, 43800 Tarragona, Spain
e-mail: pasqualipaola@gmail.com

Key Points

- Cryosurgery is a quick surgical technique with a relatively long healing process.
- The cosmetic outcome depends on following the correct instructions during the post-surgery period.
- Hypo- or hyperpigmentation and scarring tend to improve with time.

22.1 Introduction

For a surgical procedure, the post-operative wound care period is the final step of a sequence of numerous steps that need to be taken to guarantee the best results. It is the part of the process that requires the direct participation of the patient or caretaker. In cryosurgery, this is much more so the case because healing occurs by secondary intention. Wound caring will be more laborious and take a longer period of time when compared to standard surgical procedures. Patients need to know from the beginning that cryosurgery is a quick procedure with a long post-operative period, while surgery is a long procedure with a fast healing period. It is a trade-off.

Cryosurgical post-operative events can be spectacular and somehow alarming for someone not accustomed to it. Warnings are never enough when dealing with probe treatment of a large vascular lesion or the palliative treatment of a malignancy. In general, patients and/or caretakers

P. Pasquali (ed.), *Cryosurgery: A Practical Manual*,
DOI 10.1007/978-3-662-43939-5_22, © Springer-Verlag Berlin Heidelberg 2015

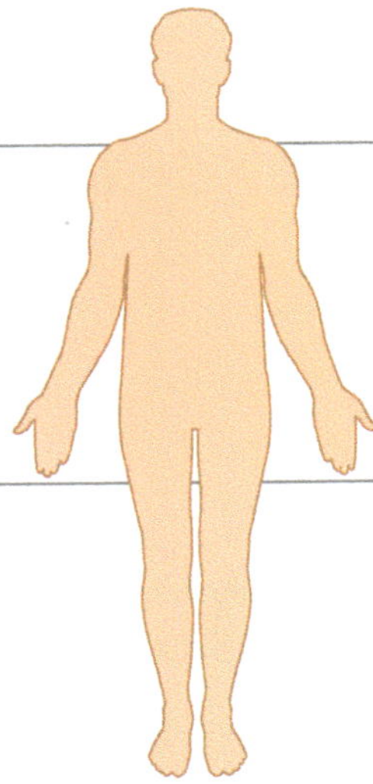

Anatomical site	Superficial	Deep	Except
	5-7	5-14	Earlobes take longer than other areas of face
	2-3 weeks	Up to 1 months	Genital area heals very fast (faster than the face)
	4-6 weeks	Over two months	Post varicose trophic changes of the skin cause even longer healing times

Fig. 22.1 Approximate healing times in relation to anatomical areas

are not familiar with the cryosurgical post-operative process; this can include many nurses and doctors. The time spent explaining what to expect and how to deal with every event as well as providing written take-home instructions is the best investment to help reduce anguish and unnecessary phone calls. It is also important to be available, personally or through a trained assistant, in case sudden unexpected events occur: knowledge of such support helps reassure patients.

Healing time will depend on many factors, the most important ones being depth of freezing and anatomical site. As a rule of thumb, superficial freezing heals faster, and deep freezing take longer; for the same type of freezing procedure, treatments of the face heal faster, while in the legs they take the longest. An approximate table of the timings is shown in Fig. 22.1. Each procedure has to be explained to avoid false expectations; for instance, a patient who has had previous cryosurgery of the face needs to know that cryosurgery of the back will take longer to heal.

The most commonly expected events are:

Immediate Events

- Transient erythema
- Discomfort/pain
- Evanescent wheals
- Oedema

Events After 24–48 h

- Bulla formation
- Exudation

Late Events

- Mummification/crust formation
- Healing
- Post-operative redness
- Hyper-/hypopigmentation
- Pseudoepitheliomatous hyperplasia

22.2 Immediate Events

Immediate events are those that begin with the procedure and will occur in the presence of the operator. They include erythema, discomfort/pain, and oedema.

22.2.1 Transient Erythema (Fig. 22.2)

As soon as the skin is frozen, it looks white. With thawing, redness appears. Intensity of freezing, skin colour, location, and cold sensitivity are

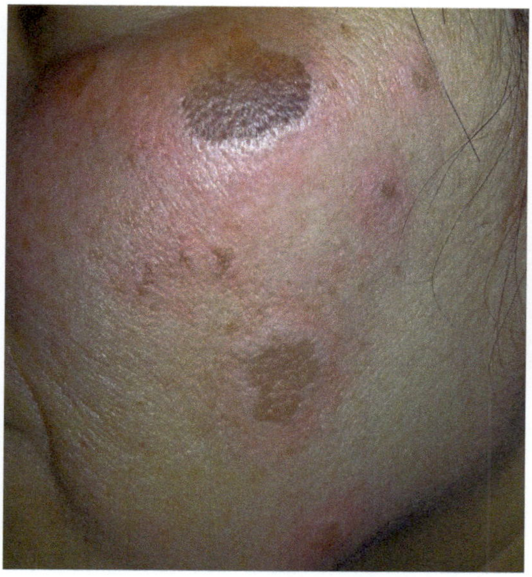

Fig. 22.2 Immediate redness after a cryosurgical spraying of lentigines solaris

some of the features that will determine the local redness.

Redness can appear immediately and last a few days. It is more obvious in fair skin and infants. It can last from several hours up to several days, depending on the depth of the procedure. For procedures of the face, make sure your patient knows about this redness: some patients feel a sudden concern about the way they will look immediately after leaving the office.

22.2.2 Discomfort/Pain

The sensation of cold is followed by discomfort and, with sufficient freezing, pain. Superficial freezing tends to be well tolerated by most people. Freezing has an anaesthetic effect. This allows multiple superficial treatments in one session or a cryobiopsy (Chap. 7). Even probe treatment in haemangiomas, which lasts a few seconds, is well tolerated by most children. Freezing larger lesions hurts more than several small ones. Face lesions tend to be very well tolerated, while scalp or earlobe lesions tend to be more painful; periungual and perianal treatments can be painful as well.

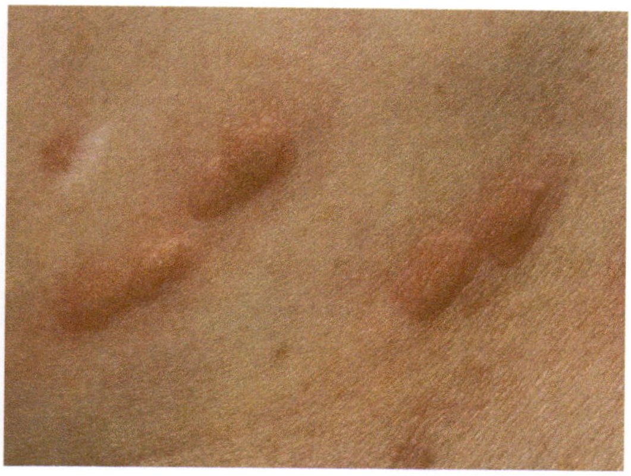

Fig. 22.3 Transient wheals immediately after cryospraying

Freezing of lesions in the temples or the scalp in general can cause a strong headache in certain patients. This pain can last 30 min or more. In general, pain sensation relates to freezing depth and freezing time, anatomical location, cultural background, and gender [1].

While freezing gives a discomfort sensation, thawing can be quite painful. In thawing, oedema sets in the nerves and gives a painful sensation. This is the reason why a patient seems to have tolerated the freezing procedure relatively well and suddenly has a painful sensation that takes seconds but can be quite annoying. Let patients sit and wait through it in order to avoid syncope or a vasovagal reaction.

Certain areas are more sensitive than others and certain patients are more sensitive in general. There are cultural differences in pain perception. Children are surprising: some are very scared just by the presence of a physician, while others will be still and quiet during a cryosurgical session.

22.2.3 Evanescent Wheals (Fig. 22.3)

Some patients present wheals immediately after freezing. These wheals include the lesion in the central area and extend a few millimetres outwardly, giving an impression of a raised lesion above the skin surface. They tend to disappear in the subsequent 2 h.

Giménez-Arnau et al. [2] have proposed the term ultra-freeze urticaria to describe an acquired localized cold urticaria in patients who develop wheals and erythema within 5–10 min of the procedure. Their group of patients presented negative standardized tests for classical cold urticaria and positive skin pathology changes of urticaria. They propose further studies to help recognize this subset of patients as well as using liquid nitrogen (LN) as a potential new tool to diagnose cold contact urticaria.

22.2.4 Oedema (Fig. 22.4)

Oedema is an expected secondary effect of cryosurgery. It directly relates to depth of freezing, skin type, age, and anatomical area differences. An 80-year-old Caucasian patient treated with a close technique in the eyelids will probably have significant oedema compared to a 30-year-old patient with Fitzpatrick skin type 3 with the same procedure done in the arm.

This can appear a few seconds after the procedure or make itself obvious gradually as time passes, reaching a maximum 24 h after the procedure. Facial oedema tends to be worse in the morning and lessen in the afternoon. It is not pain related. No matter how swollen it looks, no pain is associated with it. Warning patients of this will reduce anxiety and the number of follow-up phone calls. In areas close to orifices (e.g. nostrils, mouth, and eyelids), the oedema can be annoying, and special precautions should be taken for lesions treated in the oral mucosa. Oral anti-inflammatory drugs such as steroids are of little use.

22.3 Events After 24–48 Hours

These include bulla formation and exudation.

22.3.1 Bulla Formation (Fig. 22.5)

Bulla formation can occur 1–3 days after the procedure. If the lesion was previously curettaged, the blister can have a bloody exudate. The blister can break spontaneously or can be removed to hasten healing. There are two conditions where blisters should not be removed: in vascular tumours and in keloids. In the first, removing the blister can expose small vessels and this can cause bleeding. In the second case, it can stimulate further keloid formation.

22.3.2 Exudation

Exudation starts with rupture of the bulla/blister. It can last from a few days up to a week or more, depending on the depth of freezing and the anatomical area. Large exudates require continuous change of gauze. While exudation occurs, there is no risk of infection.

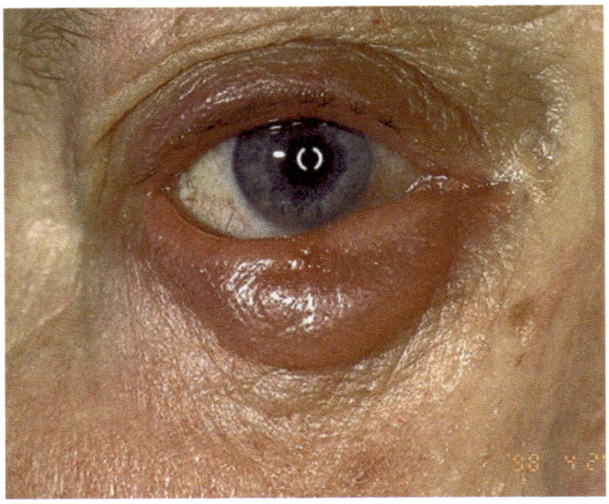

Fig. 22.4 Oedema in an area treated with cryospray

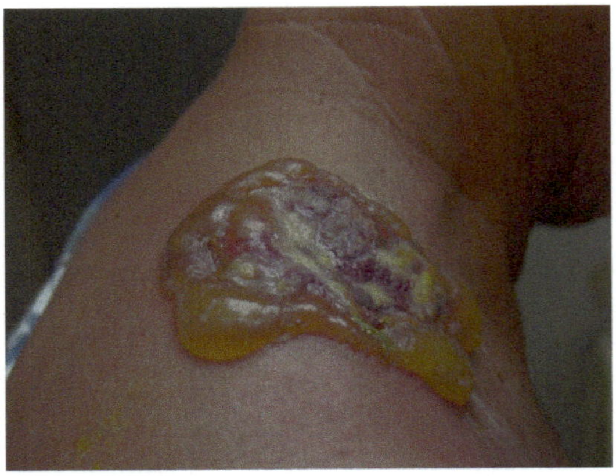

Fig. 22.5 Huge blister on the shoulder after a deep spraying of a large basal cell carcinoma (BCC)

22.4 Late Events

These include: mummification, healing, post-operative redness, hyper-/hypopigmentation, and pseudoepitheliomatous hyperplasia.

22.4.1 Mummification (Fig. 22.6)

Mummification with crust formation begins when exudation is minimal. Some cryosurgeons like to remove scabs on skin cancer lesions in order to reduce the chance of infection. Once the scab is removed, topical antibiotics or hydrocolloid dressing can speed healing. Other cryosurgeons prefer to leave the scab on.

During this period of crust formation, the wound may get infected if not properly cleaned. The first sign of alarm is the reappearance of redness and pain. Pus can be hiding under the crust.

22.4.2 Healing

Healing starts once all the tissue that has been destroyed is sloughed away. It is a delicate part of the entire process, and following the correct procedure will guarantee a good cosmetic result. After a cryosurgical procedure, the fibrous network is preserved; therefore, healing tends to leave excellent cosmetic results.

22.4.3 Post-operative Redness (Fig. 22.7)

Once the crust has fallen off, the treated area will look slightly pink. In sun-exposed areas, sun protection is of extreme importance in order to avoid hyperpigmentation. This redness is site dependent: in the face it can last a few days, while in the dorsum of the hands (i.e. lentigines treated with cryosurgery), it can last up to 3–4 weeks. It fades out with time. No treatment is required besides sun protection.

22.4.4 Hyperpigmentation (Fig. 22.8)/ Hypopigmentation (Fig. 22.9)

Once the redness has disappeared, hyper- or hypopigmentation may remain. If freezing was superficial, as in the case of benign lesions, this hypopigmentation will last just a few weeks and then improve until normal pigmentation is re-established. In deep freezing, such as for skin cancer or haemangiomas, this hypopigmentation tends to last years. In some patients, hypopigmentation can be permanent. In darker skin colours, hypopigmentation is more obvious. In sun-damaged skin, hypopigmentation is more the result of a contrast between a newly formed skin and the dyschromia caused by sun exposure. With time, the "new" skin tends to pigment due to sun exposure and the difference is less obvious.

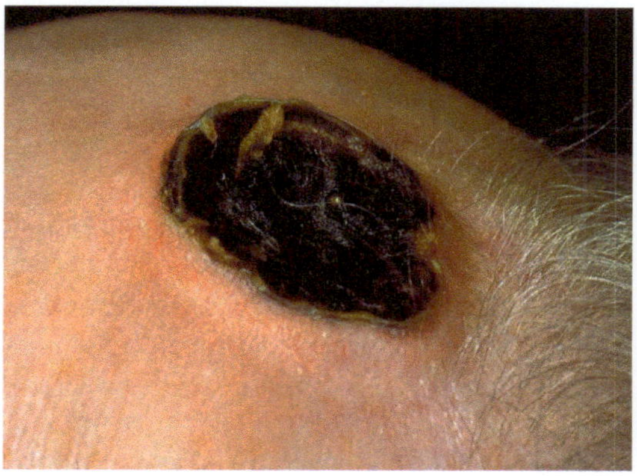

Fig. 22.6 Crust formation after a probe cryosurgery for a BCC on the scalp

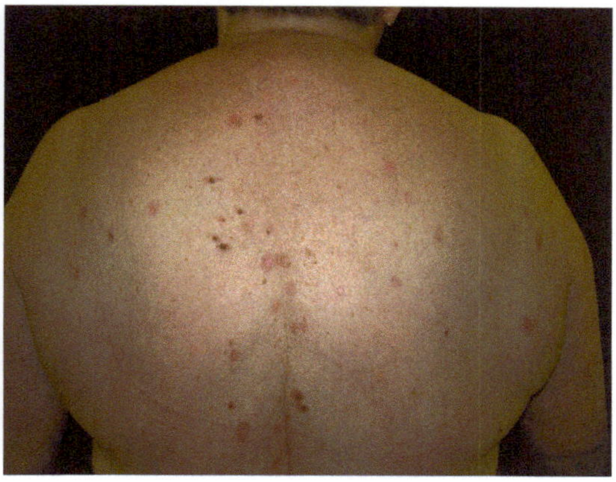

Fig. 22.7 Redness of lesions after crust detachment

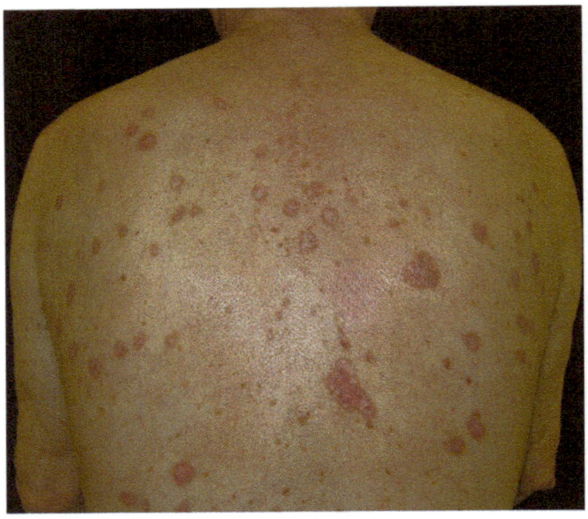

Fig. 22.8 Transient postcryosurgical hyperpigmentation

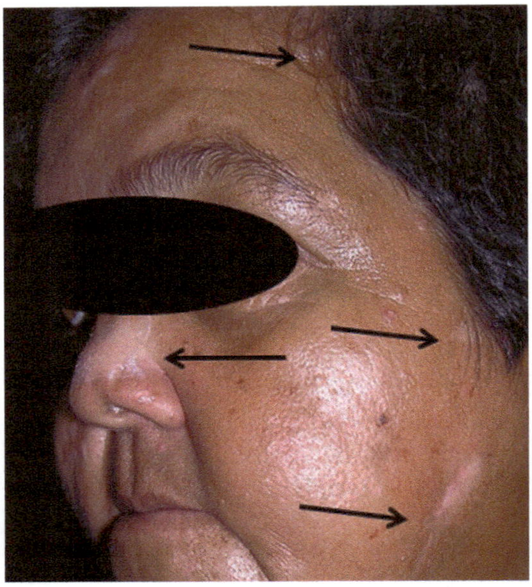

Fig. 22.9 Residual hypopigmentation (shown by *arrows*) after deep cryosurgical treatment of multiple BCCs in a skin type 4 patient with Gorlin syndrome

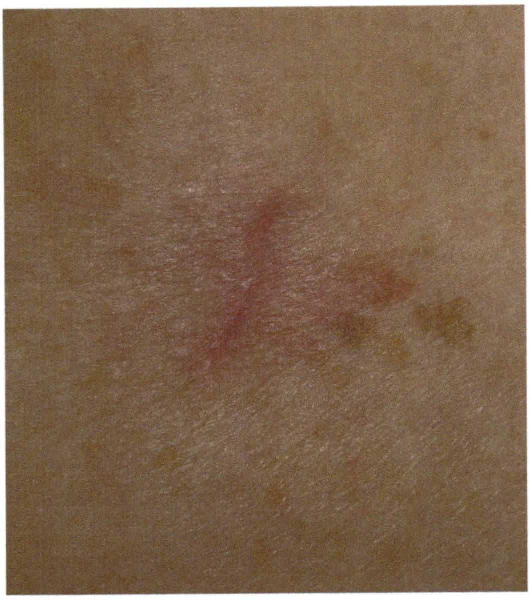

Fig. 22.10 A typical pseudoepitheliomatous hyperplasia after a cryosurgical procedure

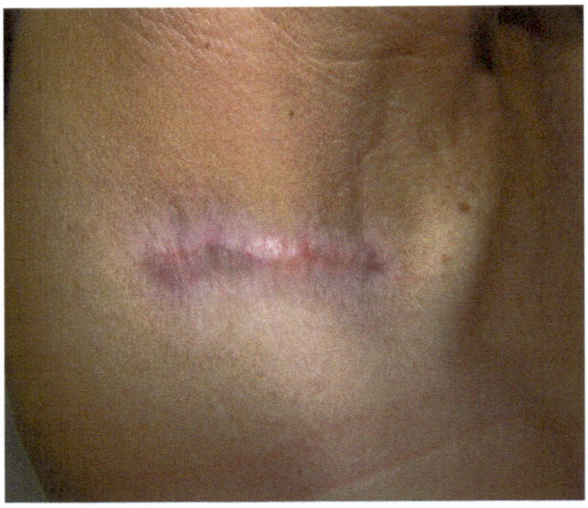

Fig. 22.11 The pseudoepitheliomatous hyperplasia on the cryosurgical procedure of patient from Fig. 22.5

22.4.5 Pseudoepitheliomatous Hyperplasia (Figs. 22.10 and 22.11)

Pseudoepitheliomatous hyperplasia is a benign condition characterized by hyperplasia of the epidermis and adnexal epithelium, and it presents in conditions characterized by a prolonged inflammation [3]. It is a secondary effect expected with deep freezing. It does not require treatment and disappears spontaneously after a few months.

Essential Tidbits

- Cryosurgery takes longer to heal than standard surgery because healing is by second intention.
- The further away from the head, the longer it will take to heal.
- Give careful oral and written instructions.
- Bullae can be removed; necrectomies in skin cancer might hasten healing and reduce the possibility of secondary infections.
- Pseudoepitheliomatous hyperplasia does not require any treatment. It disappears spontaneously with time.
- Pigmentation changes can improve with time.

Conclusions

Despite how complicated this post-operative process may seem, instructions are very simple to follow. For superficial cryosurgery, washing the area with water and soap is sufficient; for deep freezing, besides the washing, covering the area with gauze will be required to contain oozing. Eventually, some antibiotic ointment when mummification begins will help avoid heavy crust formation and prevent bacterial infection. Bacterial infection occurs rarely but is possible when deep freezing has been carried out and proper cleaning procedures were not applied. The reappearance of local pain several days or weeks after cryosurgery may suggest secondary bacterial infection.

Glossary

Mummification Refers to the process of shrivelling and drying up.

Pseudoepitheliomatous hyperplasia Is a histopathological reaction pattern rather than a disease sui generis that occurs in response to chronic irritation including cryosurgery.

References

1. Poziomczyk CS, Köche B, Dornelles Mde A, Dornelles SI. Pain evaluation in the cryosurgery of actinic keratoses. An Bras Dermatol. 2011;86(4): 645–50. [Article in English, Portuguese].
2. Giménez-Arnau A, Ali Al-Haqan E, Sacrista M, Curto L, Pujol RM. Ultra-freeze induced cold contact wheals during cryosurgery: an uncommon subset of acquired cold contact urticaria. Eur J Dermatol. 2013;23(5):694–9.
3. Zayour M, Lazova R. Pseudoepitheliomatous hyperplasia: a review. Am J Dermatopathol. 2011;33(2): 112–22.

Pitfalls and Their Management in Cryosurgery

23

Paola Pasquali and Raimo Suhonen

Contents

P. Pasquali, MD (✉)
Department of Dermatology, Pius Hospital de Valls, 43800 Tarragona, Spain
e-mail: pasqualipaola@gmail.com

R. Suhonen, MD, PhD
Department of Dermatology, Ikioma Medical Center, Kalevankatu 22, Mikkeli FI 50100, Finland
e-mail: raimos@iki.fi

Key Points

- In cryosurgery, the expected postsurgical events can be understood as pitfalls. The drawn line between the two might not be clear-cut.
- Severe post-cryosurgical events can be pitfalls and can occur if a patient's skin type, a patient's age, the anatomical area of the lesion, and the presence of a previously damaged tissue are not taken into account.
- There are pitfalls that are not specific to cryosurgery but can occur in all surgical procedures; examples of these are syncope, bleeding, and infection.

23.1 Introduction

Pitfalls can occur during or after a cryosurgical procedure just as in any other surgical technique. They are unfortunate events that have to be differentiated from expected occurrences. For instance, edema is an expected occurrence, but a paraphimosis caused by severe edema is a complication. Most postoperative cryosurgical sequelae are temporary; however, occasionally permanent damage can be caused. Pitfalls can be attributed to a cryosurgical procedure done inappropriately; other pitfalls can be attributed to a correct technique used in the wrong anatomical area or lesion. Problems can occur during the

P. Pasquali (ed.), *Cryosurgery: A Practical Manual*,
DOI 10.1007/978-3-662-43939-5_23,

procedure, immediately thereafter, or as late events.

Cryosurgical equipment is commonly available; such equipment is low cost when compared to lasers. The ease with which they are put into operation together with the lack of formal training has enabled an indiscriminate use without a proper patient selection or appropriate operator training [1].

All expected occurrences need to be discussed previously with patients. Lack of proper information can turn an expected event into a complication; if patients are aware of the intensity of inflammation and oozing, the less alarmed he/she will become when these occur. This will translate into fewer trips to the emergency room where staff not used to seeing such reactions may take incorrect measures. Forewarning patients and family with oral and written instructions will reduce alarm and help them recognize real pitfalls.

A complete medical history will help to rule out cold-sensitive individuals. Cold-associated diseases like cryoglobulinemia, Raynaud's disease, cryofibrinogenemia, cold urticaria, and general cold intolerance should preclude the use of cryosurgery [2, 3].

Cryosurgeons should be aware of reactions of the same procedure in different anatomical areas [4], in different skin types, and in different age groups. This makes the boundary between an expected side effect and a complication a blurred one sometimes. In fact, some authors consider that morbidity and side effects cannot always be treated as separate entities in cryosurgery [5]. Although this view is shared, we have preferred to separate out the complications and discuss them in a different chapter in order to emphasize those situations that should be considered as real pitfalls here and give some tips on how to manage them.

23.2 Common Pitfalls

23.2.1 LN Spattering

Occasionally, LN spatters during spraying if the releasing end is frosted. This causes a slightly burning sensation and superficial spot freezing wherever LN touches unprotected skin. If the operator notices such a situation, the procedure should be stopped at once and the equipment left to thaw completely. Another possible incident is inadvertently freezing the patient or another person (even the operator) from the released end of the hose (attached to probes or cryochambers). Care should be taken to grab the hose and begin freezing until this stays frozen firmly in place (Fig. 23.1).

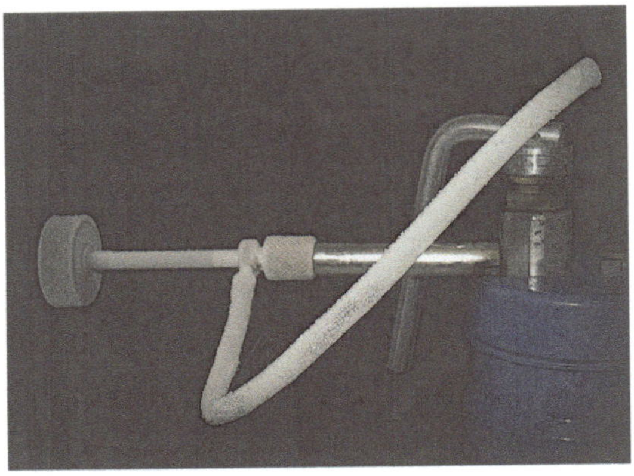

Fig. 23.1 Freeze the hose before the procedure or grab it in your hands until frozen in order to avoid freezing the patient or nearby personnel

23.2.2 Edema as Complication

Edema following cryosurgery is en expected event. There are several factors relevant to predicting its severity: (1) individual susceptibility, (2) age, (3) anatomical location, and (4) skin type. Special care should be taken in certain areas. One example is the penile foreskin: if there is a need to treat multiple lesions (i.e., condyloma) or one large plaque (i.e., Bowen's disease), it should be done by sectors, one side at a time, to avoid severe edema that might cause paraphimosis in uncircumcised males. This iatrogenic entrapment of the penis can become a urological emergency. To avoid this potential complication, it is best to plan the procedure in several sessions.

Care should also be taken to remove rings (like wedding rings) if treating lesions in fingers (like warts or myxoid cysts). The presence of the ring can cause a tourniquet effect when the

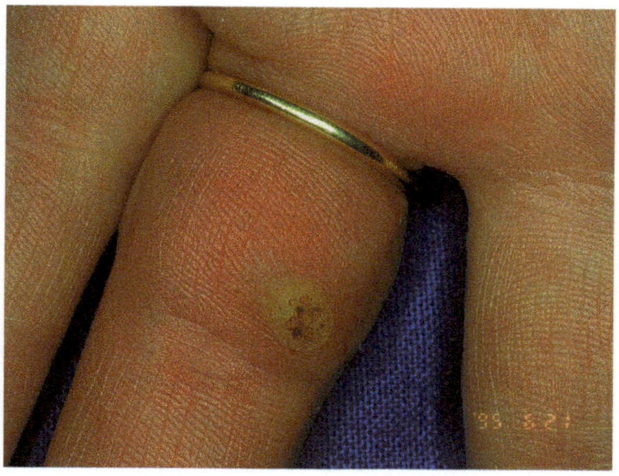

Fig. 23.2 Remove rings before freezing to avoid tourniquet effect

finger becomes edematous after a cryosurgical procedure on a finger (Fig. 23.2). Post-cryosurgical edema responds very little to steroid medication; therefore, precautions should be taken in advance.

23.2.3 Bleeding

In deep freezing or in previously curetted areas, bleeding can be a possible complication. Sometimes it can be a consequence of an underlying medical condition [6]. Once a lesion is curetted or shaved (for skin biopsy), small vessels are exposed. Topical hemostatic treatments are mandatory before freezing to avoid blood splashing (if spraying technique is going to be used) or blood contact with the probe and eventual sticking to the surface. Even when these precautions are taken, vessels dilate with thawing and occasionally bleed profusely immediately after complete thawing. One common mistake is to cover the treated area when it is still frozen and send the patient home without checking on possible post-thawing bleeding. It is thus essential that proper hemostasis be performed.

In deep freezing such as in skin cancers or vascular tumors, thick scabs can form which occasionally maintain small vessels from bleeding. Once removed (either intentionally or by accident), these vessels can start bleeding. In most cases, this bleeding is superficial and easily controlled just by pressing with gauze over the area; however, occasional profuse bleeding occurs. This is the reason why crust removal should be avoided on vascular tumors. For other lesions, it should be performed by someone with experience and the capacity to stop an eventual bleed. Hemostatic solution can suffice but occasionally electrocoagulation or even ligation of the vessel with a suture is required.

23.2.4 Pain and Syncope

Cryosurgery can cause pain. The degree of pain will depend on personal sensitivity to cold, personal pain threshold, skin type, depth of freezing, and previous pain experiences. Superficial freezing is anesthetic; as freezing continues, so does discomfort and eventually pain. During thawing pain is usually more intense than during freezing due to edema on nerve endings. This delay in the pain sensation has to be kept in mind in order to avoid having the patient leave the office before it commences; otherwise, there is a risk of feeling an unexpected (for the patient) pain sensation and the risk of syncope.

Syncope is not an exclusive event of a cryosurgical procedure: in fact, it can occur in certain patients who move too quickly from lying to standing position, particularly if he/she has been tense during the lying position. This can be avoided by changing position very slowly and allowing a few minutes between lying, sitting, and standing.

Pain sensation of cryosurgical procedures in the temple, parietal, or even frontal regions can cause headaches that last from minutes to hours and can be intense particularly in deep freezing.

23.2.5 Insufflation of Subcutaneous Tissue

A previous curettage or draining of a cystic lesion can leave an opening in the skin and exposure of subcutaneous tissue. If an open cryosurgery is performed, LN can be insufflating inside the tissue. Crepitance can be felt (heard and/or palpated). It is usually not painful nor poses any danger to the patient. It reabsorbs spontaneously. To avoid it, either probe freeze or restrain the LN with a firmly placed cone.

23.2.6 Permanent Changes in Pigmentation

Depending on the skin type and the anatomical area and the depth of the procedure, cryosurgery can leave transient or permanent discoloration of the skin. Hypopigmentation is the most common color change and it is usually temporal. However, hypopigmentation can be permanent, especially when treating skin cancers or in superficial freezing in sun-exposed areas (Fig. 23.3). The latter occurs because skin reepithelialization occurs with preservation of the original skin color which contrasts with the pigmented sun-damaged skin, which is usually discolored. The newly regenerated skin looks hypopigmented in comparison to the surrounding skin. This should be explained previously to the patient in order to avoid false expectations. Hypopigmentation can occasionally repigment in the center (Fig. 23.4) and gradually extend toward the periphery. In skin types 3 or more, light freezing can be the cause of hyperpigmentation which occasionally improves with time (Fig. 23.5). For cosmetic procedures (like in lentigines), treat a hidden area first and wait a few weeks to see the result before attempting to treat large areas. Treatment of skin cancer in very visible areas (like the nose) should be avoided in darker skin types.

23.2.7 Retraction Caused by Freezing Next to Orifices

Secondary healing in the lower lid (Figs. 23.6a–c and 23.7) or next to the nostrils can cause ectropion or nostril notch. Retraction can improve with time. Whenever a tumor has destroyed part of the tissue matrix, then a nonaesthetic scar is inevitable (Fig. 23.8a, b). A presurgical photograph is of utmost importance as presurgical graphic record of the area; the patient should have realistic expectations of the cosmetic outcome.

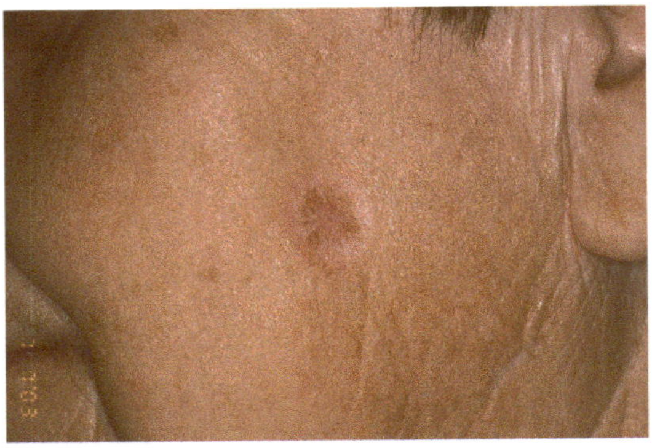

Fig. 23.4 Hypopigmentation can occasionally repigment in the center

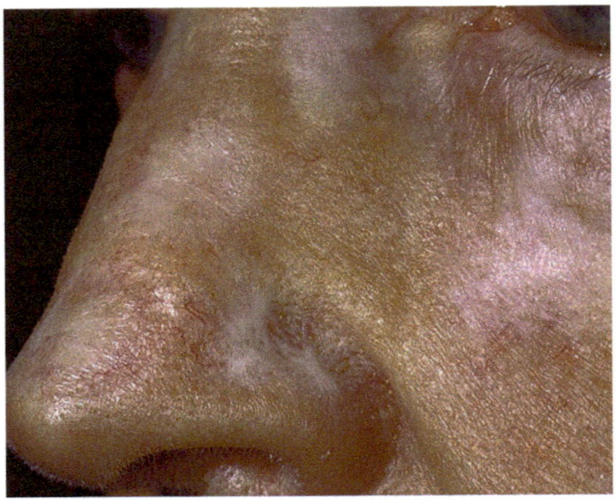

Fig. 23.3 Hypopigmentation from multiple cryosurgical procedures in a patient with sun damage

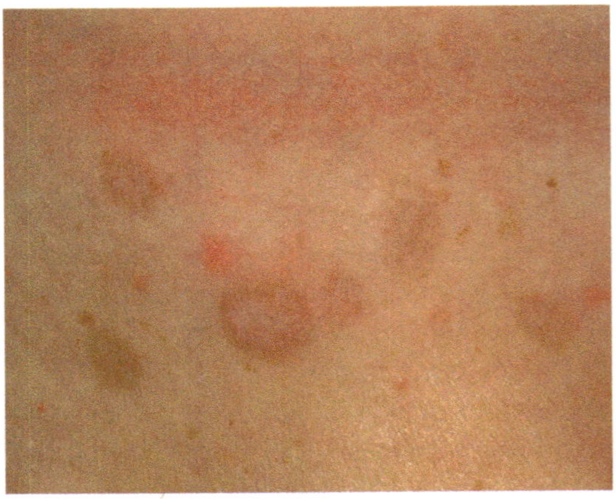

Fig. 23.5 Hyperpigmentation at the periphery of lesions (seborrheic keratosis) treated with cryosurgery

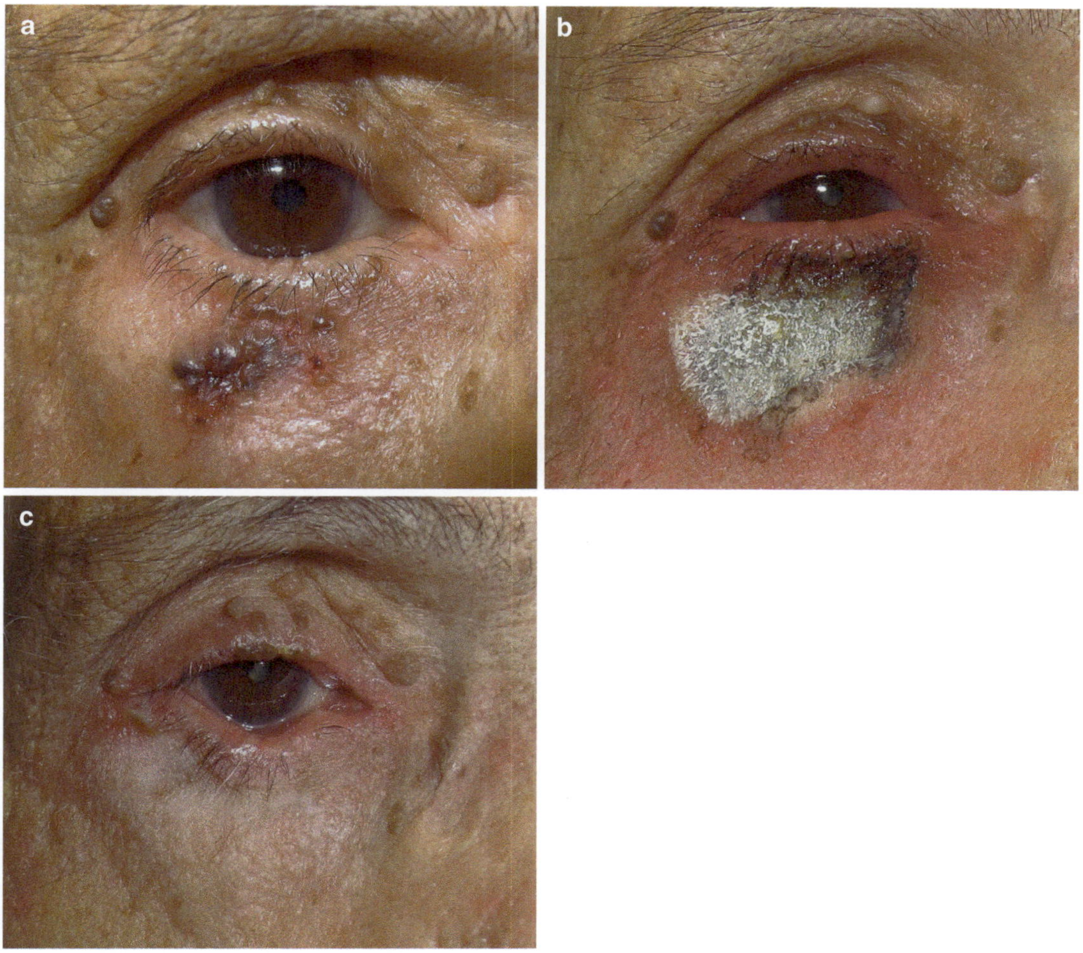

Fig. 23.6 (**a**) Basal cell carcinoma (BCC) in the lower. (**b**) Cryosurgical treatment. (**c**) Slight ectropion

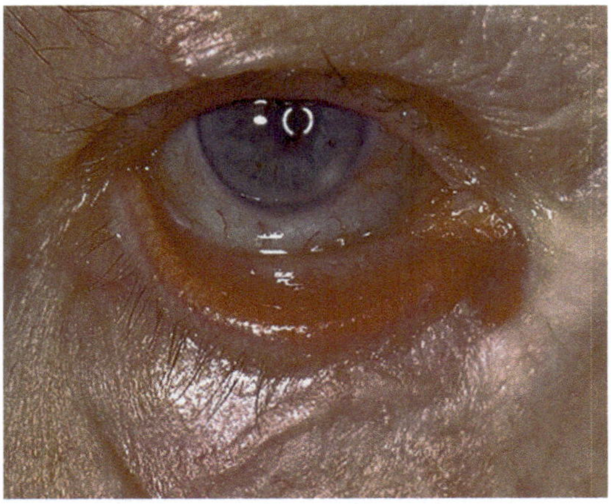

Fig. 23.7 A more pronounced ectropion after a cryosurgical procedure on a BCC of the lower eyelid

23.2.8 Cartilage Defect

Cartilage is very resistant to freezing. Cryosurgical treatment in the earlobe tends to have excellent cosmetic results. Occasionally, deep cryosurgery on large malignant earlobe tumors (especially those that have broken through the cartilage and/or extended from the retroauricular area over the helix) can leave a cartilage defect (Fig. 23.9). This possibility should be discussed before surgery with the patient in order to correct false expectations.

23.2.9 Nail Matrix Damage

Treatment of large myxoid cyst or periungual warts at the proximal nail fold can cause nail

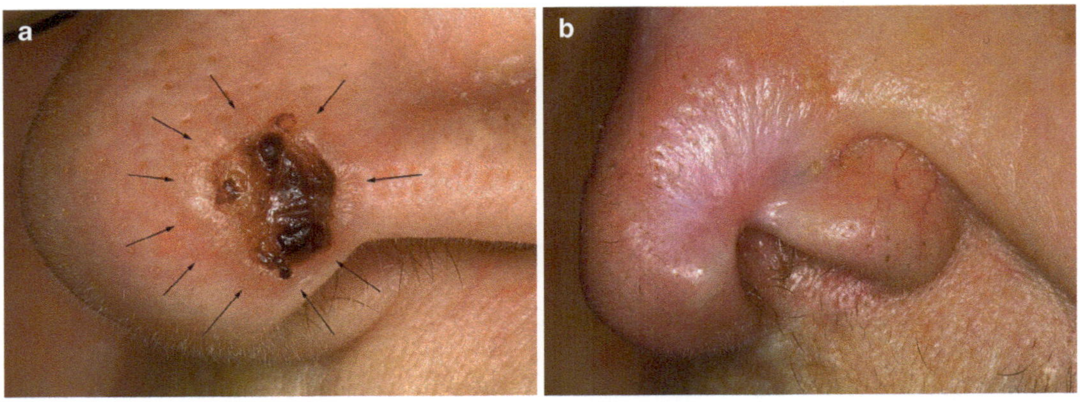

Fig. 23.8 (**a**, **b**) Notching of the nasal ala after a cryosurgical procedure on a large and ulcerated BCC, The *arrows* point at the external margins of the tumor which extends down to the nostril margin

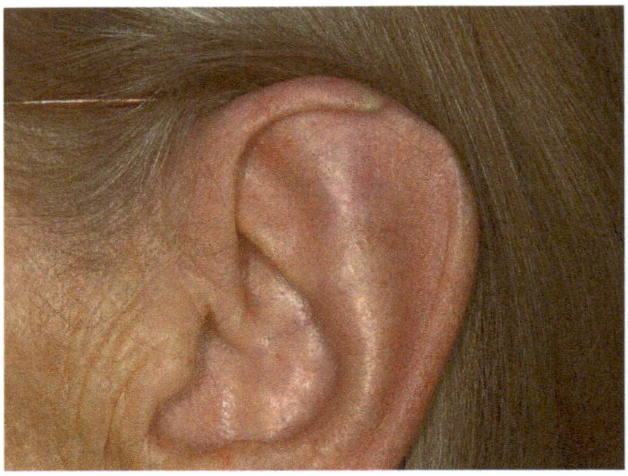

Fig. 23.9 Defect on the earlobe after cryosurgical treatment of a large BCC

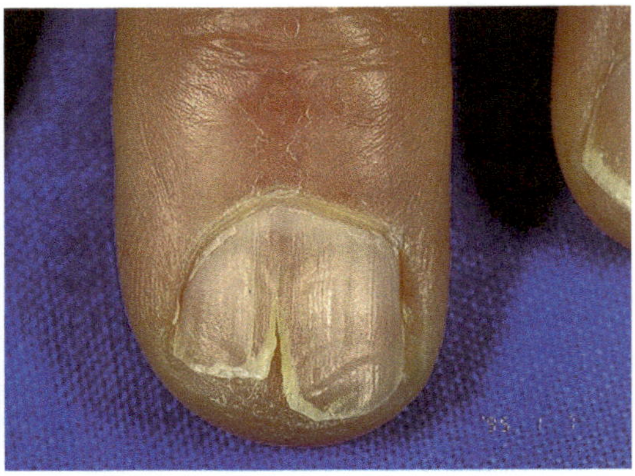

Fig. 23.10 Nail matrix damage after a cryosurgery of a myxoid cyst

matrix damage (Fig. 23.10). Avoid treating thick lesions in this area since deep freezing procedures will increase the possibility of causing permanent damage to the nail matrix.

23.2.10 Infection

A cryosurgical procedure can be painful in the first few minutes. Patients do not complain of pain the next day. If pain reappears one week or so after the procedure, during the healing period, there is probably an infection. The sudden appearance of phlogosis (redness, local pain, heat, pus secretion) in a treated area that had been involved normally is due to bacterial infection. It is a rare event and occurs more frequently in deep freezing than in superficial procedures. The best way to avoid it is by carefully instructing the patient to clean the area daily with water and soap. Postoperative care should be more meticulous in areas with lots of oozing, in areas near orifices, and in extremities. Antibiotic ointment and scar removal is usually sufficient. Oral medication is rarely needed.

23.2.11 LN Spraying in the Conjunctiva

When treating with spraying technique near the eye, it is possible to spray the conjunctiva (Fig. 23.11). Special care should be taken to protect the eyes. This can also occur if the patient suddenly moves and the spray hits the conjunctiva by error. Usually no treatment is required and spontaneous healing will occur in approximately 1 week.

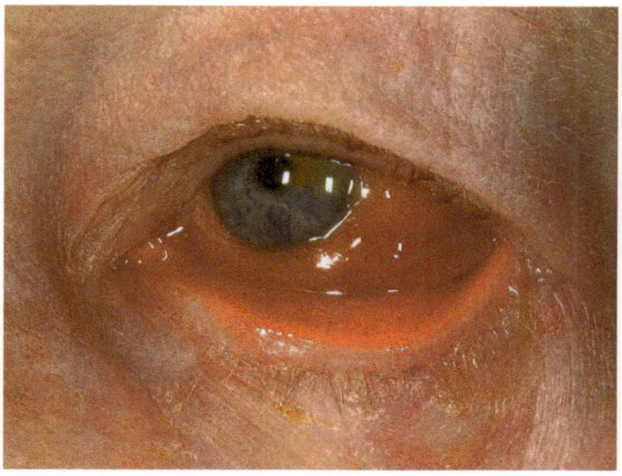

Fig. 23.11 Unintentional LN spraying of the conjunctiva

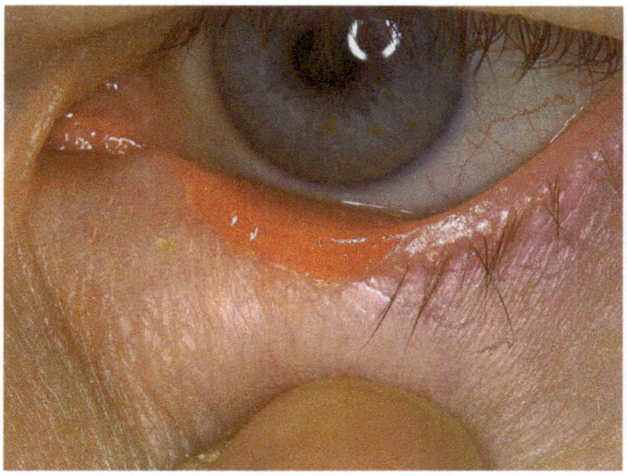

Fig. 23.12 Outgrowth of the conjunctiva over the palpebral border after a cryosurgical treatment of a carcinoma of the eyelid

23.2.12 Conjunctival Ectopy

After a cryosurgical treatment of a carcinoma of the eyelid, a rare complication is the outgrowth of the conjunctiva over the palpebral border (Fig. 23.12). It seldom needs correction, but if it is bothersome, it can be surgically corrected.

23.2.13 Milia

After deep freezing, scars can present small milia (Fig. 23.13). They have no symptoms and can be easily drained if they generate concern in the patient.

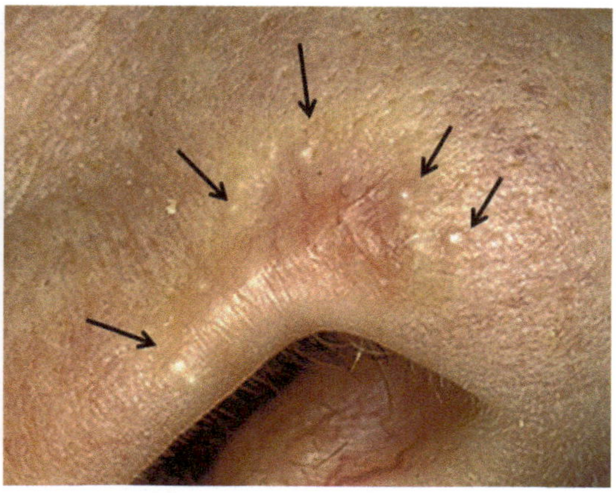

Fig. 23.13 Milia around a cryosurgical scar of a BCC treated on the nose

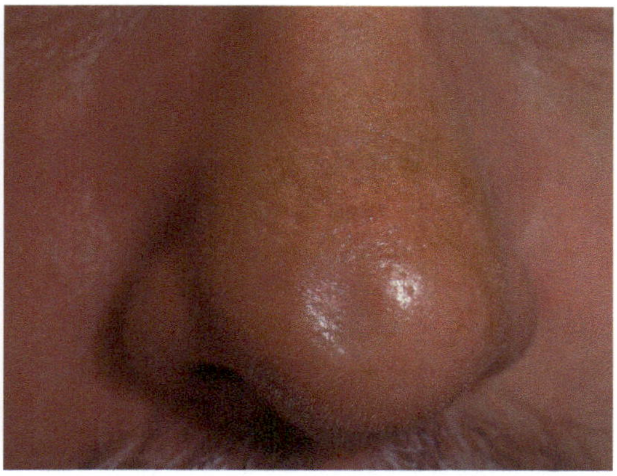

Fig. 23.14 Depressed scar of a BCC treated with cryosurgery on the tip of the nose

23.2.14 Depressed or Atrophic Scars

Deep freezing can occasionally leave a depressed scar (Fig. 23.14). It tends to improve with time but can occasionally be a permanent sign. They are more obvious in areas like the tip of the nose, cheeks, or front.

23.2.15 Hair Loss

In superficial treatment, hair loss usually does not occur. In deep freezing, there can be a permanent loss of hair (Fig. 23.15a, b). It is an expected event, but if the patient had not been warned, then it can be a complication.

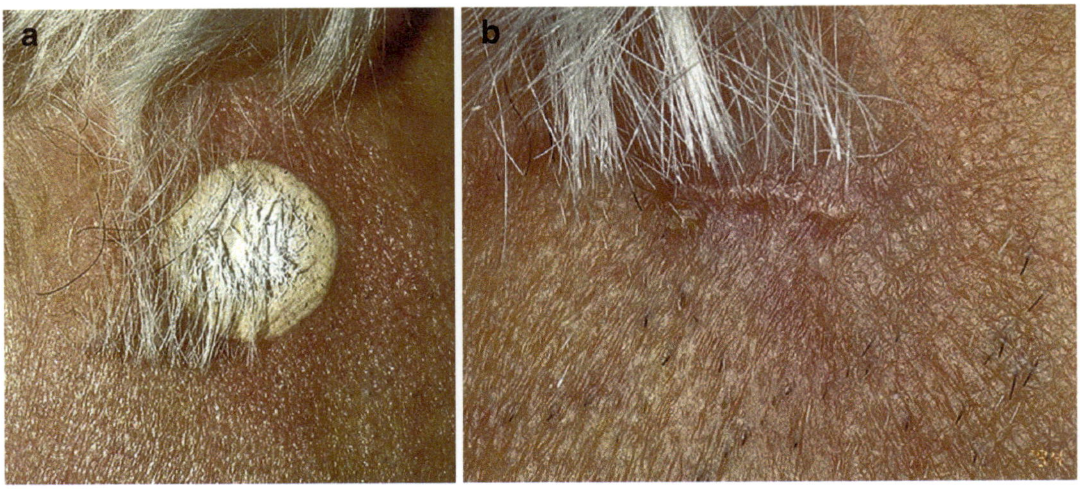

Fig. 23.15 (**a**, **b**) Permanent hair loss after a probe cryosurgery of a BCC on a hair-bearing area

23.2.16 Sensory Impairment

Cryospray is used as a local anesthesia for superficial procedures such as shave biopsy (Chap. 7). In fact, local applications of cold have been used for pain relief (cryotherapy) and pain management [7]. The works of Sonnex et al. showed that cryosurgery can cause loss of sensation that can be a cause of concern to patients. These changes are associated with the selective damage to myelin and axon cylinders [8]. Recovery can take months to years.

Faber et al. [9] found mild transient sensory loss in 28 % of treated lesions and this was site dependent. Sensory impairment after a cryosurgical procedure resolves with time. Patients should be told about this possibility, especially for procedures in the fingers.

Essential Tidbits

- Detailed information about all possible secondary effects will help patients recognize real pitfalls.
- Cryosurgery of lesions in penile foreskin should be performed in sessions. Never freeze the entire circumference in one session. This will help avoid paraphimosis secondary to edema.
- Remove rings when treating finger lesions.
- Make sure to perform complete hemostasis on curetted areas treated with cryosurgery. Bleeding can be profuse due to post-thawing vasodilation.
- The onset of pain and redness several days after the procedure can be due to infection.

Conclusions

In cryosurgery, the line between expected post-procedural events and complications sometimes can be very thin. The better the patient is informed of all possible occurrences, the lower the number of events considered as complications and the easier it will be for him/her to recognize a real complication.

In addition to the events mentioned in this chapter, many pitfalls presenting in the literature are anecdotal. In cryosurgery as in any surgical procedure, proper training and experience will reduce the possibility of complications.

Glossary

Cold urticaria An allergy in which hives form after exposure to a cold stimulus

Crepitance A crackling or popping sound or feeling caused by LN trapped under the skin

Skin LN insufflation Refers to the act of blowing LN into the skin

LN Liquid nitrogen

Phlogosis Inflammation of external parts of the body; its cardinal signs are redness, heat, pain, and swelling.

References

1. Pasquali P. The cryosurgery alternative. Int J Dermatol. 2007;46(5):511–3.
2. Elton RF. Complications of cutaneous cryosurgery. J Am Acad Dermatol. 1983;8(4):513–9.
3. Zacarian S. Complications, indications and contraindications in cryosurgery. In: Roenigk R, Roenigk H, editors. Dermatologic surgery principles and practice. New York: Marcel Dekker Inc; 1989. p. 241–61.
4. Ahmed I, Berth-Jones J, Charles-Holmes S, O'Callaghan CJ, Ilchyshyn A. Comparison of cryotherapy with curettage in the treatment of Bowen's disease: a prospective study. Br J Dermatol. 2000;143(4):759–66.
5. Colver GB, Jackson A, Dawber RPR. Cutaneous Cryosurgery: Principles and Clinical Practice. London: CRC Press Taylor and Francis group. 2005.
6. Hancox JG, Graham GF, Yosipovitch G. Hemorrhagic bullae after cryosurgery in a patient with hemophilia A. Dermatol Surg. 2003;29(10):1084–6.
7. Campos NA, Chiles JH, Plunkett AR. Ultrasound-guided cryoablation of genitofemoral nerve for chronic inguinal pain. Pain Physician. 2009;12(6):997–1000.
8. Sonnex TS, Jones RL, Weddell AG, Dawber RP. Long term effects of cryosurgery on cutaneous sensation. Br Med J (Clin Res Ed). 1985;290(6463):188–90.
9. Faber WR, Naafs B, Smitt JH. Sensory loss following cryosurgery of skin lesions. Br J Dermatol. 1987; 117(3):343–7.

Future Considerations for Cryosurgery

24

Paola Pasquali

Contents

Però comprender puoi che tutta morta
fia nostra conoscenza de quel punto
che del futuro fia chiusa la porta
Dante Alighieri
(Inferno X, 103–108)
(Thus you can understand how all our knowledge will be completely dead at that time when the door to future things is closed forever.)

24.1 Introduction

As we approach the end of this book, we need to stop and think: What does the future hold for cutaneous cryosurgery? What has been done correctly? Where can improvements take place?

The overwhelming evidence of the clinical effectiveness of this technique needs to rely on more and better research. We need to promote the integration of what is known as the knowledge triangle: education, research, and innovation.

24.2 Education

It seems clear that any procedure requires training. Formal instruction in cryosurgery should be included in all training surgical programs for all those specialists who will be working with this technique. Although this might sound like an obvious suggestion, there are many programs that do not include cryosurgery as part of their surgical training or have left such training in the hands of willing professors.

P. Pasquali, MD
Department of Dermatology, Pius Hospital de Valls, 43800 Tarragona, Spain
e-mail: pasqualipaola@gmail.com

P. Pasquali (ed.), *Cryosurgery: A Practical Manual*,
DOI 10.1007/978-3-662-43939-5_24, © Springer-Verlag Berlin Heidelberg 2015

Congress courses are important as continuous medical education but do not substitute for the need for the abovementioned formal training during residency programs. The presence of cryosurgical focus and forum sessions, workshops, and symposia at congresses worldwide has been able to offset some of this lack of formal training.

In surgical workshops, it is important to show different options in relation to all others. Efforts should be made to give courses in which participants can compare different treatment alternatives and understand the advantages and disadvantages of each one. The best treatment is the one tailored to patient's needs. The best surgeons should know all treatment alternatives in order to offer the best solution. The lack of knowledge of one technique closes a door.

24.3 Research

In recent years, research in cryobiology has centered mostly on cryoimmunology. This knowledge is opening a whole new way of understanding and applying cryosurgery, especially in the field of premalignant and malignant lesions.

Further clinical studies will require a standardized cryosurgical technique. Many efforts have been made in the past to establish formal parameters of treatment. The idea was to systematize procedures to make them reproducible and not operator dependent. There were serious attempts at standardization using time, thermocouple needles to measure temperature at the bottom of the lesion, and distance of freezing front.

The present possibility of measuring skin temperature by infrared sensoring technology will allow cryosurgery to be done in a consistent manner by determining exactly the required temperature needed for each type of lesion. This will avoid under- or overtreatments. Temperature measuring at the skin surface has the enormous advantage of being noninvasive, unlike thermocouples.

Combination treatments for skin cancerization are showing amazing results, and additional studies aimed to establish best treatment schedules are warranted.

24.4 Noninvasive Imaging Technologies

Digital photography with imaging processing, dermoscopy, high-frequency ultrasound, confocal microscopy, optical coherence tomography, and nuclear magnetic resonance are some of the new and not-so-new imaging technologies that show us different and better ways to look at the skin.

Time will show that we need to support our medical decisions on information that goes beyond what simply meets the eye.

High-frequency ultrasound (HFUS) has been underutilized thus far, although important research has shown that, with the knowledge of volume/depth of tumors, better therapeutic decisions can be made.

It seems inconceivable that in the age of HFUS a superficial basal cell carcinoma (BCC) is removed with Mohs micrographic surgery under the guise of being the gold standard, when a simple, inexpensive, and noninvasive HFUS image could have spared the patient and the system time and money. Although for different reasons, overtreating needs to be avoided just as much as undertreating.

Pairing temperature controlled cryosurgery and HFUS for skin cancer seems to be a winning combination. Visualizing the tumor and monitoring the freezing front will help correct the lack of a histologic specimen for margin control. The future most likely will bring new equipment that incorporates different imaging technologies within the cryosurgical unit.

With more research and new technologies, better cryosurgical procedures and new applications in combination treatments will be possible. Education will train future generations of cryosurgeons who will guarantee a promising and long life to this compelling specialty.

Part VI

Atlases

25 Histopathologic Events of Cryolesion: An Atlas

Miroslava Zolano Orozco, Consuelo García Silva, and Mercedes Hernández-Torres

The following atlas shows the histopathologic changes present in each stage of the cryolesion.

M.Z. Orozco, MD (✉)
Department of Dermatology, Civil Hospital of Guadalajara Fray Antonio Alcalde, Hospital 268, Col. El Retiro, Guadalajara 45235, Mexico
e-mail: miros_derm16@hotmail.com

C.G. Silva, MD
Department of Cryosurgery, Dr. José Barba Rubio Dermatological Institute of Jalisco, Av Federalismo Norte 3121, Zapopan 44190, Mexico
e-mail: mdcongs@yahoo.com.mx

M. Hernández-Torres, MD
Department of Dermatopathology, Dr. José Barba Rubio Dermatological Institute of Jalisco, Av Federalismo Norte 3120, Zapopan 44190, Mexico
e-mail: mmhdezt@gmail.com

P. Pasquali (ed.), *Cryosurgery: A Practical Manual*,
DOI 10.1007/978-3-662-43939-5_25,

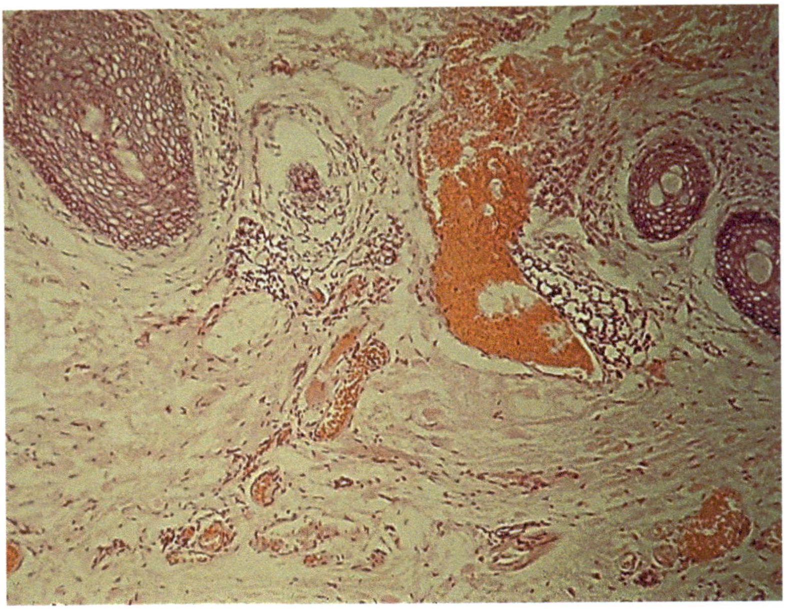

Fig. 25.1 During the first minutes of performing cryosurgery, there is an immediate reaction that is clinically manifest as burning pain of short duration, formation of a white block of ice, and edema. Histologically, this corresponds with vasodilation or dilated blood vessels, congestion (many erythrocytes inside the vessel lumen). Some epithelial cells begin to show changes

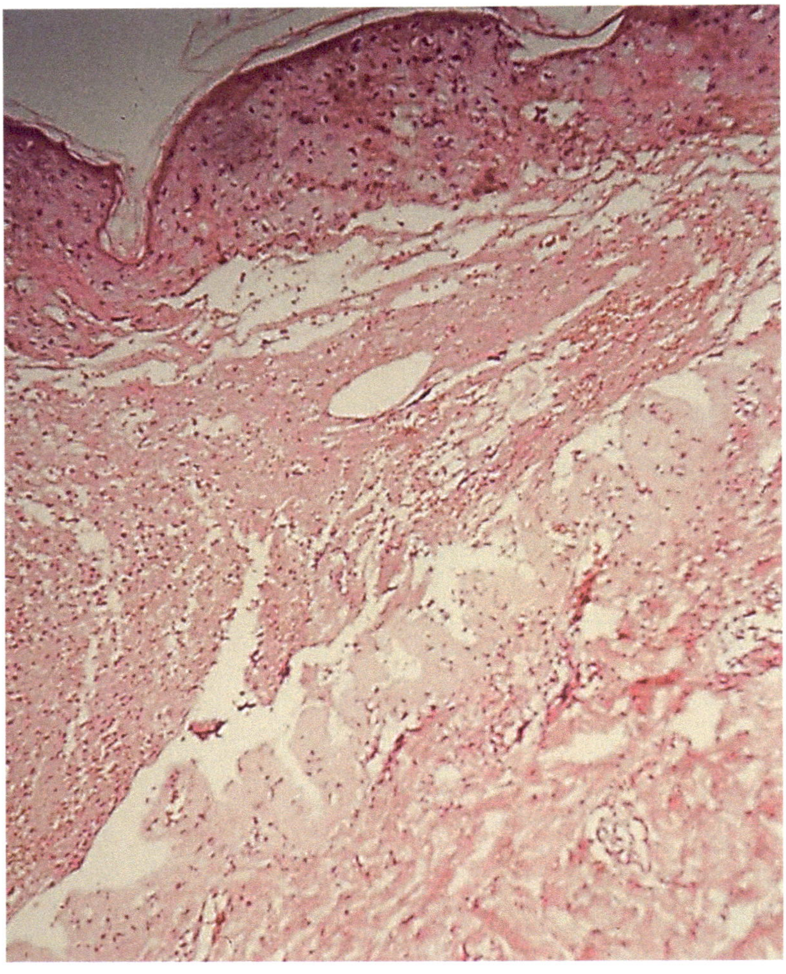

Fig. 25.2 In the first 24 h, a blister formation was clinically observed. Most cases presented serum or blood serum content. Microscopically, epithelial necrosis was seen as well as subepidermal blister formation

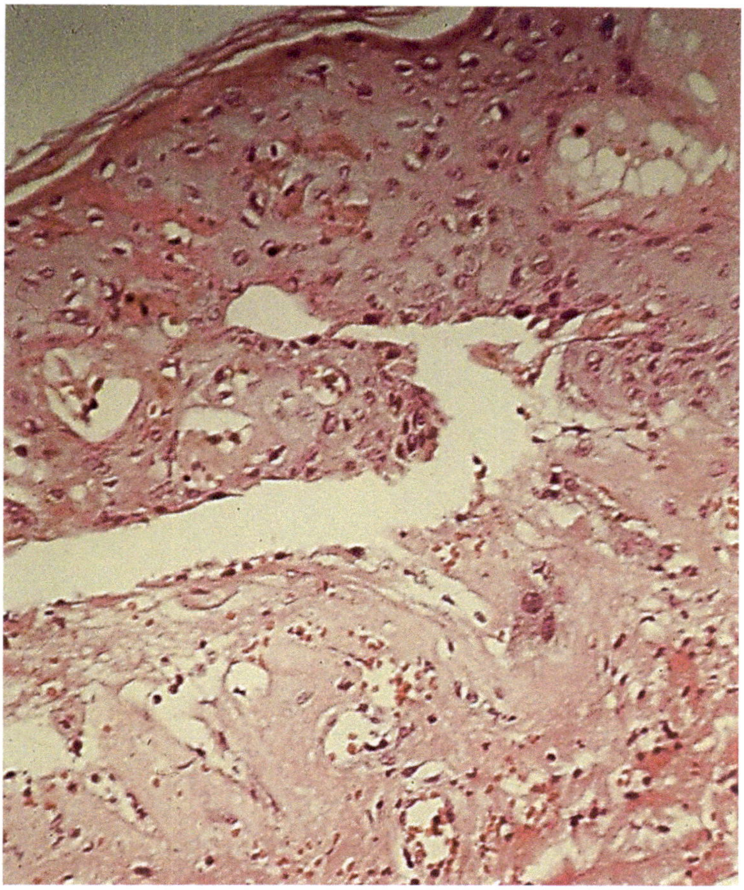

Fig. 25.3 Upon a closer look, necrotic keratinocytes could be seen. An eosinophilic material was present inside the blister as well as inflammatory cells and erythrocytes

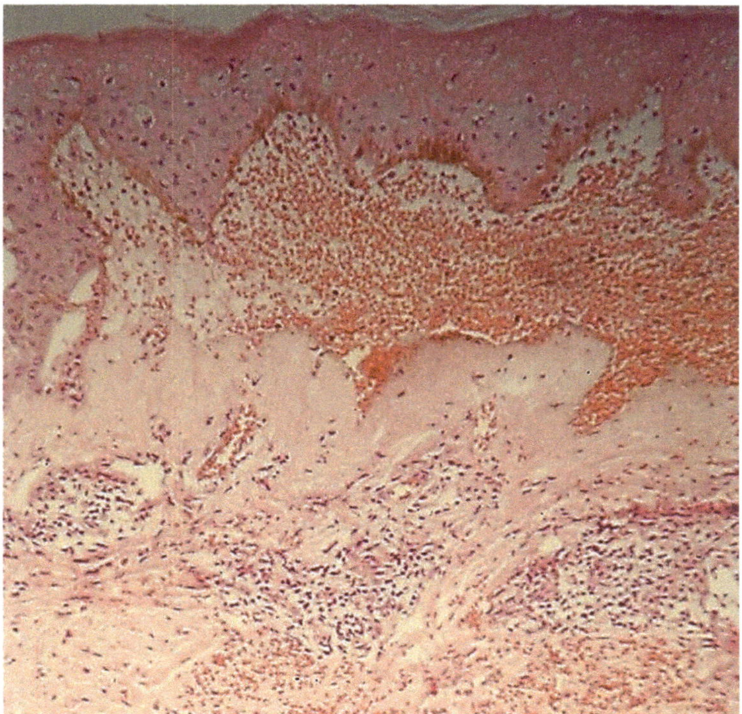

Fig. 25.4 Clinically, some blisters can be hemorrhagic. Histopathologically, one can observe the same subepidermal blister with countless erythrocytes in its cavity and dense lymphocytic inflammatory infiltrate

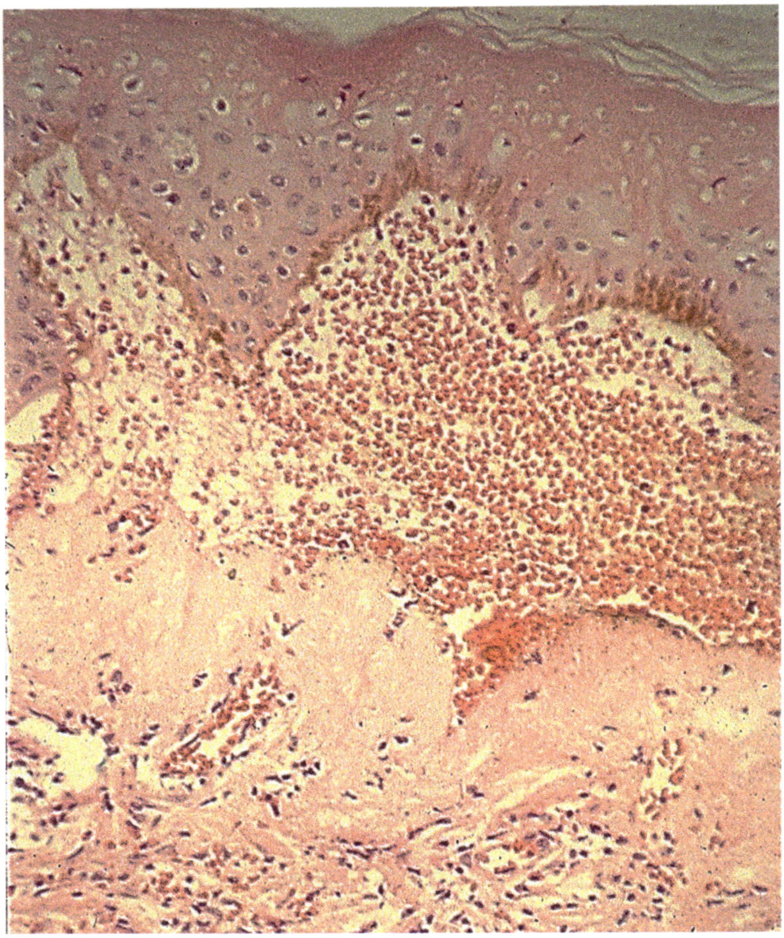

Fig. 25.5 Upon a closer view, one can observe necrosis affecting most of the epithelium

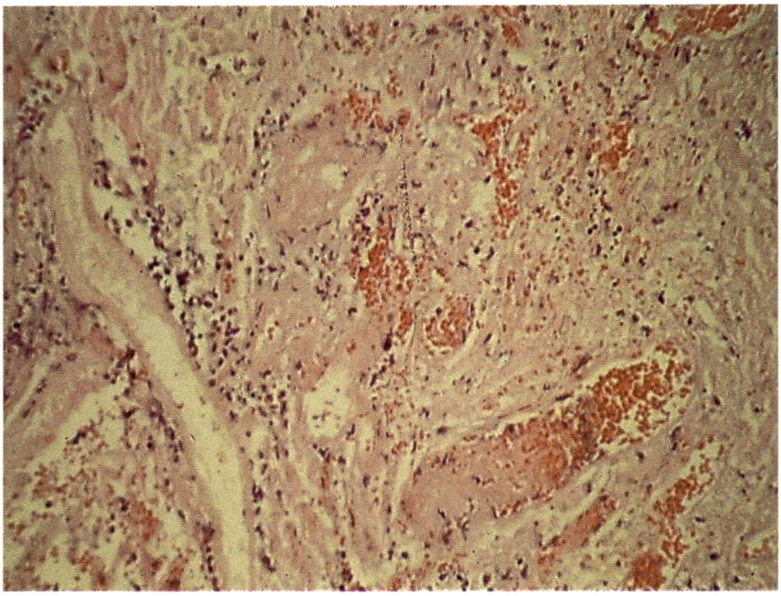

Fig. 25.6 On the third day, one can clinically observe a sloughing blister and a yellowish serous secretion which later will be replaced by a yellowish necrotic membrane. From a histopathology point of view, one can see many thrombi, extravasated erythrocytes, and an inflammatory infiltrate predominantly of lymphocytes

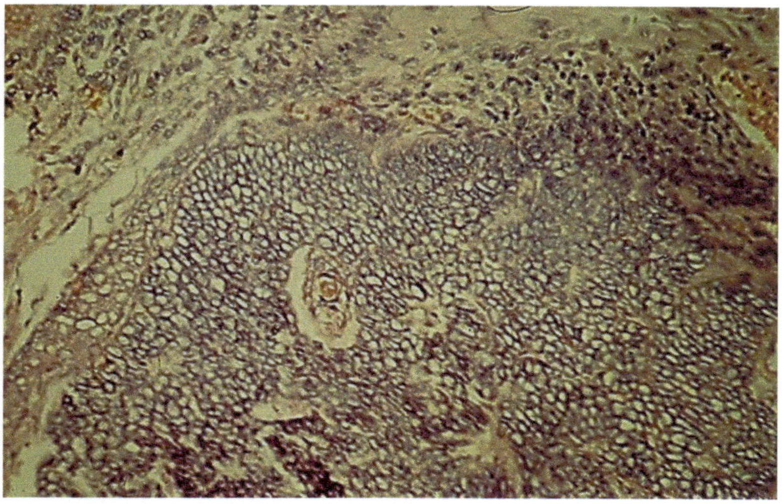

Fig. 25.7 This image corresponds to a basal cell carcinoma treated with cryosurgery. One can observe the onset of cellular changes in these basaloid cells

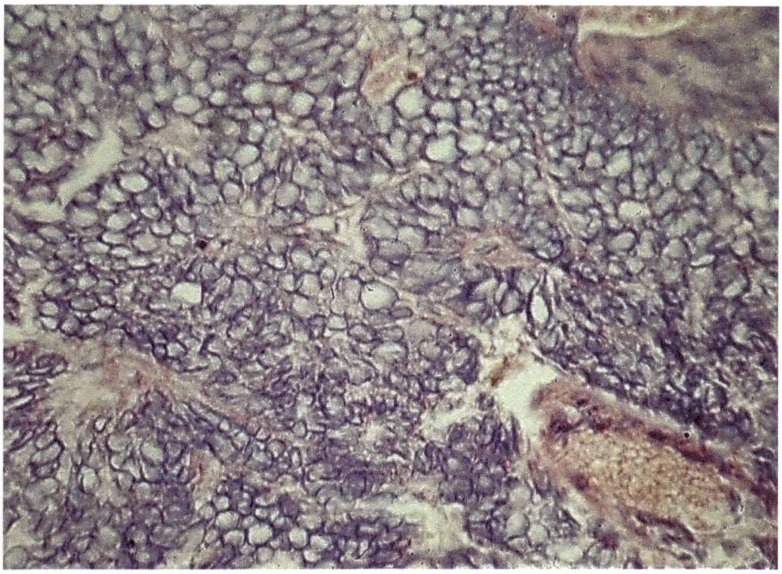

Fig. 25.8 Upon a closer view, one observes nuclei of different sizes and changes in staining affinity which can be interpreted as cell death

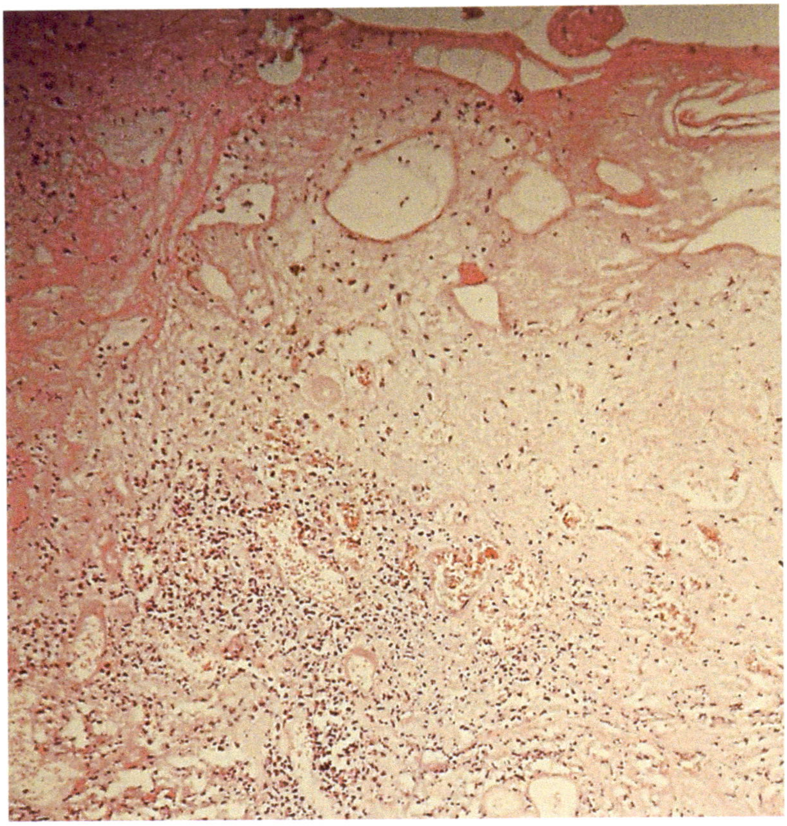

Fig. 25.9 A week later, one can see clinically evident ulceration. Histologically, ulceration is also present as well as many dilated blood vessels and inflammatory infiltrate

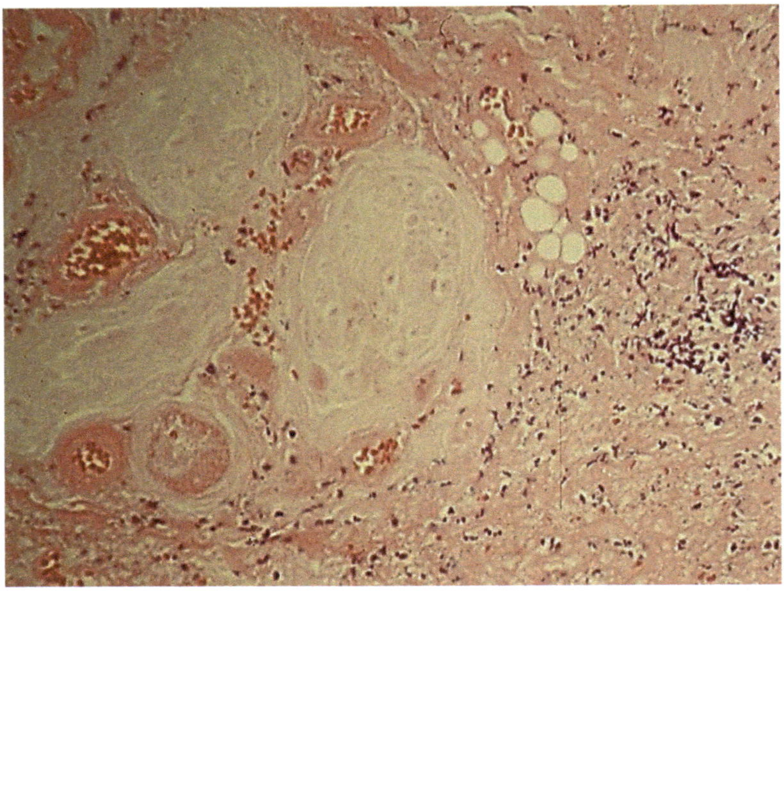

Fig. 25.10 This histological picture shows damage to the neural structures, which may manifest as prolonged anesthesia. It is always usually transient damage

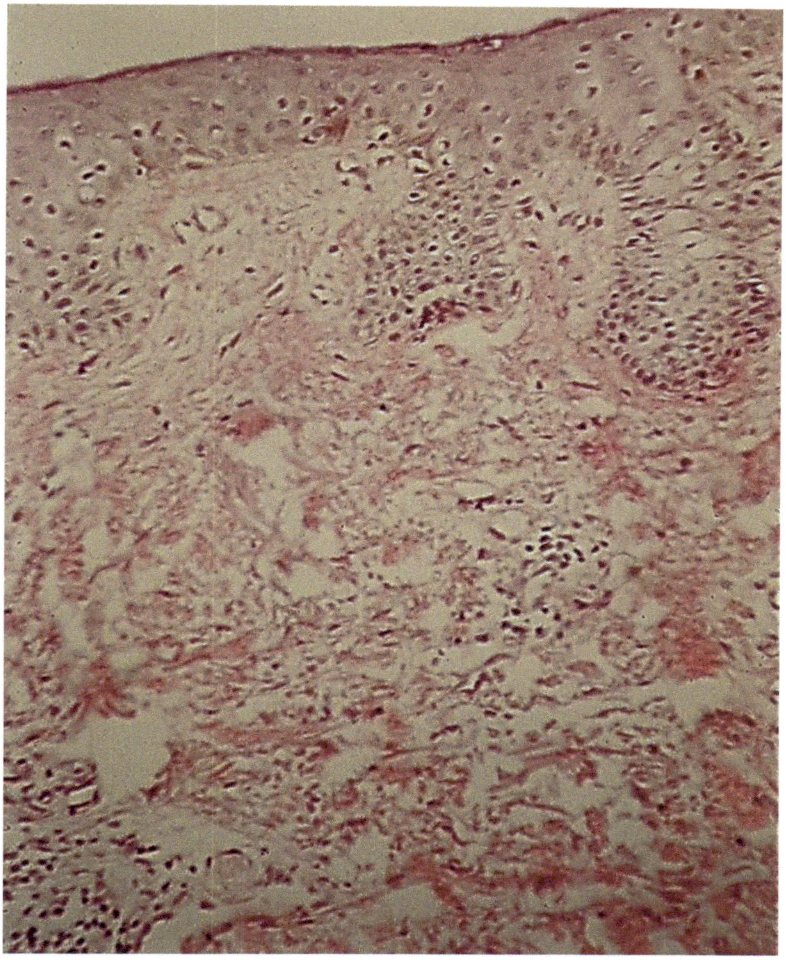

Fig. 25.11 After the third week, there is scab followed by scar formation. Scars are usually visible at the end of the fourth week. Microscopically, there is reepithelialization, elongation of the rete processes, and thickening of collagen fibers

In Vivo Reflectance Confocal Microscopy Assessment of Wound Induction and Repair of a Skin Injury Produced by Liquid Nitrogen: An Atlas

26

Melissa Chu and Nikiforos Kollias

With the advent of reflectance confocal microscopy, it has become possible to study in vivo the responses of human skin to injury and the ensuing repair process. In the present study we wanted to follow the process of epidermal necrosis and ensuing repair following a cryo-injury using reflectance confocal microscopy. A contact probe was placed on the chosen skin site, either on a solar lentigo or on normal skin, and the skin was treated for 20 s with liquid nitrogen. Both the treated site and a control site chosen from the surrounding control skin at a distance of 5 cm from the exposed skin site were measured with laser scanning confocal microscopy and with digital imaging. Time points for this study included baseline and Days 1, 2, 3, 7, 10, 14, 17, 21, 24, 28, and 31. We have developed a technique that enables us to study the exact same spot (within a 2–3 μm) on the skin at the cellular level, using glyphic lines, hair follicles, sweat glands, and dermal papillae as reference. It is important to note that some of these features that one might assume as permanent landmarks have been found to change dramatically in 28 days.

This work was originally presented as a poster at the Society for Investigative Dermatology 2011 meeting and prepared while the authors were employed by Johnson & Johnson Consumer Co.

M. Chu
292 Kingbird Ct, Three Bridges, NJ 08887, USA
e-mail: melissa.r.chu@gmail.com

N. Kollias, PhD (✉)
Department of Dermatology, University of British Columbia, Vancouver, BC, Canada
e-mail: nik@kollias.net

P. Pasquali (ed.), *Cryosurgery: A Practical Manual*,
DOI 10.1007/978-3-662-43939-5_26, © Springer-Verlag Berlin Heidelberg 2015

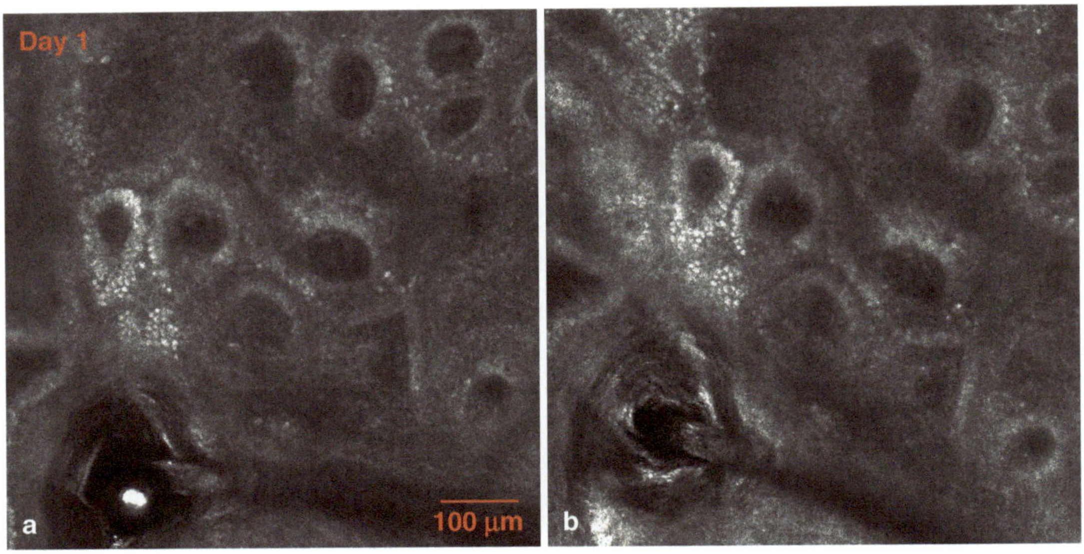

Fig. 26.1 Two confocal images obtained from the same skin site and from the same depth (approximately 80 µm) on Day 1 (**a**) and on Day 3 (**b**). Papillae and some keratinocytes loaded with melanin granules can be seen

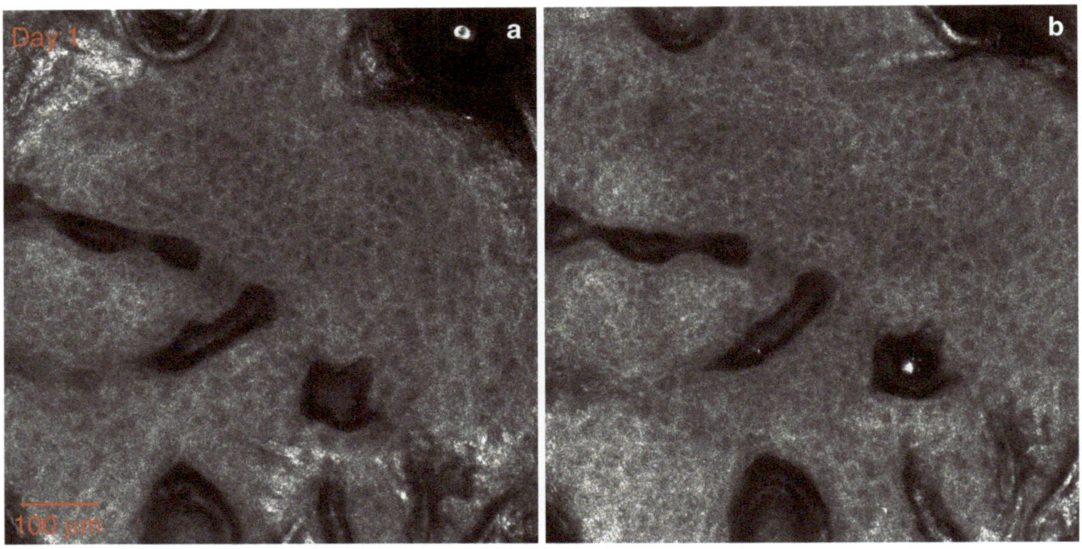

Fig. 26.2 Two confocal images obtained at the same depth of the stratum granulosum on Day 1 (**a**) and Day 5 (**b**). The scale is the same as in Fig. 26.1a, b. We show the alignment of skin sites at the level of the granulocytes. In this case the undulations of the surface of the stratum corneum and sweat glands as well as hair follicles play a role in the alignment of images. It is difficult to follow individual cells in these images or their migration from day to day although the alignment would cause us to assume that it might be possible

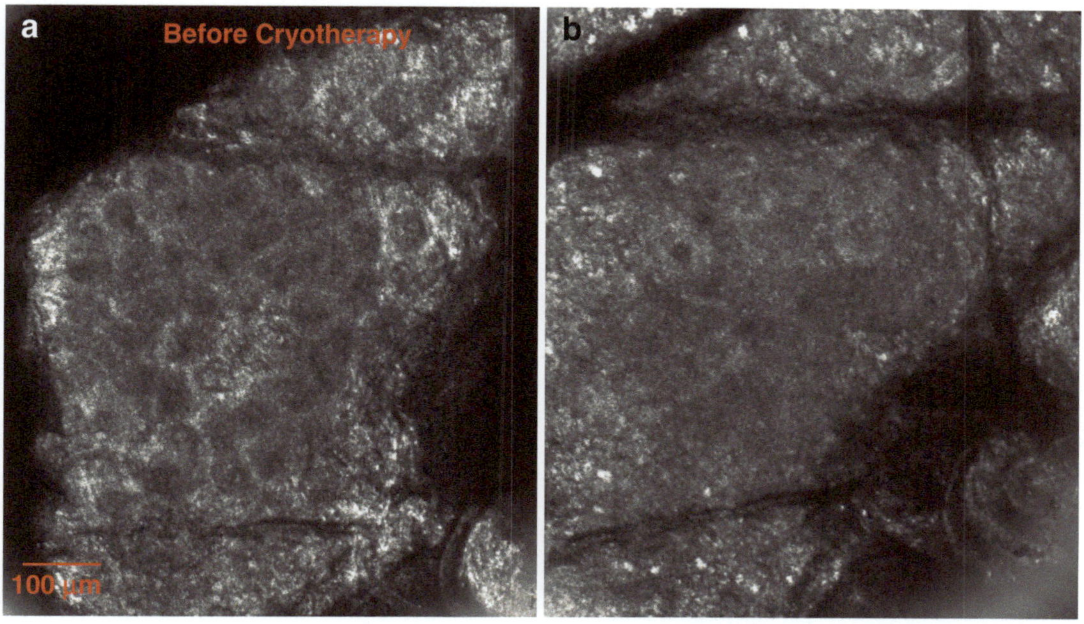

Fig. 26.3 Imaging the same location on the skin allows us to study morphological changes after cryotherapy. The two images were captured just below the stratum corneum on Day 1 (**a**) and Day 3 (**b**). The cell outlines in the image on the left correspond to keratinocytes within the granular layer. Post-injury, cellular membranes lost definition and glyphic islands flattened. What we found to be surprising in the confocal images immediately after freezing was that the cell membranes in the stratum granulosum and stratum spinosum remained intact contrary to the assumption that the cells rupture upon freezing because of the expansion of ice crystals as the temperature is lowered. The cell outlines became imperceptible at Day1 after freezing

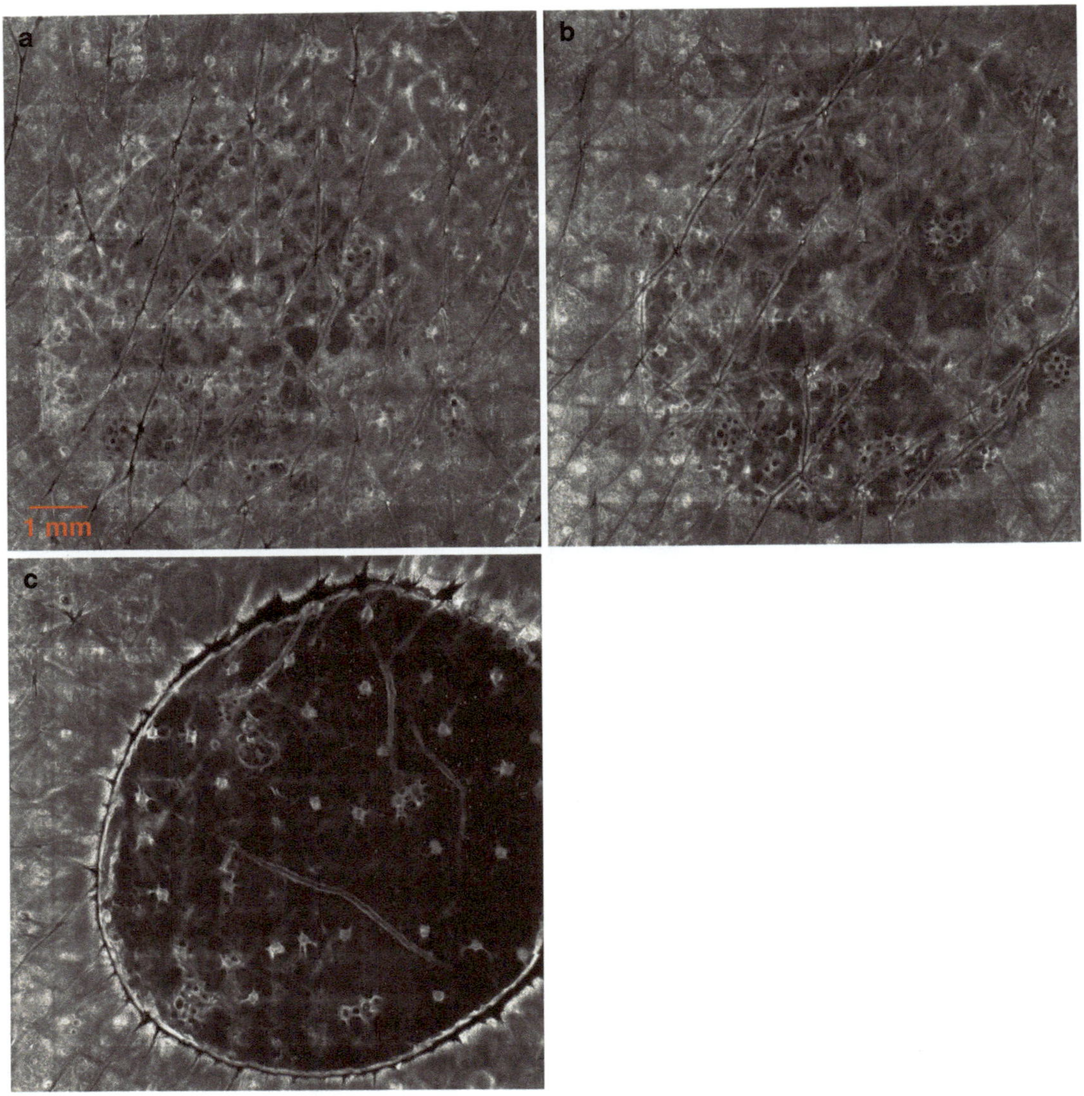

Fig. 26.4 Each of the microimages is a composite of 10 × 10 individual microscopic fields (0.5 × 0.5 mm). The area that was frozen is distinguishable in each image. The three images were obtained from the same site on Days 1 (**a**), 3 (**b**), and 7 (**c**) after freezing. Depth of the image mosaics is 70 μm below the surface of the stratum corneum. Soon after freezing a blister forms due to the separation of the epidermis from the dermis. Evidence of the blister may be documented from Day 1 after freezing and becomes fully separated by Day 2 to Day 3. The papillae may be seen in the image from Day 1, and they become imperceptible as full separation is achieved

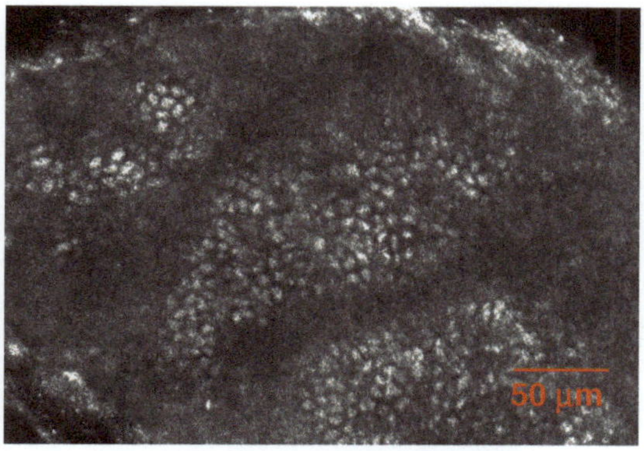

Fig. 26.5 A confocal image obtained from within the blister roof – the damaged epidermis – on Day 7 after freezing with liquid nitrogen. The melanin granules at or close to where the basal layer was remain intact and have not diffused beyond the original cellular boundaries. There is no longer evidence of cell boundaries. As full epidermal separation occurred, the sweat glands remain intact, connecting the dead epidermis to the underlying dermis with blister fluid in between the two which serves as a good optical coupling medium. The epidermis of lentigines is found to contain a large number of refractive cells believed to be bright because of scattering by the melanin granules in the melanin-bearing keratinocytes. We were interested to find out the extent to which the melanin granules would migrate to the intercellular space once the keratinocyte membranes were ruptured. There was no redistribution of melanin granules following the disappearance of the cell membranes. This finding was consistent for all volunteers with lentigines

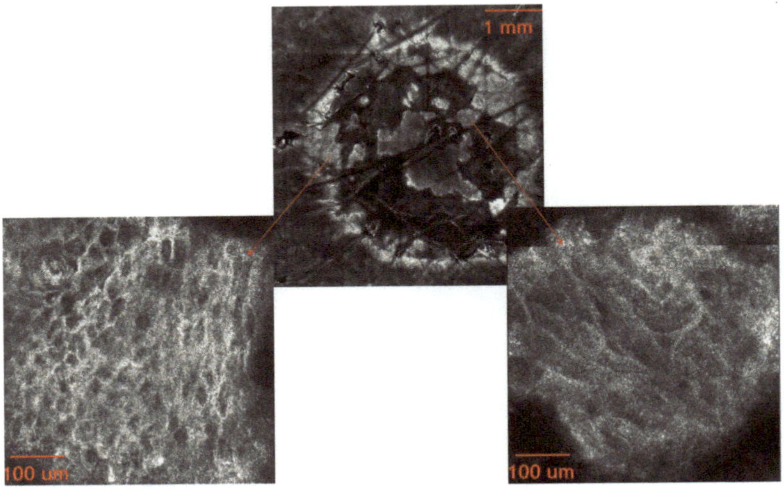

Fig. 26.6 Major tissue repair events in the repair process became evident after Day 5 following the cryo-injury. The three confocal images have different magnifications – the central image covers an area of 5×5 mm, while the side images cover each an area of 0.5×0.5 mm. On Days 7 and 10, keratinocytes generated by the wound healing response were observed and are found to have very bright cell boundaries. The wound was found to repair from the periphery toward the center, with new keratinocytes appearing elongated (50–100 μm on their long axis), much larger than those in normal skin and with very bright cell membranes and dark nuclei. Repair was also found in central regions of the wound around hair follicles as seen in the confocal image on the right. The migrating cells appeared on selected sites of the periphery of the wound and from the periphery of the hair follicle. We found a great deal of activity in some sites and little activity in others along the periphery

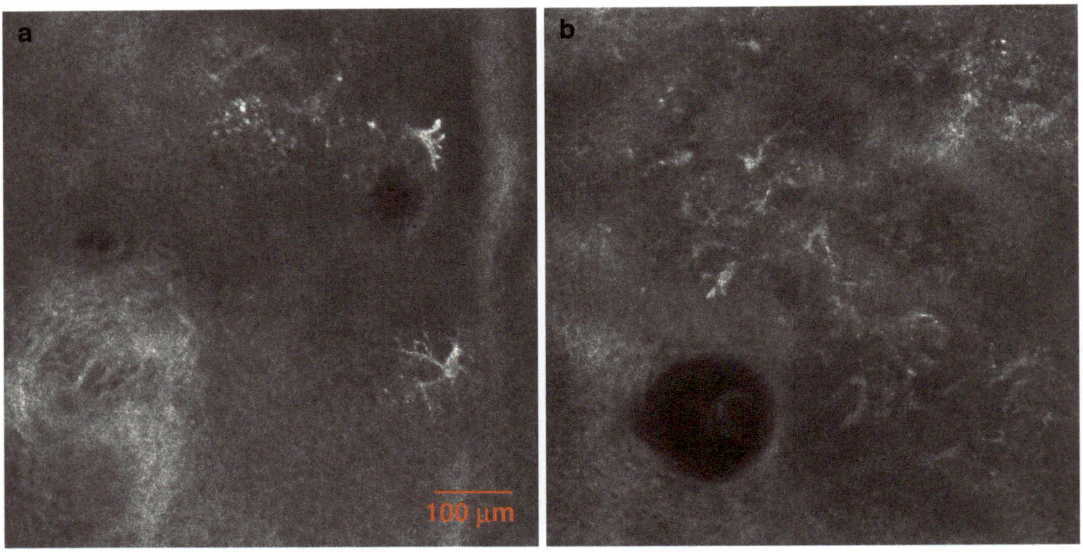

Fig. 26.7 Approximately 14 days post-injury, the invaginations of the papillae are absent, and papillae appear devoid of the typical cellular assembly that makes up their tops and walls (**a, b**). They are found in the images as dark holes; with time (in days) capillaries appear within these "holes" with a great deal of flow of erythrocytes in streams of single cells. At later time points, brightly scattering dendritic cells appear (**a, b**). These dendritic cells are located near the dermal-epidermal junction, extending both into the epidermis and dermis. At times, it is unclear if the cell body lies in the epidermis or the dermis. These cells scatter light very strongly and have been reported to be melanocytes

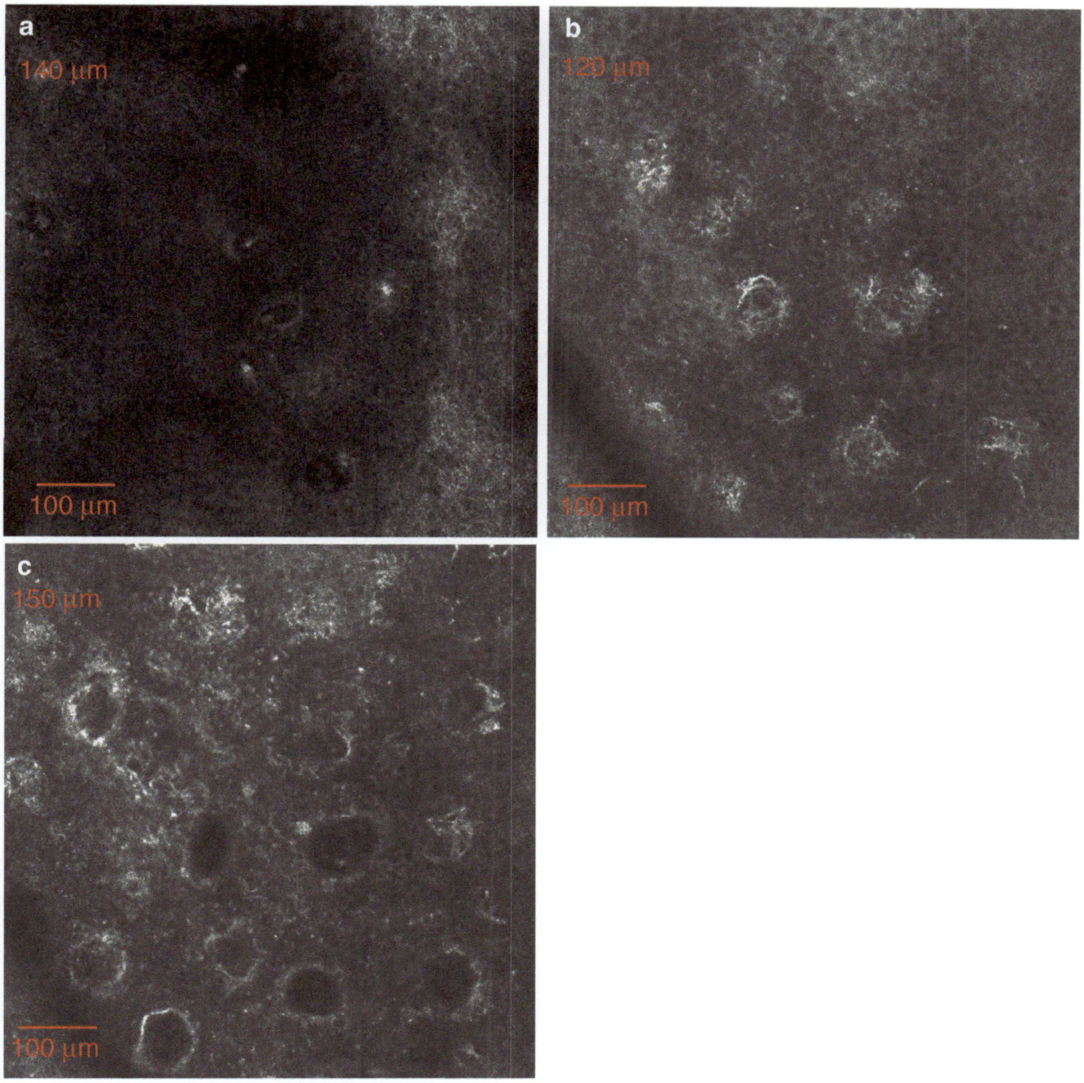

Fig. 26.8 The confocal images were obtained on Days 10 and 30. On Day 10 (**a**), the prominent features in the superficial dermis are the tops of the capillary loops that appear as bright spots due to the large erythrocyte flow, within a collagen matrix that scatters very little indicative of fine collagen fibrils. On Day 30 (**b**, **c**), we see prominent dendritic cells that are often associated with dermal papillae in an almost 1:1 relationship. In B at a depth of ~120 μm, the upper part of the papillae is shown, and in (**c**) at a depth of 150 μm, the presence of dendritic cells in the papillae walls is evident. We found the same type of cells at 15 days after solar-simulated-radiation-induced injury as well; their presence did not appear to correlate with the appearance of UV-induced pigmentation. In observing one such cell for approximately 20 min, we followed 12 bright granules in their movement from the end of one dendrite toward the cellular center – the nucleus. We never found any clinical evidence for postinflammatory hyperpigmentation in the present experiments. While these dendritic cells are present, the papillae appear to grow and develop the typical invaginations of the epidermal-dermal junction

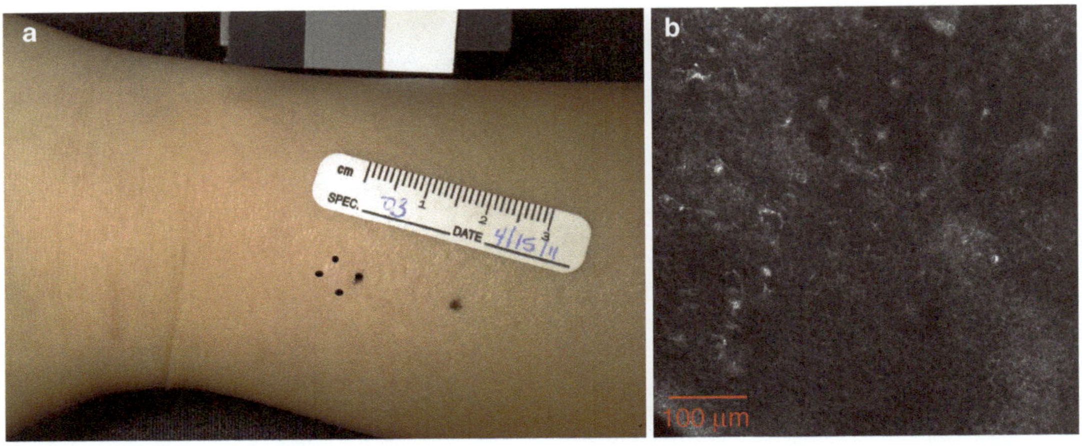

Fig. 26.9 By Day 30 following the cryo-injury and while the clinical appearance of the injured skin site is indistinguishable from the surrounding normal skin, we found large numbers of large dendritic cells often associated with papillae but not exclusively. The image on the *left* is of a volunteer's forearm with the liquid nitrogen-exposed site marked with *four dots* (**a**): the skin shows no signs of the injury. The image on the *right* (**b**) of a confocal section 0.5 × 0.5 mm in area shows many dendritic cells, although at a lower concentration than at earlier time points

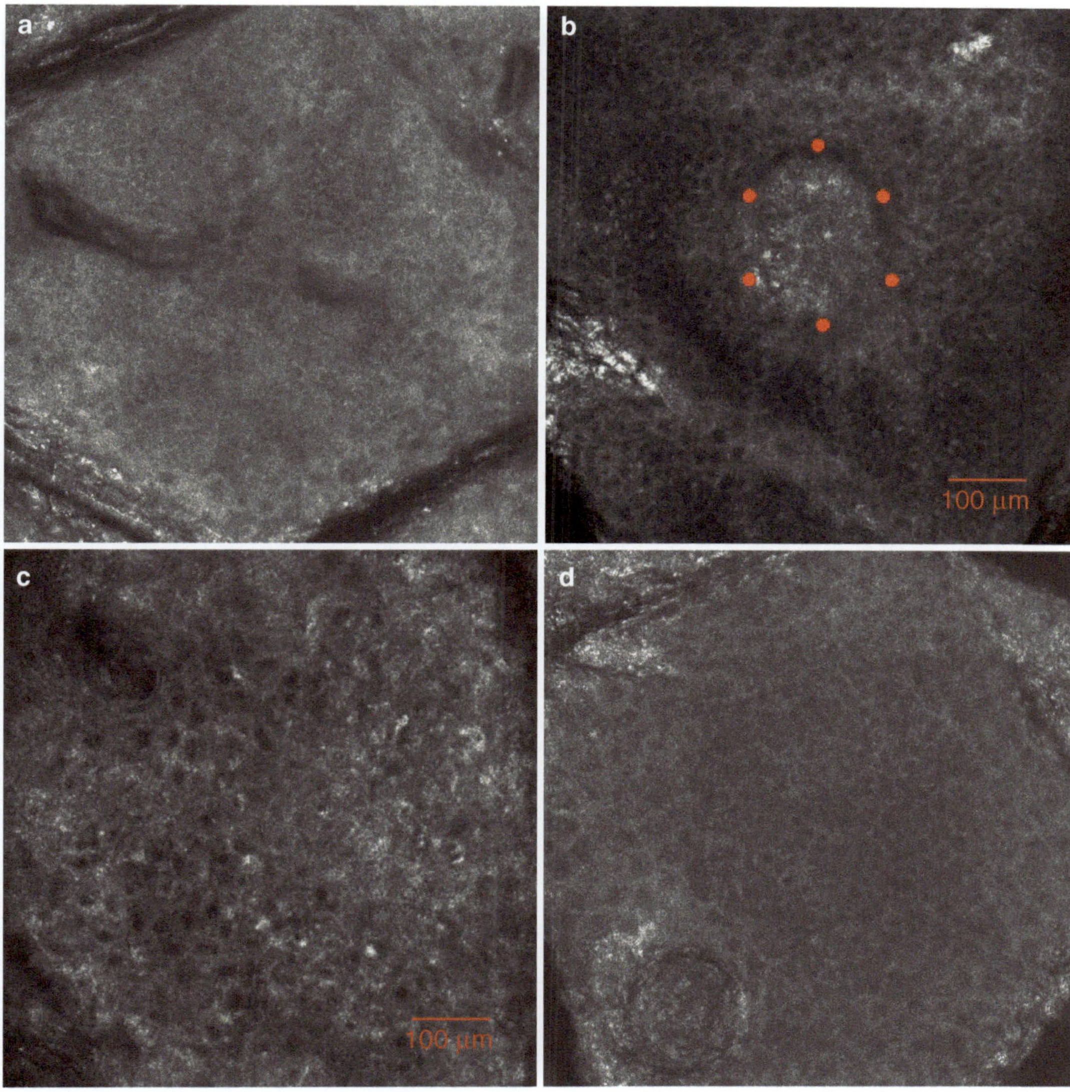

Fig. 26.10 Comparison with other types of micro-injury. In injuries produced by liquid nitrogen, by fractional laser absorbed by water, and by exposure to UVB radiation (sunburning), the epidermal cell boundaries disappear, and in the latter two, the tissue at the depth of the spinous layer appears occupied by cellular debris. In cryo-injury the damage extends to the papillary dermis, while in the fractional laser treatment, it extends into the reticular dermis and it remains confined within the exposed area. In the case of the cryo-injury, the tissue repairs in a favorable environment provided by the encapsulation of the injured site by the blister roof and the eventual formation of a new and well-organized epidermis and dermis and the formation of stratum corneum once the roof of the blister is removed. In this study we show an interesting class of dendritic cells that appear to play an important role in the repair and that although the tissue may appear clinically normal at the microscopic level, the repair continues for several weeks. (**a**) shows epidermal damage at Day 3 at the spinous level due to cryo-injury. (**b**) shows epidermal damage produced by a fractional laser (1,540 nm) – the area of the microbeam is outlined, epidermal damage by exposure to 3MED of UVB radiation. (**c**) shows the area exposed to a microbeam is to the right of the center, and (**d**) shows normal, unpigmented skin

Index

P. Pasquali (ed.), *Cryosurgery: A Practical Manual*,
DOI 10.1007/978-3-662-43939-5, © Springer-Verlag Berlin Heidelberg 2015

Kolibri 360 GmbH
Ferdinand-Jühlke-Straße 7
99095 Erfurt, Deutschland
produktsicherheit@kolibri360.de